BMA

Infectious Disease and Pharmacology

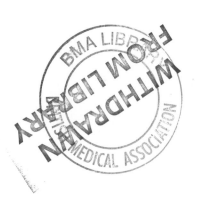

Infectious Disease and Pharmacology

Series Editor

Richard A. Polin, MD
William T. Speck Professor of Pediatrics
College of Physicians and Surgeons
Columbia University
Director Division of Neonatology
New York Presbyterian
Morgan Stanley Children's Hospital
New York, New York

Other Volumes in the Neonatology Questions and Controversies Series

GASTROENTEROLOGY AND NUTRITION

HEMATOLOGY, IMMUNOLOGY AND GENETICS

HEMODYNAMICS AND CARDIOLOGY

NEPHROLOGY AND FLUID/ELECTROLYTE PHYSIOLOGY

NEUROLOGY

THE NEWBORN LUNG

Infectious Disease and Pharmacology

William E. Benitz, MD
Philip Sunshine Professor of Neonatology
Division of Neonatal and Developmental Medicine
Stanford University School of Medicine
Lucile Packard Children's Hospital
Palo Alto, California

P. Brian Smith, MD MPH MHS
Professor of Pediatrics
Division of Neonatal-Perinatal Medicine
Duke University Medical Center
Duke Clinical Research Institute
Durham, North Carolina

Consulting Editor

Richard A. Polin, MD
William T. Speck Professor of Pediatrics
College of Physicians and Surgeons
Columbia University
Director Division of Neonatology
New York Presbyterian
Morgan Stanley Children's Hospital
New York, New York

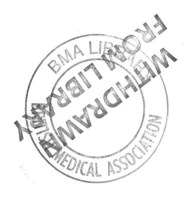

ELSEVIER

ELSEVIER

1600 John F. Kennedy Blvd.
Ste 1800
Philadelphia, PA 19103-2899

INFECTIOUS DISEASE AND PHARMACOLOGY   ISBN: 978-0-323-54391-0

Notices

Practitioners and researchers must always rely on their own experience and knowledge in evaluating and using any information, methods, compounds or experiments described herein. Because of rapid advances in the medical sciences, in particular, independent verification of diagnoses and drug dosages should be made. To the fullest extent of the law, no responsibility is assumed by Elsevier, authors, editors or contributors for any injury and/or damage to persons or property as a matter of products liability, negligence or otherwise, or from any use or operation of any methods, products, instructions, or ideas contained in the material herein.

Library of Congress Cataloging-in-Publication Data

Names: Benitz, William E., editor.
Title: Infectious disease and pharmacology : neonatology questions and controversies / [edited by] William E. Benitz, MD, Division of Neonatal and Developmental Medicine, Stanford University School of Medicine, Palo Alto, California, Brian Smith, MD MPH MHS, Professor of Pediatrics, Division of Neonatal-Perinatal Medicine, Duke University Medical Center, Duke Clinical Research Institute, Durham, North Carolina ; consulting editor, Richard A. Polin, MD, William T. Speck Professor of Pediatrics, College of Physicians and Surgeons, Columbia University, Director Division of Neonatology, New York Presbyterian, Morgan Stanley Children's Hospital, New York, New Yor.
Description: Philadelphia, PA : Elsevier, [2019]
Identifiers: LCCN 2018007172 | ISBN 9780323543910 (pbk.)
Subjects: LCSH: Newborn infants–Diseases–Examinations, questions, etc. | Neonatology–Examinations, questions, etc. | Anti-infective agents–Side effects.
Classification: LCC RJ254 .I54 2019 | DDC 618.92/01076–dc23 LC record available at https://lccn.loc.gov/2018007172

Content Strategist: Sarah E. Barth
Content Development Specialist: Lisa M. Barnes
Publishing Services Manager: Deepthi Unni
Project Manager: Beula Christopher
Designer: Paula Catalano

Printed in China

Last digit is the print number: 9   8   7   6   5   4   3   2   1

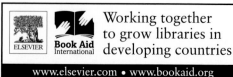

Working together to grow libraries in developing countries

www.elsevier.com • www.bookaid.org

Contributors

Julie Autmizguine, MD, MHS, FRCPC
Assistant Professor
Department of Pharmacology and
    Physiology
Université de Montréal
CHU Sainte-Justine
Montreal, Quebec, Canada
    *Antibiotic Considerations for
    Necrotizing Enterocolitis*

Daniel K. Benjamin Jr., MD, MPH, PhD
Kiser-Arena Distinguished Professor
    of Pediatrics
Duke University Medical Center;
Faculty Associate Director
Duke Clinical Research Institute
Durham, North Carolina
    Candida Prophylaxis

Sonia L. Bonifacio, MD
Clinical Associate Professor of
    Pediatrics
Department of Pediatrics
Division of Neonatal and
    Developmental Medicine
Stanford University
Palo Alto, California
    Neuroprotective Therapies in Infants

Ninfa M. Candela, MD
Assistant Professor of Pediatrics
Department of Pediatrics
Division of Pediatric Gastroenterology,
    Hepatology and Nutrition
University of Massachusetts Medical
    School
Worcester, Massachusetts
    *Therapies for Gastroesophageal
    Reflux in Infants*

Michael Cohen-Wolkowiez, MD, PhD
Professor of Pediatrics
Duke University Medical Center
Duke Clinical Research Institute
Durham, North Carolina
    *Antibiotic Dosing Considerations for
    Term and Preterm Infants*

Charles Michael Cotten, MD, MHS
Professor
Department of Pediatrics
Duke University
Durham, North Carolina
    Antibiotic Stewardship

Samantha Dallefeld, MD
Fellow
Department of Pediatrics
Duke University Medical Center
Duke Clinical Research Institute
Durham, North Carolina
    *Antibiotic Dosing Considerations for
    Term and Preterm Infants*

Mihai Puia Dumitrescu, MD, MPH
Fellow, Neonatology
Department of Pediatrics
Duke University Medical Center
Durham, North Carolina
    Candida Prophylaxis

Jessica E. Ericson, MD, MPH
Assistant Professor
Department of Pediatrics
Pennsylvania State College of
    Medicine
Hershey, Pennsylvania
    *Empiric Antimicrobials for Neonatal
    Sepsis*

Adam Frymoyer, MD
Clinical Assistant Professor
Division of Neonatal and
  Developmental Medicine
Department of Pediatrics
Stanford University
Palo Alto, California
  *Pharmacokinetic Considerations in
  Neonates*

**Rachel G. Greenberg, MD, MB,
MHS**
Assistant Professor
Department of Pediatrics
Duke University Medical Center
Duke Clinical Research Institute
Durham, North Carolina
  *When to Perform Lumbar Puncture
  in Infants at Risk for Meningitis in
  the Neonatal Intensive Care Unit*

Tamara I. Herrera, MD
Physician
University of the Republic, School of
  Medicine
Department of Neonatology
Centro Hospitalario Pereira Rossell
Montevideo, Uruguay
  *Antibiotic Stewardship
  When to Perform Lumbar Puncture
  in Infants at Risk for Meningitis in
  the Neonatal Intensive Care Unit*

**William Hope, BMBS, FRACP,
FRCPA, PhD**
Professor of Therapeutics and
  Infectious Diseases
Department of Antimicrobial
  Pharmacodynamics and Therapeutics
University of Liverpool
Liverpool, United Kingdom
  *Antifungal Dosing Considerations
  for Term and Preterm Infants*

Chi Dang Hornik, PharmD, BCPS
Assistant Professor
Department of Pediatrics and Pharmacy
Duke University Medical Center
Duke Clinical Research Institute
Durham, North Carolina
  *Antibiotic Dosing Considerations for
  Term and Preterm Infants*

Nazia Kabani, MD, BS
Fellow
Pediatric Infectious Diseases and
  Perinatal-Neonatal Medicine
Department of Pediatrics
Division of Pediatric Infectious
  Diseases
Division of Neonatology
University of Alabama at Birmingham
Birmingham, Alabama
  *Neonatal Herpes Simplex Virus
  Infection*

David Kaufman, MD
Professor
Department of Pediatrics
University of Virginia School of
  Medicine
Charlottesville, Virginia
  *Diagnosis, Risk Factors, Outcomes,
  and Evaluation of Invasive Candida
  Infections*

David W. Kimberlin, MD
Professor of Pediatrics
University of Alabama at Birmingham;
Sergio Stagno Endowed Chair in
  Pediatric Infectious Diseases
University of Alabama at Birmingham;
Co-Director, Division of Pediatric
  Infectious Diseases
University of Alabama at Birmingham
Birmingham, Alabama
  *Neonatal Herpes Simplex Virus
  Infection*

Prabhakar Kocherlakota, MD
Associate Professor of Pediatrics
Division of Neonatology, Department
  of Pediatrics
Maria Fareri Children's Hospital at
  Westchester Medical Center
New York Medical College
Valhalla, New York
  *Pharmacologic Therapy for
  Neonatal Abstinence Syndrome*

**Jodi Lestner, MBChB, MRes,
MRCPCH**
Clinical Fellow
Antimicrobial Pharmacodynamics and
  Therapeutics
Department of Molecular and Clinical
  Pharmacology
Institute of Translational Medicine
Liverpool, Great Britain
  *Antifungal Dosing Considerations
  for Term and Preterm Infants*

Tamorah Lewis, MD, PhD
Assistant Professor
Department of Pediatrics
University of Missouri Kansas City
  School of Medicine
Kansas City, Missouri
  Neonatal Pharmacogenetics

Jenifer R. Lightdale, MD, MPH
Division Chief, Pediatric
  Gastroenterology and Nutrition
Department of Pediatrics
UMass Memorial Children's Medical
  Center;
Professor of Pediatrics
University of Massachusetts Medical
  School
Worcester, Massachusetts
  *Therapies for Gastroesophageal
  Reflux in Infants*

Hillary Liken, MD
Department of Pediatrics
University of North Carolina
Chapel Hill, North Carolina
  *Diagnosis, Risk Factors, Outcomes,
  and Evaluation of Invasive Candida
  Infections*

Maria Elisabeth Moreira, MD
Pediatrician Researcher
Oswaldo Cruz Foundation/Fiocruz;
Neonatal Researcher
Clinica Perinatal Laranjeiras
National Institute of Women, Children,
  and Adolescent Health Fernandes
Figueira, Oswaldo Cruz Foundation
Rio de Janeiro, RJ, Brazil
  Congenital Zika Syndrome

**Ahmed Moussa, MD, MMed,
FRCPC**
Neonatologist
Clinical Assistant Professor,
  Department of Pediatrics
CHU Sainte-Justine
Université de Montréal
Montréal, Québec, Canada
  *Antibiotic Considerations for
  Necrotizing Enterocolitis*

Sagori Mukhopadhyay, MD, MMSc
Assistant Professor
Department of Pediatrics
University of Pennsylvania Perelman
  School of Medicine;
Attending Physician Neonatology
Pennsylvania Hospital and Children's
  Hospital of Philadelphia
Philadelphia, Pennsylvania
  *Management of the Asymptomatic
  Newborn at Risk for Sepsis*

Namrita J. Odackal, DO
Neonatology Fellow
Division of Neonatal-Perinatal
  Medicine
Department of Pediatrics
University of Virginia Health System
Charlottesville, Virginia
  *Diagnosis, Risk Factors, Outcomes,
  and Evaluation of Invasive Candida
  Infections*

Olivia B. Payne, BS
University of Virginia School of
  Medicine
Charlottsville, Virginia
  *Empiric Antimicrobials for Neonatal
  Sepsis*

Sallie R. Permar, MD, PhD
Professor
Department of Pediatrics, Immunology,
  and Molecular Genetics and
  Microbiology
Duke Human Vaccine Institute
Durham, North Carolina
  *When and How to Treat Neonatal
  CMV Infection*

Karen Marie Puopolo, MD, PhD
Associate Professor
Department of Pediatrics
University of Pennsylvania Perelman
  School of Medicine;
Section Chief
Newborn Medicine
Pennsylvania Hospital;
Attending Physician
Neonatology
Children's Hospital of Philadelphia
Philadelphia, Pennsylvania
  *Management of the Asymptomatic
  Newborn at Risk for Sepsis*

Rosana Richtmann, MD
Physician
Emilio Ribas-Institute of Infectious
  Diseases-São Paulo;
Infections Disease Chief
Santa Joana Hospital and Maternity
  and Pro-Matre Paulista
São Paulo, SP, Brazil
  Congenital Zika Syndrome

**Marie-Eve Rochon, MD, MSc,
FRCPC**
Fellow, Neonatology
CHU Sainte-Justine
Université de Montréal
Montreal, Québec, Canada
  *Antibiotic Considerations for
  Necrotizing Enterocolitis*

J. Lauren Ruoss, MD
Department of Pediatrics
Division of Neonatal-Perinatal
  Medicine
University of Florida
Gainesville, Florida
  *Biomarkers in the Diagnosis of
  Neonatal Sepsis*

Amanda G. Sandoval Karamian, MD
Child Neurology Resident Physician
Stanford University, Lucile Packard
  Children's Hospital
Palo Alto, California
  *Antiepileptic Drug Therapy in
  Neonates*

Krisa VanMeurs, MD
Rosemarie Hess Professor in Neonatal
  and Developmental Medicine
Department of Pediatrics
Division of Neonatal and
  Developmental Medicine
Stanford University
Palo Alto, California
  Neuroprotective Therapies in Infants

Kelly C. Wade, MD, PhD, MSCE
Associate Professor of Clinical
  Pediatrics
Associate Director of Therapeutics and
  Education
CHOP Newborn Care at Pennsylvania
  Hospital
Perelman School of Medicine
Children's Hospital of Philadelphia
Philadelphia, Pennsylvania
  *Antiviral Dosing Considerations for
  Term and Preterm Infants*

Kristin E.D. Weimer, MD, PhD
Fellow, Neonatology
Department of Pediatrics
Duke University Hospital
Durham, North Carolina
  *When and How to Treat Neonatal
  CMV Infection*

Courtney J. Wusthoff, MD, MS
Neurology Director
Lucile Packard Children's Hospital
  NeuroNICU;
Assistant Professor of Neurology and
  Neurological Sciences and Pediatrics-
  Neonatal and Developmental
  Medicine
Stanford Division of Child Neurology
Palo Alto, California
  *Antiepileptic Drug Therapy in
  Neonates*

James Lawrence Wynn, MD
Associate Professor of Pediatrics
Department of Pediatrics
University of Florida;
Associate Professor of Experimental
  Medicine
Department of Pathology, Immunology,
  and Laboratory Medicine
University of Florida;
Associate Director, Neonatal-Perinatal
  Fellowship Program
Department of Pediatrics
University of Florida
Gainesville, Florida
  *Biomarkers in the Diagnosis of
  Neonatal Sepsis*

Kanecia Zimmerman, MD, MPH
Assistant Professor
Department of Pediatrics
Duke University Medical Center
Duke Clinical Research Institute
Durham, North Carolina
  *Antibiotic Dosing Considerations for
  Term and Preterm Infants*

Series Foreword

"To study the phenomena of disease without books is to sail an uncharted sea, while to study books without patients is not to go to sea at all"

William Osler

Physicians in training generally rely upon the spoken word and clinical experiences to bolster their medical knowledge. There is probably no better way to learn how to care for an infant than to receive teaching at the bedside. Of course, that assumes that the "clinician" doing the teaching is knowledgeable about the disease, wants to teach and can teach effectively. For a student or intern, this style of learning is efficient because the clinical service demands preclude much time for other reading. Over the course of one's career, it becomes clear that this form of education has limitations because of the fairly limited number of disease conditions one encounters even in a lifetime of clinical rotations and the diminishing opportunities for teaching moments.

The next educational phase generally includes reading textbooks and qualitative review articles. Unfortunately, both of those sources are often outdated by the time they are published and represent one author's opinions about management. Systematic analyses (meta-analyses) can be more informative, but more often than not the conclusion of the systematic analysis is that "more studies are needed" to answer the clinical question. Furthermore, it has been estimated that if a subsequent large randomized clinical trial had not been performed, the meta-analysis would have reached an erroneous conclusion more than one-third of the time.

For practicing clinicians, clearly the best way to keep abreast of recent advances in a field is to read the medical literature on a regular basis. However, that approach is problematic given the multitude of journals, unless one reads only the two or three major Pediatric journals published in the United States. That approach however, will miss many of the outstanding articles that appear in more general medical journals (e.g., Journal of the American Medical Association, New England Journal of Medicine, Lancet and the British Medical Journal) subspecialty journals and the many Pediatric Journals published in other countries.

While there is no substitute to reading journal articles on a regular basis, the "Questions and Controversies" series of books provides an excellent alternative. This third edition of the series was developed to highlight the clinical problems of most concern to practitioners. The series has been increased from six to seven volumes and includes new sections on genetics and pharmacology. In total, there are 70 new chapters not included previously. The editors of each volume (Drs. Bancalari, Davis, Keszler, Oh, Baum, Seri, Ohls, Christensen. Maheshwari, Neu, Benitz, Smith, Poindexter, Cilio and Perlman) have done an extraordinary job in selecting topics of clinical importance to everyday practice. Unlike traditional review articles, the chapters not only highlight the most significant controversies, but when possible, have incorporated basic science and physiological concepts with a rigorous analysis of the current literature.

As with the first edition, I am indebted to the exceptional group of editors who chose the content and edited each of the volumes. I also wish to thank Lisa Barnes (content development specialist at Elsevier) and Judy Fletcher (global content development director at Elsevier), who provided incredible assistance in bringing this project to fruition.

Richard A. Polin, MD

Preface

Because of their immature immune system, infants are frequently affected by a broad array of infections, which are frequently associated with lifelong consequences. In addition, their immature renal and hepatic function often led to profound differences in drug exposures relative to older children and adults. Even when drug exposures are similar to older children and adults, infants may experience differences in safety and efficacy. In this first edition of the Infectious Diseases and Pharmacology volume of "Neonatology: Questions and Controversies," we provide an update of the epidemiology, clinical manifestations, and treatment and outcomes for neonatal-perinatal infections. This volume will also expose readers to the latest information on dosing of antibiotics, antivirals, and antifungals. Additionally, therapies for neonatal reflux, seizures, neuroprotection, and neonatal abstinence syndrome are discussed and updates on pharmacokinetic and pharmacogenetic considerations in neonatal care are provided. This information is critical in the infant population, given the rapid changes in physiology, metabolic pathways, and renal elimination that occur over the first months of life. Contributors include pediatricians, neonatologists, and experts in pediatric infectious disease, neurology, and pharmacology, with a wide variety of research interests. We hope that these updates will prove valuable to our colleagues who are responsible for the management of newborn babies as they navigate the often-hazardous transition to extrauterine life.

William E. Benitz, MD
P. Brian Smith, MD, MPH, MHS

Contents

Corresponding color figures for select images are available on Expert Consult. 🌐

Infectious Disease

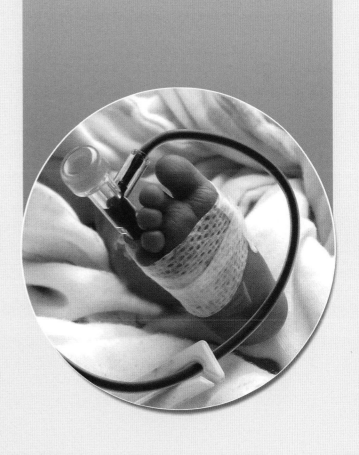

CHAPTER 1

Management of the Asymptomatic Newborn at Risk for Sepsis

Sagori Mukhopadhyay, MD, MMSc, Karen Marie Puopolo, MD, PhD

- The current incidence of neonatal early-onset sepsis (EOS) among infants born ≥37 weeks is relatively low (≈1/2000) and as much as 10-fold lower among well-appearing term infants.
- There are three major approaches to EOS risk assessment among term infants: categorical consideration of risk factors, multivariate consideration of risk factors in combination with clinical condition, and consideration of the clinical condition alone as it evolves in the first 48 hours after birth.
- Currently available laboratory tests lack sensitivity for predicting culture-confirmed EOS among term infants.
- EOS-associated clinical activities have significant impact on early mother–newborn interaction and initiation of breastfeeding.
- Depending on the local structure of care, EOS risk assessment activities are costly in terms of caregiver time, resource allocation, and monetary expenditures.
- Preclinical animal and clinical human studies demonstrate an impact of perinatally administered antibiotics on the initial composition of the newborn gut microbiome.
- Retrospective human epidemiologic studies associate perinatal and early infancy antibiotics with multiple morbidities in early childhood.

Introduction

Management of newborns at risk of early-onset bacterial sepsis (EOS) is one of the most common clinical tasks conducted by perinatal clinicians. Depending on the local structure of care, decisions are made by midwives, community pediatricians, resident house staff, newborn hospitalists, or neonatal intensive care specialists. EOS risk management begins with an assessment of whether the newborn is at a higher-than-average risk for EOS, continues to a decision to administer empiric antibiotic therapy, and ends with the decision to stop or extend empiric therapies, if given. Caregivers engage in this management to protect newborns from what may be a serious and even life-threatening infection. However, as the incidence of EOS has declined in the United States, risk management has become increasingly controversial, especially among initially well-appearing infants born at term.[1,2] The incidence of EOS among all infants born ≥37 weeks' gestation is now ≈1 case per 2000 live births[3]; among well-appearing term infants born to mothers without concern for intrapartum infection, the incidence may be as low as 1 case in 25,000 births.[4] Faced with a low-incidence, high-consequence condition, neonatal caregivers are challenged to determine the best approach to ensure newborn health. The difficulty of this task was brought forward in a recent national survey of EOS practices in American newborn nurseries. Wide variation was identified in most aspects of EOS risk management, with significant impact on the newborn and on the maternal–infant dyad.[5]

Two newborn characteristics can be used to identify categories of infants at markedly higher risk of EOS compared with infants without such characteristics. The first is gestational age (or birth weight used as a surrogate for gestational age). Centers for Disease Control and Prevention (CDC) multistate surveillance data in the United States demonstrate that the incidence among infants born <37 weeks' gestation is five to six times higher compared with the incidence among infants born ≥37 weeks' gestation. The incidence of EOS among those born with birth weight <1500 g is ≈20 times higher than among those born at term.[1] The microbiology of EOS also differs among premature infants: Despite widespread application of intrapartum antibiotic prophylaxis to prevent group B streptococcus (GBS)–specific EOS,[6] GBS is the most common organism isolated in term infants with EOS.[1] In contrast, *Escherichia coli* is the most common isolate among premature infants. The second characteristic predictive of EOS is infant clinical presentation. Escobar and colleagues evaluated the outcomes of EOS evaluation among 2875 newborns evaluated for EOS. Roughly half of the infants were evaluated due to clinical symptoms, and the other half were evaluated based on the presence of specific risk factors (e.g., maternal chorioamnionitis, rupture of membranes >18 hours). The unadjusted incidence of EOS was 10-fold higher among infants who were critically ill compared with those who were initially asymptomatic; on multivariate analysis, initial asymptomatic status predicted ≈60% lower risk of EOS compared with presentation with any degree of instability.[7]

Despite a high relative risk of infection, not all premature infants are infected, and not all symptomatic term infants are infected. The challenge among such infants is to determine which infants *may not* require EOS evaluation and empiric antibiotics. Among term, well-appearing infants, in contrast, the primary challenge is to determine who, despite initial reassuring clinical condition, is at highest risk to develop symptomatic EOS. For these infants, the task is to determine which infants *may* require EOS evaluation and empiric antibiotics. In this chapter, we will evaluate the merits and limitations of different approaches to assessing the risk of EOS among term, well-appearing newborns.

Approaches to EOS Risk Assessment Among Well-Appearing Term Infants

Categorical approaches to EOS risk assessment: The first national consensus guidelines for EOS were issued by the American Academy of Pediatrics (AAP) in 1992,[8] by the CDC in 1996,[9] and by the American College of Obstetricians and Gynecologists in 1996.[10] These guidelines were directed at reducing GBS-specific EOS incidence by interrupting mother-to-infant GBS transmission during labor. The evidence for specific chemoprophylaxis approaches to mediate such interruption and effectiveness of the various approaches were reviewed in each subsequent revision.[11–18] Universal GBS screening and intrapartum chemoprophylaxis was recommended in the revised CDC guideline in 2002[17] and reaffirmed in the 2010 recommendations.[18]

These guidelines also contain recommendations for the management of infants after delivery with the goal of early identification of EOS cases and early initiation of antibiotics to halt the progression of disease. These recommendations use decision trees to direct management with a series of categorical consideration of risk factors, using these factors in dichotomous fashion with clear cutoff values. Decision trees ensure ease of clinical use and direct immediate decision making and are often used where time is a critical factor in determining success of outcome.[19] This approach does not require computation or longitudinal monitoring. The aim of the categorical approach is to maximize sensitivity at the expense of specificity. With the goal to "not miss" EOS cases, a wide margin for categorizing infants as "at risk" is seen as beneficial, and the likelihood of overtreatment is judged to be acceptable. Whereas the CDC largely focuses on management strategies for infants in context of maternal

Table 1.1 CDC AND AAP GUIDELINES FOR EOS RISK ASSESSMENT AMONG INFANTS BORN AT ≥37 WEEKS' GESTATION

Clinical Risk Factor	Recommendations
Obstetric clinical diagnosis of chorioamnionitis	Blood culture at birth CBC and differential (± CRP) at birth and/or at 6–12 hr age Administer empiric antibiotics
Inadequate indicated GBS IAP and ROM ≥18 hr	± Blood culture at birth ± CBC and differential, ± CRP at birth and/or at 6–12 hr age Observation for minimum 48 hr
Inadequate indicated GBS IAP and ROM <18 hr	Clinical observation for minimum 48 hr
Adequate indicated GBS IAP	Clinical observation for minimum 24–48 hr

GBS-specific chemoprophylaxis, AAP guidelines have evolved to provide more holistic guidance for all bacterial causes of EOS.[20–22] The specific criteria and tests recommended by the most recent guidelines are outlined in Table 1.1.

Multivariate risk assessment: This approach utilizes established risk factors and newborn clinical condition to estimate the individual infant's risk of EOS. In their study of infants being evaluated for EOS using a CDC-recommended categorical approach, Escobar and colleagues demonstrated that a limited number of risk factors could be used to predict infection.[7] Subsequently, these investigators used a cohort of 608,000 infants born at ≥34 weeks' gestation to develop predictive models for culture-confirmed EOS based on objective data known at the moment of birth[23] and the evolving newborn condition in the first 6 to 12 hours after birth.[24] The objective data used include gestational age, highest intrapartum maternal temperature, maternal GBS status, duration of rupture of membranes (ROM), and type and duration of intrapartum antibiotics. The models were used to develop a web-based Sepsis Risk Calculator (SRC) with recommended clinical algorithms based on the final risk estimate.[25] Blood culture and enhanced clinical observation are recommended for infants with EOS risk estimated at ≥1/1000, and blood culture and empiric antibiotics are recommended for infants with EOS risk estimated at ≥3/1000. The primary advantage of the multivariate approach is that it accounts for interactions between risk factors, providing differential information on an individual infant's risk rather than placing infants in categories with a wide range of risk. A further advantage is that it uses only objective data, including maternal fever, without requiring obstetric clinical judgment with respect to clinical chorioamnionitis. If needed, the risk estimated can be recalculated during the first 6 to 12 hours as the newborn clinical condition evolves. Care pathways must be established to ensure that the risk estimate is accurately calculated and recorded at birth. The clinical care algorithms rely on enhanced clinical surveillance for infants with estimates 1/1000 requiring birth hospitalization for a minimum of 48 hours, as well as frequent vital signs and clinical nursing assessments. Institutions opting for this approach may set different risk thresholds for specific actions if local resources mandate more conservative algorithms (for example, setting the threshold for antibiotics at a risk estimate of 2/1000), but the use of more liberal thresholds has not been validated.

Risk assessment based primarily on newborn clinical condition: A third strategy for evaluating risk among well-appearing term infants consists of reliance on clinical signs of illness to identify infants with EOS. Such an approach is based on the observation that among term infants, asymptomatic condition at birth is associated with an ≈60% to 70% reduction in risk for EOS.[7,24] EOS in persistently asymptomatic infants is uncommon. In their prospective SRC validation report, only 1/56,261 infants managed using the SRC had bacteremia despite never manifesting signs of illness.[25] Other centers report the convergence of EOS with symptoms: In one report of 19,320 infants born at ≥35 weeks' gestation, all 8 infants with EOS had clinical signs of illness at birth or developed illness before 48 hours of age.[26] In another, 11 of 53,788 newborns of all gestational ages developed GBS-specific EOS; 5 of 11 were symptomatic at birth, and 6 became ill between 6 and 48 hours of age.[27] Two

Table 1.2 CLINICAL OBSERVATION FOR WELL-APPEARING INFANTS AT RISK FOR EOS

Reference #	Screening Policy	Years	Infants Included	Laboratory Tests (%)	Antibiotics (%)	EOS Rate (%)
28	*First period*: Laboratory tests (blood culture, CRP, CBC) for infants born to mothers with intrapartum fever or inadequate GBS IAP. Antibiotics for intrapartum fever or abnormal laboratory tests	2005–2007	Well at birth ≥35 weeks n = 9832	11.6	2.8	0.21
	Second period: Laboratory tests for infants born to mothers with intrapartum fever or neonates with inadequate IAP and ≥2 additional risk factors	2009–2011	Well at birth ≥35 weeks n = 10,569	1.6	0.6	0.05
29	*First period*: Laboratory tests (blood culture, CBC) and serial physical exam for infants born to mothers who are GBS positive (or have risk factors) and inadequate IAP	2004–2005	Well at birth ≥37 weeks n = 7625	6.9	1.2	0.17
	Second period: Serial physical exam alone for infants born to mothers who are GBS positive (or have risk factors) and inadequate IAP	2005–2006	≥37 weeks n = 7611	0.6	0.5	0.03

centers in Italy have reported experience with strategies based on identification of at-risk newborns using categorical approaches to risk, accompanied by laboratory tests and serial examinations of at-risk newborns (Table 1.2).[28,29] Both of these reports demonstrate decreases in laboratory test utilization and empiric antibiotic administration, with strategies relying on serial clinical examination of at-risk newborns.

Areas of Controversy

EOS risk assessment for initially well-appearing term infants is a matter of considerable controversy among newborn caregivers, with debate centered on four main issues: (1) how many newborns is it acceptable to evaluate and empirically treat to identify one case of EOS; (2) what is the best way to use available laboratory tests to assess risk; (3) what are the economic and social costs of EOS risk assessment; and (4) what unintended consequences result from perinatal antibiotic administration?

How many infants should be empirically evaluated and empirically treated for risk of EOS? This judgment is perhaps the most controversial aspect of the categorical risk approach. The impact of using the recommendations contained within the CDC or AAP recommendations has been described in a variety of reports (Table 1.3). Depending on which categorical approach is taken, 5% to 20% of term and late preterm infants are evaluated with laboratory tests, and 5% to 10% are administered neonatal antibiotics for risk of EOS. The multivariate risk approach was predicted to result in fewer newborns evaluated and empirically treated with antibiotics.[23,24] A prospective validation report including 204,685 infants born at ≥35 weeks' gestation cared for in an integrated health care system demonstrates that blood culture testing declined by 66% and empiric antibiotic administration declined by 48% (to 2.6%) with use of the multivariate risk approach, compared with the use of a risk algorithm

Table 1.3 OUTCOMES OF CATEGORICAL APPROACHES TO EOS RISK ASSESSMENT

Reference #	Policy	Years	Infants Included	Laboratory Tests (%)	Antibiotics (%)	EOS Rate (%)
26	CDC 1996	1996–1999	≥35 weeks n = 19,320	10.0	N/A	0.07
33	CDC 2002	2008–2009	Well-appearing ≥35 weeks n = 7943	24	7	0.03
34	CDC 2010	2013–2014	≥36 weeks n = 6544	13	12	0.04
25	CDC 2010	2010–2012	≥35 weeks n = 95,354	14	5	0.06
35	AAP 2013	2006–2012	≥35 weeks n = 12,121	4.6	4.6	0.03

Laboratory testing defined as some combination of blood culture and/or CBC and/or CRP. Report includes only infants born in setting of chorioamnionitis.

based on CDC 2010 recommendations. No adverse impacts of the multivariate risk approach were noted during the birth hospitalization or after-birth hospital discharge. Hospital readmissions within 7 days of birth for culture-confirmed EOS were rare, occurring at a rate of ≈5/100,000 births, regardless of the approach taken for risk assessment at birth.[25] Strategies based on clinical observation are predicted to result in very low rates of empiric antibiotic administration. In the two reports of using clinical observation for well-appearing infants deemed at risk for EOS on the basis of inadequate GBS intrapartum antibiotic prophylaxis (IAP), <1% of such infants were treated with empiric antibiotics for development of symptoms; neither of these reports provide data on use of antibiotics among infants symptomatic from birth.

Both the multivariate model and observation-based approach provide significant practical challenges compared with the categorical decision-tree approach. The SRC was designed for use with all live births ≥34 weeks; it is not validated for secondary assessment of infants flagged at risk by categorical approaches as has been done in retrospective studies.[30,31] It does not rely on categorical risk flags but uses objective risk data to provide an estimated risk of EOS at the moment of birth. This estimate is subsequently adjusted based on the evolving newborn clinical condition. Centers adopting this approach must develop processes for ensuring that the data required for the multivariate risk estimate are available and that the SRC output is properly calculated, recorded, and communicated to caregivers. The SRC provides guidance on specific actions that can be taken at specific levels of risk. Observation-based approaches require centers to decide who is eligible for observation versus intervention; how to screen for risk (using a categorical or multivariate approach, with or without laboratory testing); and how serial clinical examinations will be conducted, recorded, and communicated. Furthermore, centers would need to develop explicit guidance for intervention based on specific changes in the newborn clinical condition. A National Institute of Child Health and Human Development–sponsored expert panel recently advocated for clinical observation of asymptomatic term infants born to mothers with suspected intrauterine infection,[32] whereas the reports detailed in Table 1.3 and Table 1.4 used this approach for infants born in the context of intrapartum maternal fever, as well those born to mothers with inadequate indicated GBS IAP.[33–36] Theoretically, a center could dispense with all EOS risk assessment and implement serial clinical observation for all well-appearing term newborns, intervening with laboratory testing and/or empiric antibiotics only when signs of illness became apparent. Such an approach would be predicted to result in very low utilization of laboratory testing and empiric antibiotic administration, but would significantly affect the structure of well-nursery care. The need for frequent clinical assessments and vital sign measurements would affect mother/infant couplet care and could result in increased labor costs resulting from increased demands on both nursing and pediatric providers.

Table 1.4 WBC TESTING AMONG WELL-APPEARING NEWBORNS AT RISK FOR EOS

Reference #	Years	Infants With CBC	CBC Timing (hours)	Abnormal CBC Definition	Abnormal CBC (#)	EOS among Tested Infants, # (%)
26	1996–1999	≥35 weeks All EOS Risk n = 1665	<4	WBC ≤5000 or ≥30,000 ANC <1500 I/T >0.2	454/1665	0 (0.0)
33	2008–2009	≥35 weeks All EOS risk n = 1062	0–2	WBC ≤5000 I/T >0.2	32/1062	3 (0.3)[a]
35	2011–2012	≥35 weeks Exposed to CAM n = 692	0, 12, and 24	At least one value abnormal of ANC, ATI, or I/T	686/692	3 (0.4)
36	2006–2012	≥35 weeks Exposed to CAM n = 535	0 and 12	I/T >0.2[b]	185/535	3 (0.6)[c]
29	2004–2005	≥35 weeks All EOS risk n = 477	0–48	WBC ≤5000 or ≥15,000[b]	327/477	3 (0.6)

For each study, number of infants includes only those for whom the whole CBC was obtained. *ANC,* absolute neutrophil count; *ATI,* absolute immature neutrophil count; *CAM,* chorioamnionitis; *CBC,* complete blood count; *EOS,* early-onset sepsis; *I/T,* ratio of immature to total neutrophil forms; *WBC,* white blood count.
[a]None of the 3 cases of EOS were among the 32 infants with abnormal CBC.
[b]In both reports clinicians also variably obtained CRP levels.
[c]Although three cases of EOS were well appearing by 6 to 8 hours of age, all were depressed at birth, requiring positive pressure ventilation, continuous positive airway pressure (CPAP), or bag/mask ventilation.

Most importantly, clinicians using an observation-based approach to EOS risk assessment will need to view newborn transition from well appearing to symptomatic as an expected outcome and not a failure of care.

   What is the best way to use available laboratory tests to assess EOS risk? Clinicians seek to use laboratory tests to both predict and diagnose EOS. Bacterial culture; the white blood cell (WBC) count and differential (including absolute neutrophil count [ANC] and the ratio of immature to total neutrophil forms [I/T]); proinflammatory cytokines such as interleukins 1β, 6, 8, and 10 and tumor necrosis factor alpha; acute-phase reactants such as procalcitonin and C-reactive protein (CRP); and cell surface markers such as CD64 have been variably correlated with culture-proven, clinical, and viral sepsis. Most recently, molecular methods such as microarray and proteome analysis have sought to characterize molecular signatures that correlate with culture-confirmed infection.

- *Bacterial culture and the definition of EOS*: Epidemiologic studies of EOS are based on culture-confirmed isolation of pathogenic bacterial species from normally sterile compartments, most commonly blood and cerebrospinal fluid, and rarely in some circumstances, pleural or peritoneal fluid. Neonatal surface cultures taken at birth are generally considered to represent colonization; although used to test the efficacy of GBS IAP, cultures of the nares, inner ear, periumbilical and perianal regions, or swallowed amniotic fluid do not reflect invasive infection. Among symptomatic infants, evidence of surface colonization has been used to justify the diagnosis of "culture-negative sepsis" by arguing that blood cultures are sterile due to the use of maternally administered intrapartum antibiotic administration. Currently available blood culture systems use optimized enriched culture media with antimicrobial-inactivating elements that efficiently neutralize commonly used beta-lactam antibiotics as well as gentamicin. These culture systems detect bacteremia at a level of 1 to 10 colony-forming units if a minimum of 1 milliliter of blood is inoculated.[37–40] Studies report no impact of intrapartum antibiotics on blood culture time to positivity among bacteremic infants.[41,42] Nonetheless, concern for culture-negative infection drives variable definitions of "clinical sepsis" or "culture-negative sepsis." Some authors have advocated for a neonatal consensus diagnosis of EOS, based on the presence of symptoms and elevations of specific inflammatory markers.[43] Both epidemiologic studies and clinical intervention trials may benefit from a neonatal consensus definition of EOS that extends beyond culture-confirmed disease, particularly among studies conducted in low-resource settings. Among adult patients, early recognition of sepsis syndrome and prompt initiation of volume resuscitation as well as antibiotics is critical to intact survival. However, there is no equivalent clinical imperative among well-appearing term newborns. The most straightforward approach to evaluating the predictive performance of laboratory tests is to use the outcome of culture-confirmed infection.

- **Complete blood count (CBC)**: The most commonly used laboratory test to evaluate risk of EOS among newborns is the CBC and its components.[5] Recent studies suggest this practice should be reconsidered. Multiple single centers have reported the poor sensitivity of total WBC and differential for identifying culture-confirmed EOS among initially well-appearing infants. The rates at which newborns are flagged with "abnormal" WBC vary widely, influenced by metric chosen, the definition of abnormal, and the time at which the test is obtained (see Table 1.4). Newman et al. addressed each of these issues in a multicenter study including 67,623 CBC/differential tests obtained within 1 hour of a blood culture, with 245 cases of culture-confirmed infection (incidence of EOS, 0.4% among tested infants).[44] Test performance was analyzed using multiple approaches, including determining the mean values and distribution of values comparing infected and uninfected infants and sensitivity, specificity, and likelihood ratios for infection at different thresholds of "abnormal." In addition, multiple models were built to determine if adjusting for age, birth weight, birth facility, year of birth, maternal diagnosis of preeclampsia, mode of delivery, and 5-minute Apgar score would improve test performance. The best test performance was obtained by accounting for age in hours after birth. The poorest test performance associated with values obtained immediately after birth was particularly notable: the receiver–operator curve for total WBC was 0.52 at <1 hour of age. Platelet count was also nonpredictive, even for values obtained >4 hours of age. The best test performance was obtained for extremely low WBC and ANC values obtained after 4 hours of age; the I/T^2 (essentially the I/T divided by the ANC) was the only test characteristic with good performance independent of newborn age.[44,45] A larger multicenter study including 293 centers in the Pediatrix Medical Group performed similar analyses: 168,604 blood cultures from infants admitted to a neonatal intensive care unit were matched to CBC obtained within 24 hours of the blood culture, including 2001 cases of culture-confirmed EOS.[46] This study included infants of all gestational ages, with results provided in gestational age categories. Poor sensitivity was again found for WBC, the differential components, and the platelet count. Among infants born at ≥37 weeks' gestation, the highest likelihood ratios were associated with WBC <5000, ANC <1500, and I/T >0.5, and platelet counts were nonpredictive. Despite this evidence, U.S. national recommendations continue to advocate for use of the WBC and differential in EOS risk assessment.

- **CRP and other markers of inflammation**: Most studies of inflammatory molecules and biomarkers have been performed on infants who are symptomatic and being evaluated for sepsis. None of these has yet proven useful in predicting infection in initially well-appearing infants. Nonetheless, CRP was the second most common laboratory test used to identify infants at risk for EOS in a national survey of neonatal providers.[5] CRP is one of several acute-phase reactant proteins synthesized in the liver in response to proinflammatory cytokines. CRP is documented to rise and fall over the course of neonatal GBS infection with a variable course.[47] A single measurement of CRP sent at the same time as blood culture lacks sensitivity for EOS, although serial measurements have a likelihood ratio of ≈3 for predicting culture-confirmed infection.[48] CRP is particularly problematic for use in the immediate neonatal period, as it rises in response to other common neonatal conditions such as bruising and cephalohematoma and in generalized conditions of fetal distress that lead to meconium-stained amniotic fluid.[49] Similarly, procalcitonin is an acute-phase reactant that increases earlier than CRP in the course of infection, but also rises in response to asphyxia, respiratory distress syndrome, and pneumothorax; procalcitonin also appears to naturally rise and decline in the first 48 hours after birth.[50] A review of 18 neonatal procalcitonin studies demonstrated a wide range of cutoff values, definitions for outcomes, and ultimately variable test performance.[51] Most recently, molecular methods have been utilized to identify a "molecular signature" of EOS. Sweeney and colleagues employed an 11-gene microarray to identify culture-confirmed early- and late-onset infection in retrospective analysis of three different study cohorts including a wide range of gestational ages. The study found high diagnostic accuracy in distinguishing culture-confirmed infection.[52]

What are the economic and social costs of EOS risk assessment? Many reports have focused on the economic impact of maternal GBS screening and IAP, but few have addressed the costs of neonatal assessment and treatment. Economic analysis of EOS risk activities is complicated by variation across centers in the both diagnostic and therapeutic approach and, importantly, whether newborns are admitted to higher-cost intensive care units or primarily cared for in well-nursery settings. We performed an economic analysis addressing the costs associated with EOS risk assessment among well-appearing infants born at ≥36 weeks' gestation who were ultimately found to be uninfected. We estimated that a local algorithm aligned with the categorical approach recommended in the 2010 CDC GBS guidelines results in $110,000 to $150,000 in costs per 1000 live births.[34] Extrapolated to ≈3.6 million term births per year in the United States, approximately $400 to $500 million is spent annually on EOS-associated procedures. The social costs are also considerable. In most perinatal centers, blood tests, intravenous line placement, and antibiotic administration are performed in neonatal care settings separate from maternal care settings, resulting in mother–infant separation after birth. In a survey of national EOS, 95% of respondents separate mother and infant to perform laboratory testing, and ≈40% of newborns receiving antibiotics for EOS are separated from the mother for the duration of care.[5] Such separation has a significantly negative effect on the establishment of breastfeeding. In a study of 692 asymptomatic term infants separated from the mother for the evaluation of EOS, separation during the first 2 hours after birth resulted in significantly lower incidence of exclusive breastfeeding and increased use of formula in the absence of a medical indication.[53] This unintended consequence of EOS evaluation among well-appearing newborns may have long-term child health implications.

Are there long-term consequences that result from perinatal antibiotic administration? Microbial exposure has been shown to have a role in determining host immune behavior as early as prenatal life, via the maternal microflora.[54] This is followed by a postnatal period when the increase in microbial exposure at birth overlaps with the critical developmental window of immune cell programming.[55–58] The roles of commensal microflora exposure in innate and adaptive immune pathways, including induction of toll-like receptor tolerance to exogenous endotoxin and production of short-chain fatty acid (SCFA) that stimulate the regulatory T-cell population, have been demonstrated in multiple studies.[59,60] In preclinical studies, disruption of the early host microflora—either absolutely (as in germ-free mice) or partially by antibiotic exposure—results in an increased proinflammatory response in host gut to environmental irritants and an increased mortality when fighting invasive pathogens.[61,62] Mice given subtherapeutic levels of antibiotics after weaning exhibit increased adiposity and increased bacterial SFCA metabolism and energy extraction.[63,64] Early low-dose antibiotics combined with a high-fat diet cause even greater increases in adiposity.[65,66] Many of these effects occur only during the newborn period, highlighting the importance of early-life microbiota and the potential for disruption to cause lasting adverse health outcomes. Intrapartum antibiotics are administered with the intent of altering colonization of the newborn with pathogenic bacterial species. An unintended consequence may be more global alteration of the early microbiota in both diversity and composition. Recently, multiple studies have documented the

Table 1.5 STUDIES ADDRESSING PERINATAL ANTIBIOTICS AND NEONATAL MICROBIOME

Reference #	Infant Population (#)	Exposure	Microbiota Source and Timing	Impact on IAP-Exposed Compared With Unexposed
67–70	Term (52)	IAP (ampicillin)	Infant gut at 7 and 30 days	↑ *Enterobacteriaceae* and ↓ *Bifidobacterium* at both 7 and 30 days BF impact
71	Term (198)	IAP/VD (96) No IAP/VD (40) IAP/CS/P (17) IAP/CS/E (23)	Infant gut at 3 months and 1 year	↑ *Proteobacterium* and *Clostridia* (especially CS) ↓ *Bacteroidetes* BF impact
72	Term dyads (262)	GBS status IAP	Infant gut at 1 and 6 months	↑ *Clostridiaceae*, *Ruminococcoceae*, *Enterococcaceae* in infants born to GBS + mothers when adjusting for IAP
73	Women at <32 weeks' gestation (27)	IAP for GBS + and GBS unknown	Maternal vaginal microbiota	Most *Lactobacillus* in GBS+/ no IAP Most *Pseudomonas* in GBS –/+ IAP
74	Term dyads (36) Mothers with elevated BMI	IAP (cefazolin or penicillin G)	Placenta Oral (mother and infant) Gut (mother)	↑ *Proteobacteria* ↓ *Streptococcaceae*, *Gemellaceae*, and *Lactobacilli* ↓ Maternal–infant similarity
75	Term dyads (45)	Observational	Vertical transmission of *Lactobacillus*	Both IAP and PROM ↓ *Lactobacillus* in infant
76	Term (50)	IAP for GBS	Stool culture at day 3	↓ *Clostridia*
77, 78	Preterm (27) Term (13)	Prematurity	Longitudinal over 3 months	↑ *Enterobacteriaceae* even when adjusting for prematurity

BF, Breastfeeding; *BMI*, body mass index; *CS/P*, planned cesarean section delivery; *CS/E*, emergent cesarean section delivery; *GBS*, group B streptococcus; *IAP*, intrapartum antibiotic prophylaxis; *PROM*, premature rupture of membranes; *VD*, vaginal delivery.

impact of intrapartum antibiotics, with effects extending days to months (Table 1.5).[67–78] Neonatal antibiotics administered for risk of EOS have not been as well studied to date, but are anticipated to have some impact on the developing microbiota as well. Epidemiologic studies have reported an association of early-life antibiotics with increased risk of multiple adverse outcomes, including obesity, diabetes, asthma, eczema and food allergies, altered response to subsequent infections, and decreased vaccine responses.[55,79–89] Whether intrapartum and neonatal antibiotics specifically have enduring health consequences for the infant is a source of active research that will affect the risk/benefit balance of EOS risk assessment practices.

REFERENCES

1. Taylor JA, Opel DJ. Choriophobia: a 1-act play. *Pediatrics*. 2012;130:342–346.
2. Benitz WE, Wynn JL, Polin RA. Reappraisal of guidelines for management of neonates with suspected early-onset sepsis. *J Pediatr*. 2015;166:1070–1074.
3. Schrag SJ, Farley MM, Petit S, et al. Epidemiology of invasive early-onset neonatal sepsis, 2005 to 2014. *Pediatrics*. 2016;138:e20162013.
4. Kaiser Permanente Division of Research. Neonatal Early-Onset Sepsis Calculator. Kaiser Permanente Division of Research; 2017 [cited February 2, 2017]. Available from https://neonatalsepsiscalculator .kaiserpermanente.org.
5. Mukhopadhyay S, Taylor JA, Von Kohorn I, et al. Variation in sepsis evaluation across a national network of nurseries. *Pediatrics*. 2017;139:e20162845.
6. Van Dyke MK, Phares CR, Lynfield R, et al. Evaluation of universal antenatal screening for group B *Streptococcus*. *N Engl J Med*. 2009;360:2626–2636.

7. Escobar GJ, Li DK, Armstrong MA, et al. Neonatal sepsis workups in infants ≥ 2000 grams at birth: A population-based study. *Pediatrics*. 2000;106:256–263.

8. Committee on Infectious Diseases. Committee on Fetus and Newborn: Guidelines for prevention of group B streptococcal (GBS) infection by chemoprophylaxis. *Pediatrics*. 1992;90:775–778.

9. Centers for Disease Control and Prevention. Prevention of perinatal group B streptococcal disease: A public health perspective. *MMWR Recomm Rep*. 1996;45(RR–7):1–24.

10. Prevention of early-onset group B streptococcal disease in newborns. *Int J Gynaecol Obstet*. 2003;81:115–122.

11. Boyer KM, Gadzala CA, Burd LI, et al. Selective intrapartum chemoprophylaxis of neonatal group B streptococcal early-onset disease. I. Epidemiologic rationale. *J Infect Dis*. 1983;148:795–801.

12. Boyer KM, Gadzala CA, Kelly PD, et al. Selective intrapartum chemoprophylaxis of neonatal group B streptococcal early-onset disease. II. Predictive value of prenatal cultures. *J Infect Dis*. 1983;148:802–809.

13. Boyer KM, Gadzala CA, Kelly PD, et al. Selective intrapartum chemoprophylaxis of neonatal group B streptococcal early-onset disease. III. Interruption of mother-to-infant transmission. *J Infect Dis*. 1983;148:810–816.

14. Boyer KM, Gotoff SP. Prevention of early-onset neonatal group B streptococcal disease with selective intrapartum chemoprophylaxis. *N Engl J Med*. 1986;314:1665–1669.

15. Schrag SJ, Zywicki S, Farley MM, et al. Group B streptococcal disease in the era of intrapartum antibiotic prophylaxis. *N Engl J Med*. 2000;342:15–20.

16. Schrag SJ, Zell ER, Lynfield R, et al. A population-based comparison of strategies to prevent early-onset group B streptococcal disease in neonates. *N Engl J Med*. 2002;347:233–239.

17. Schrag S, Gorwitz R, Fultz-Butts K, et al. Prevention of perinatal group B streptococcal disease. Revised guidelines from CDC. *MMWR Recomm Rep*. 2002;51:1–22.

18. Verani JR, McGee L, Schrag SJ. Prevention of perinatal group B streptococcal disease—revised guidelines from CDC, 2010. *MMWR Recomm Rep*. 2010;59:1–36.

19. Penaloza-Ramos MC, Sheppard JP, Jowett S, et al. Cost-effectiveness of optimizing acute stroke care services for thrombolysis. *Stroke*. 2014;45:553–562.

20. Polin RA, Papile L, Baley J, et al. Management of neonates with suspected or proven early-onset bacterial sepsis. *Pediatrics*. 2012;129:1006–1015.

21. Brady MT, Polin RA. Prevention and management of infants with suspected or proven neonatal sepsis. *Pediatrics*. 2013;132:166–168.

22. Polin RA, Watterberg K, Benitz W, et al. The conundrum of early-onset sepsis. *Pediatrics*. 2014;133:1122–1123.

23. Puopolo KM, Draper D, Wi S, et al. Estimating the probability of neonatal early-onset infection on the basis of maternal risk factors. *Pediatrics*. 2011;128:e1155–e1163.

24. Escobar GJ, Puopolo KM, Wi S, et al. Stratification of risk of early-onset sepsis in newborns ≥34 weeks' gestation. *Pediatrics*. 2014;133:30–36.

25. Kuzniewicz MW, Puopolo KM, Fischer A, et al. A quantitative, risk-based approach to the management of neonatal early-onset sepsis. *JAMA Pediatr*. 2017;171:365–371.

26. Ottolini MC, Lundgren K, Mirkinson LJ, et al. Utility of complete blood count and blood culture screening to diagnose neonatal sepsis in the asymptomatic at risk newborn. *Pediatr Infect Dis J*. 2003;22:430–434.

27. Hashavya S, Benenson S, Ergaz-Shaltiel Z, et al. The use of blood counts and blood cultures to screen neonates born to partially treated group B *Streptococcus*-carrier mothers for early-onset sepsis: is it justified? *Pediatr Infect Dis J*. 2011;30:840–843.

28. Berardi A, Fornaciari S, Rossi C, et al. Safety of physical examination alone for managing well-appearing neonates ≥ 35 weeks' gestation at risk for early-onset sepsis. *J Matern Fetal Neonatal Med*. 2014;1–5.

29. Cantoni L, Ronfani L, Da Riol R, et al. Physical examination instead of laboratory tests for most infants born to mothers colonized with group B *Streptococcus*: support for the Centers for Disease Control and Prevention's 2010 recommendations. *J Pediatr*. 2013;163:568–573.

30. Shakib J, Buchi K, Smith E, et al. Management of newborns born to mothers with chorioamnionitis: is it time for a kinder, gentler approach? *Acad Pediatr*. 2015;15:340–344.

31. Warren S, Garcia M, Hankins C. Impact of neonatal early-onset sepsis calculator on antibiotic use within two tertiary healthcare centers. *J Perinatol*. 2017;37:394–397.

32. Higgins RD, Saade G, Polin RA, et al. Evaluation and management of women and newborns with a maternal diagnosis of chorioamnionitis: summary of a workshop. *Obstet Gynecol*. 2016;127:426–436.

33. Mukhopadhyay S, Eichenwald EC, Puopolo KM. Neonatal early-onset sepsis evaluations among well-appearing infants: projected impact of changes in CDC GBS guidelines. *J Perinatol*. 2013;33:198–205.

34. Mukhopadhyay S, Dukhovny D, Mao W, et al. 2010 perinatal GBS prevention guideline and resource utilization. *Pediatrics*. 2014;133:196–203.

35. Jackson GL, Engle WD, Sendelbach DM, et al. Are complete blood cell counts useful in the evaluation of asymptomatic neonates exposed to suspected chorioamnionitis? *Pediatrics*. 2004;113:1173–1180.

36. Kiser C, Nawab U, McKenna K, et al. Role of guidelines on length of therapy in chorioamnionitis and neonatal sepsis. *Pediatrics*. 2014;133:992–998.

37. Jorgensen JH, Mirrett S, McDonald LC, et al. Controlled clinical laboratory comparison of BACTEC plus aerobic/F resin medium with BacT/Alert aerobic FAN medium for detection of bacteremia and fungemia. *J Clin Microbiol*. 1997;35:53–58.

A

38. Flayhart D, Borek AP, Wakefield T, et al. Comparison of BACTEC PLUS blood culture media to BacT/Alert FA blood culture media for detection of bacterial pathogens in samples containing therapeutic levels of antibiotics. *J Clin Microbiol*. 2007;45:816–821.

39. Dunne WM Jr, Case LK, Isgriggs L, et al. In-house validation of the BACTEC 9240 blood culture system for detection of bacterial contamination in platelet concentrates. *Transfusion*. 2005;45:1138–1142.

40. Nanua S, Weber C, Isgriggs L, et al. Performance evaluation of the VersaTREK blood culture system for quality control testing of platelet units. *J Clin Microbiol*. 2009;47:817–818.

41. Garcia-Prats JA, Cooper TR, Schneider VF, et al. Rapid detection of microorganisms in blood cultures of newborn infants utilizing an automated blood culture system. *Pediatrics*. 2000;105:523–527.

42. Sarkar SS, Bhagat I, Bhatt-Mehta V, et al. Does maternal intrapartum antibiotic treatment prolong the incubation time required for blood cultures to become positive for infants with early-onset sepsis? *Am J Perinatol*. 2015;32:357–362.

43. Wynn JL, Wong HR, Shanley TP, et al. Time for a neonatal-specific consensus definition for sepsis. *Pediatr Crit Care Med*. 2014;15:523–528.

44. Newman TB, Puopolo KM, Wi S, et al. Interpreting complete blood counts soon after birth in newborns at risk for sepsis. *Pediatrics*. 2010;126:903–909.

45. Newman TB, Draper D, Puopolo KM, et al. Combining immature and total neutrophil counts to predict early onset sepsis in term and late preterm newborns: use of the I/T2. *Pediatr Infect Dis J*. 2014;33:798–802.

46. Hornik CP, Benjamin DK, Becker KC, et al. Use of the complete blood cell count in early-onset neonatal sepsis. *Pediatr Infect Dis J*. 2012;31:799–802.

47. Philip AG. Response of C-reactive protein in neonatal Group B streptococcal infection. *Pediatr Infect Dis*. 1985;4:145–148.

48. Benitz WE, Han MY, Madan A, et al. Serial serum C-reactive protein levels in the diagnosis of neonatal infection. *Pediatrics*. 1998;102:E41.

49. Pourcyrous M, Bada HS, Korones SB, et al. Significance of serial C-reactive protein responses in neonatal infection and other disorders. *Pediatrics*. 1993;92:431–435.

50. Benitz WE. Adjunct laboratory tests in the diagnosis of early-onset neonatal sepsis. *Clin Perinatol*. 2010;37:421–438.

51. Chiesa C, Pacifico L, Osborn JF, et al. Early-onset neonatal sepsis: still room for improvement in procalcitonin diagnostic accuracy studies. *Medicine (Baltimore)*. 2015;94:e1230.

52. Sweeney TE, Wynn JL, Cernada M, et al. Validation of the Sepsis MetaScore for diagnosis of neonatal sepsis. *J Pediatric Infect Dis Soc*. 2018;15;7(2):129–135.

53. Mukhopadhyay S, Lieberman ES, Puopolo KM, et al. Effect of early-onset sepsis evaluations on in-hospital breastfeeding practices among asymptomatic term neonates. *Hosp Pediatr*. 2015;5:203–210.

54. Gomez de Aguero M, Ganal-Vonarburg SC, Fuhrer T, et al. The maternal microbiota drives early postnatal innate immune development. *Science*. 2016;351:1296–1302.

55. Vangay P, Ward T, Gerber JS, et al. Antibiotics, pediatric dysbiosis, and disease. *Cell Host Microbe*. 2015;17:553–564.

56. Dominguez-Bello MG, Costello EK, Contreras M, et al. Delivery mode shapes the acquisition and structure of the initial microbiota across multiple body habitats in newborns. *Proc Natl Acad Sci USA*. 2010;107:11971–11975.

57. Chu DM, Ma J, Prince AL, et al. Maturation of the infant microbiome community structure and function across multiple body sites and in relation to mode of delivery. *Nat Med*. 2017;23:314–326.

58. Renz H, Brandtzaeg P, Hornef M. The impact of perinatal immune development on mucosal homeostasis and chronic inflammation. *Nat Rev Immunol*. 2011;12:9–23.

59. Lotz M, Gutle D, Walther S, et al. Postnatal acquisition of endotoxin tolerance in intestinal epithelial cells. *J Exp Med*. 2006;203:973–984.

60. Smith PM, Howitt MR, Panikov N, et al. The microbial metabolites, short-chain fatty acids, regulate colonic Treg cell homeostasis. *Science*. 2013;341:569–573.

61. Deshmukh HS, Liu Y, Menkiti OR, et al. The microbiota regulates neutrophil homeostasis and host resistance to Escherichia coli K1 sepsis in neonatal mice. *Nat Med*. 2014;20:524–530.

62. Olszak T, An D, Zeissig S, et al. Microbial exposure during early life has persistent effects on natural killer T cell function. *Science*. 2012;336:489–493.

63. Cho I, Yamanishi S, Cox L, et al. Antibiotics in early life alter the murine colonic microbiome and adiposity. *Nature*. 2012;488:621–626.

64. Samuel BS, Shaito A, Motoike T, et al. Effects of the gut microbiota on host adiposity are modulated by the short-chain fatty-acid binding G protein-coupled receptor, Gpr41. *Proc Natl Acad Sci USA*. 2008;105:16767–16772.

65. Cox LM, Yamanishi S, Sohn J, et al. Altering the intestinal microbiota during a critical developmental window has lasting metabolic consequences. *Cell*. 2014;158:705–721.

66. Ridaura VK, Faith JJ, Rey FE, et al. Gut microbiota from twins discordant for obesity modulate metabolism in mice. *Science*. 2013;341:1241214.

67. Corvaglia L, Tonti G, Martini S, et al. Influence of intrapartum antibiotic prophylaxis for group B Streptococcus on gut microbiota in the first month of life. *J Pediatr Gastroenterol Nutr*. 2016;62:304–308.

68. Mazzola G, Murphy K, Ross RP, et al. Early gut microbiota perturbations following intrapartum antibiotic prophylaxis to prevent group B streptococcal disease. *PLoS ONE*. 2016;11:e0157527.

69. Aloisio I, Mazzola G, Corvaglia LT, et al. Influence of intrapartum antibiotic prophylaxis against group B *Streptococcus* on the early newborn gut composition and evaluation of the anti-Streptococcus activity of Bifidobacterium strains. *Appl Microbiol Biotechnol*. 2014;98:6051–6060.

70. Aloisio I, Quagliariello A, De Fanti S, et al. Evaluation of the effects of intrapartum antibiotic prophylaxis on newborn intestinal microbiota using a sequencing approach targeted to multi hypervariable 16S rDNA regions. *Appl Microbiol Biotechnol*. 2016;100:5537–5546.
71. Azad MB, Konya T, Persaud RR, et al. Impact of maternal intrapartum antibiotics, method of birth and breastfeeding on gut microbiota during the first year of life: a prospective cohort study. *BJOG*. 2016;123:983–993.
72. Cassidy-Bushrow AE, Sitarik A, Levin AM, et al. Maternal group B Streptococcus and the infant gut microbiota. *J Dev Orig Health Dis*. 2016;7:45–53.
73. Roesch LF, Silveira RC, Corso AL, et al. Diversity and composition of vaginal microbiota of pregnant women at risk for transmitting Group B Streptococcus treated with intrapartum penicillin. *PLoS ONE*. 2017;12:e0169916.
74. Gomez-Arango LF, Barrett HL, McIntyre HD, et al. Antibiotic treatment at delivery shapes the initial oral microbiome in neonates. *Sci Rep*. 2017;7:43481.
75. Keski-Nisula L, Kyynarainen HR, Karkkainen U, et al. Maternal intrapartum antibiotics and decreased vertical transmission of Lactobacillus to neonates during birth. *Acta Paediatr*. 2013;102:480–485.
76. Jaureguy F, Carton M, Panel P, et al. Effects of intrapartum penicillin prophylaxis on intestinal bacterial colonization in infants. *J Clin Microbiol*. 2004;42:5184–5188.
77. Arboleya S, Sanchez B, Solis G, et al. Impact of prematurity and perinatal antibiotics on the developing intestinal microbiota: a functional inference study. *Int J Mol Sci*. 2016;17:e649.
78. Arboleya S, Sanchez B, Milani C, et al. Intestinal microbiota development in preterm neonates and effect of perinatal antibiotics. *J Pediatr*. 2015;166:538–544.
79. Metsala J, Lundqvist A, Virta LJ, et al. Mother's and offspring's use of antibiotics and infant allergy to cow's milk. *Epidemiology*. 2013;24:303–309.
80. Marrs T, Bruce KD, Logan K, et al. Is there an association between microbial exposure and food allergy? A systematic review. *Pediatr Allergy Immunol*. 2013;24:311–320, e8.
81. McKeever TM, Lewis SA, Smith C, et al. Early exposure to infections and antibiotics and the incidence of allergic disease: a birth cohort study with the West Midlands General Practice Research Database. *J Allergy Clin Immunol*. 2002;109:43–50.
82. Tsakok T, McKeever TM, Yeo L, et al. Does early life exposure to antibiotics increase the risk of eczema? A systematic review. *Br J Dermatol*. 2013;169:983–991.
83. Murk W, Risnes KR, Bracken MB. Prenatal or early-life exposure to antibiotics and risk of childhood asthma: a systematic review. *Pediatrics*. 2011;127:1125–1138.
84. Kummeling I, Stelma FF, Dagnelie PC, et al. Early life exposure to antibiotics and the subsequent development of eczema, wheeze, and allergic sensitization in the first 2 years of life: the KOALA Birth Cohort Study. *Pediatrics*. 2007;119:e225–e231.
85. Penders J, Kummeling I, Thijs C. Infant antibiotic use and wheeze and asthma risk: a systematic review and meta-analysis. *Eur Respir J*. 2011;38:295–302.
86. Alm B, Erdes L, Mollborg P, et al. Neonatal antibiotic treatment is a risk factor for early wheezing. *Pediatrics*. 2008;121:697–702.
87. Kuppala VS, Meinzen-Derr J, Morrow AL, et al. Prolonged initial empirical antibiotic treatment is associated with adverse outcomes in premature infants. *J Pediatr*. 2011;159:720–725.
88. Salt P, Banner C, Oh S, et al. Social mixing with other children during infancy enhances antibody response to a pneumococcal conjugate vaccine in early childhood. *Clin Vaccine Immunol*. 2007;14:593–599.
89. Bjorksten B. Diverse microbial exposure - consequences for vaccine development. *Vaccine*. 2012;30:4336–4340.

CHAPTER 2

Empiric Antimicrobials for Neonatal Sepsis

Olivia B. Payne, BS, Jessica E. Ericson, MD, MPH

2

- Most early-onset infections are caused by group B *Streptococcus* and *E. coli.*
- Ampicillin + gentamicin is an appropriate empiric antibiotic regimen for early-onset sepsis in most settings.
- Most late-onset infections are caused by gram-positive organisms.
- Nafcillin + gentamicin balances the need for a narrow spectrum with the risks of potentially providing inadequate empiric treatment in most cases.
- Empiric antimicrobials targeting MRSA, *Pseudomonas*, yeast, and viruses should be considered if risk factors are present, but are unnecessary in most cases.

Neonatal sepsis refers to an onset of systemic symptoms due to infection during the first month of age and is associated with high morbidity and mortality.[1,2] Although neonatal sepsis can be due to bacteria, viruses, or fungi, bacterial infections account for the vast majority of cases.[3] Neonatal infections are differentiated into early onset and late onset based on the age of the infant when symptoms develop.[3]

Clinical signs of neonatal sepsis are often nonspecific and can include lethargy, poor feeding, irritability, and temperature instability.[4] Furthermore, blood culture results are often not available for 48 to 72 hours, prolonging the amount of time before an infection can be proven and targeted treatment can be initiated. Delaying treatment for infants with bacterial infections may increase their risk of morbidity and mortality.[5] For this reason, empiric treatment is often started while awaiting culture results. Due to the changing epidemiology of neonatal sepsis, as well as the growing number of cases due to antibiotic-resistant pathogens, the optimal antibiotic combination for empiric treatment in the modern era is uncertain.[6,7] This review will discuss the relative risks and benefits of antibiotics currently used for empiric treatment of neonatal sepsis.

Early-Onset Sepsis

Pathogens responsible for early-onset infections are typically acquired from the mother's genital tract during delivery and cause symptoms within the first 3 days after birth.[8] Prolonged membrane rupture, chorioamnionitis, and prematurity each increase the risk of early onset sepsis (EOS).[9] Premature infants are at higher risk with as many as 11/1000 infants developing EOS; <1/1000 term infants develop EOS.[8,9] Approximately 70% of EOS cases are due to *Streptococcus agalactiae* (group B *Streptococcus* [GBS]) or *Escherichia coli* (Table 2.1).[8,9] The risk of specific organisms as a cause of EOS varies by gestational age: GBS is the most common organism among term infants, and *E. coli* is the most common organism among preterm infants.[9] Other bacteria that cause EOS include viridans group *Streptococci, Enterococcus* species, enteric gram-negative bacilli, and *Listeria monocytogenes.*[8] Mortality due

Table 2.1 ORGANISMS FREQUENTLY CAUSING EARLY-ONSET SEPSIS IN INFANTS[8]

Organism	% of Cases
≥37 weeks gestational age	
Streptococcus agalactiae	45
Escherichia coli	13
Staphylococcus aureus	6
<37 weeks gestational age	
Escherichia coli	39
Streptococcus agalactiae	27
Staphylococcus aureus	1

Adapted from Weston EJ, Pondo T, Lewis MM, et al. The burden of invasive early-onset neonatal sepsis in the United States, 2005-2008. *Pediatr Infect Dis J.* 2011;30(11):937–941.

to EOS varies by gestational age, but can be as high as 38%.[9] For this reason, antibiotics are typically started empirically while awaiting culture results.

Ampicillin and Gentamicin

The American Academy of Pediatrics and the World Health Organization recommend empiric treatment with ampicillin or penicillin in combination with gentamicin for infants with suspected EOS.[6,10,11] Ampicillin provides coverage against many gram-positive infections, including GBS and *L. monocytogenes*, as well as some gram-negative pathogens.[12] The addition of gentamicin allows for coverage of a greater number of gram-negative bacteria, including ampicillin-resistant *E. coli*.[12] Other advantages include relatively low cost and extensive experience with this specific combination.[13]

Ampicillin

Penicillins, such as ampicillin, are relatively nontoxic in infants.[13] Rare side effects include allergic reactions, neutropenia and, with high exposures, seizures.[14] Furthermore, GBS remains the leading cause of EOS, despite widespread implementation of intrapartum antibiotic prophylaxis (IAP) for pregnant women colonized with GBS.[15] GBS isolates remain fully susceptible to beta-lactams, including penicillin and ampicillin.[9,16,17]

Ampicillin is additionally the drug of choice for susceptible infections due to *Enterococcus* species and *L. monocytogenes*.[18,19] *L. monocytogenes* is a well-known but uncommon cause of maternal and neonatal infection.[9,20] EOS develops in the infant when transplacental transmission of listeriosis occurs after maternal infection or through acquisition of maternal gastrointestinal and vaginal flora during the birth process.[21] Despite its rarity, EOS due to *L. monocytogenes* is associated with a high mortality and significant sequelae in survivors.[22] Although no study has demonstrated superior effectiveness of early effective therapy for this particular condition, given the available evidence, it seems prudent to provide optimal empiric therapy for this organism until it has been ruled out.

Gentamicin

Aminoglycosides, such as gentamicin, provide exceptional activity against gram-negative bacilli and provide synergy with penicillins against GBS, *S. aureus*, enterococci, and *L. monocytogenes*.[18,23] Additional advantages of gentamicin treatment include infrequent resistance and low cost compared with many newer antibiotics.[24]

Although infections due to ampicillin-resistant *E. coli* have increased, gentamicin-resistant *E. coli* infections are rare.[12] A recent study surveyed the antibiotic susceptibilities of neonatal *E. coli* isolates from 221 German hospitals.[25] They found that although 45% of the 158 invasive *E. coli* infections were resistant to ampicillin, 96% were susceptible to gentamicin.[25] Another prospective surveillance study conducted by 16 Eunice Kennedy Shriver National Institute of Child Health and Human Development Neonatal Research Network (NRN) institutions similarly demonstrated that 78% of the 102 *E. coli* isolates obtained were ampicillin resistant but only 4% were gentamicin resistant.[9] A prospective surveillance study that included 12 neonatal units in England reported that 95% of the 125 identified EOS infections were susceptible to a gentamicin/penicillin combination.[26] These studies suggest that the specific combination of ampicillin and gentamicin remains an appropriate empiric therapy for EOS in most centers.

Limitations of Ampicillin and Gentamicin

Although ampicillin plus gentamicin is the most common antibiotic combination used for EOS, the continued appropriateness of this antibiotic strategy has been questioned by several investigators who argue that other agents may be more advantageous.

Ampicillin Concerns

A commonly noted emerging deficiency of ampicillin as empiric treatment for EOS is the trend of increasing ampicillin resistance among EOS cases due to *E. coli*.[7,9,27,28] Since widespread IAP with ampicillin was recommended in 1996, the proportion of EOS *E. coli* infections resistant to ampicillin has increased, especially among premature and very-low-birth-weight infants.[28–30] Prolonged durations of IAP with ampicillin before birth also appears to increase the risk of EOS due to ampicillin-resistant *E. coli*.[31] In a study of 35 deaths due to culture-confirmed EOS, those with ampicillin-resistant *E. coli* had exposure to a mean of 18 doses of ampicillin before delivery; those with other organisms had a mean of 5 doses ($P < 0.001$).[31] As many as 78% to 85% of early-onset *E. coli* infections are due to ampicillin-resistant strains.[32,33]

Gentamicin Concerns

The greatest concerns with gentamicin, as with all aminoglycosides, are the risks of ototoxicity and nephrotoxicity.[34] High doses of aminoglycosides can damage the sensory hair cells, leading to irreversible hearing loss.[34] Nephrotoxicity typically presents as a reversible inability to concentrate urine, along with proteinuria.[13] These risks can be reduced with careful therapeutic drug monitoring of blood levels, but toxicity sometimes occurs even at low concentrations and short durations.[13] In particular, an estimated 1 in 500 individuals has a mitochondrial DNA mutation that increases the risk of hearing loss with aminoglycoside therapy, even when blood concentrations are within the target range.[35] Additionally, aminoglycosides may potentiate the effect of environmental noise on the developing cochlea such that low concentrations of gentamicin may lead to ototoxicity if administered in a noisy environment, such as a neonatal intensive care unit (NICU).[36]

Unfortunately, it has been difficult to determine the true risk of these toxicities for infants exposed to aminoglycosides because there are many potential confounding factors, including NICU admission itself, sepsis, and other comorbidities. A recent case-control study comparing children presenting with sensorineural hearing loss at <5 years of age who had been born at ≤32 weeks gestational age found no difference in the proportions of children exposed to gentamicin between the groups with and without hearing loss.[37] There were also no differences seen in the total cumulated gentamicin dosages, predicted trough serum levels, or duration of gentamicin exposure between cases and controls.[37] A systematic review that included 11 studies and 946 infants with suspected serious bacterial infections found that 3% of infants exposed to gentamicin developed hearing impairment.[35] However, there was no comparison group, so this does not necessarily reflect aminoglycoside-attributable hearing loss. The long-term adverse effects of early-life gentamicin exposure remain unclear.

Although uncommon, cases of ampicillin and gentamicin–resistant *E. coli* have been reported; therefore, although the ampicillin/gentamicin combination appears to currently be the most rational empiric regimen for EOS, the incidence of resistant infections should be closely monitored.[25,27]

Timing of Antibiotic Initiation

In addition to weighing the potential risks and benefits, regional microbiology and individual risk factors when selecting an antibiotic for empiric therapy, the timing of antibiotic initiation should be considered. For symptomatic infants, prompt initiation of empiric antibiotics is warranted.[10,15] However, for asymptomatic infants at risk for EOS, the optimal timing of antibiotic initiation is less clear. The NRN found that, of 229 chorioamnionitis-exposed infants with EOS, 21 (9%) were asymptomatic during the first 72 hours after birth.[38] Term infants with EOS were more likely to have been asymptomatic than were preterm infants, 22% vs. 2%.[38] Although beginning empiric antibiotics for all infants with chorioamnionitis exposure allows even asymptomatic infants to be treated promptly, asymptomatic EOS is so rare that the NRN investigators estimated that 60 to 1400 infants would be exposed to antibiotics unnecessarily to provide treatment for each asymptomatic infected infant.[38] Another study failed to find EOS in any of 1413 asymptomatic infants.[39] These observations suggest that deferral of antibiotic therapy and close monitoring for development of clinical signs of sepsis may be an option for asymptomatic infants.

Late-Onset Sepsis

In contrast to EOS, late onset sepsis (LOS) pathogens are acquired from the environment after parturition, resulting in the development of symptoms between days 4 and 120 after birth.[40] Gram-positive organisms predominate in LOS cases (Table 2.2).[40,41] For hospitalized infants, invasive procedures such as the placement of intravascular catheters, chest tubes and other drains, mechanical ventilation, parenteral nutrition, and surgical procedures interfere with the infant's immune barriers, making them more susceptible to infection.[41] Coagulase-negative staphylococci (CoNS) is the most common cause of LOS (45%–53%), followed by *S. aureus* (11%–13%), *E. coli* (5%–7%), and GBS (2%–7%).[11,41]

As with EOS infections, cases of suspected LOS should be treated empirically. Because the pathogen distribution is different for LOS compared with EOS, there is greater variability among centers and clinicians regarding the preferred antibiotic regimen.[42,43] A common strategy is to use one antibiotic with predominantly gram-positive activity (i.e., ampicillin, nafcillin, vancomycin) and another with predominantly gram-negative activity (gentamicin or cefotaxime). Given that a substantial percentage of LOS infections are nosocomial, it is crucial to consider local and institutional epidemiology when determining the most appropriate empiric treatment.[11,12]

Ampicillin

Ampicillin is often used as empiric treatment of LOS for the same reasons that it is used for EOS: good coverage of GBS, *Enterococcus* species, and *L. monocytogenes*, along with some coverage of *E. coli* and other gram-negative bacteria. However, LOS is more likely to be due to CoNS or *S. aureus* than these organisms, and ampicillin

Table 2.2   ORGANISMS FREQUENTLY CAUSING LATE-ONSET SEPSIS IN INFANTS[40,41]

Organism	% of Cases
≥37 weeks gestational age	
Escherichia coli	20
Coagulase-negative staphylococci	19
Staphylococcus aureus	18
Streptococcus agalactiae	8
Pseudomonas aeruginosa	2
<37 weeks gestational age	
Coagulase-negative staphylococci	53
Staphylococcus aureus	11
Streptococcus agalactiae	2
Escherichia coli	5
Pseudomonas aeruginosa	2

Adapted from Testoni D, Hayashi M, Cohen-Wolkowiez M, et al. Late-onset bloodstream infections in hospitalized term infants. *Pediatr Infect Dis J.* 2014;33(9):920–923 and Boghossian NS, Page GP, Bell EF, et al. Late-onset sepsis in very low birth weight infants from singleton and multiple-gestation births. *J Pediatr.* 2013;162(6):1120–1124, 1124.

is only rarely effective against CoNS and *S. aureus*. GBS does still cause disease, but is much less common than in the first 3 days after birth, accounting for <10% of LOS cases.[40,41] For these reasons, many clinicians limit empiric ampicillin use to the first 3 days after birth and use broader-spectrum agents thereafter.

Vancomycin

Vancomycin is commonly used as the gram-positive antibiotic of choice for empiric treatment of LOS because of its broad spectrum. CoNS and *S. aureus* are the most common causes of LOS, and ≈50% of CoNS and 28% of *S. aureus* are resistant to beta-lactams.[44-46] Vancomycin is also effective against GBS, *Enterococcus,* and *L. monocytogenes*, less common causes of LOS. For this reason, some centers use vancomycin empirically for infants with signs of LOS.[42,47]

However, early initiation of empiric vancomycin treatment has not been shown to be beneficial in most cases of bacteremia due to these organisms. A retrospective study of 4364 infants with CoNS bacteremia found that the 2848 infants who received empiric vancomycin treatment had similar mortality when compared with 1516 infants who received vancomycin 1 to 3 days after the first positive blood culture was collected (9% vs. 8%; adjusted odds ratio [aOR] 1.06; 95% confidence interval [CI]: 0.81, 1.39).[48] The duration of bacteremia and duration of hospital stay were also similar.[48] Although this study did not compare other important sequelae of CoNS bacteremia, including neurodevelopmental impairment, it did suggest that for infants with beta-lactam–resistant CoNS infections, definitive therapy with vancomycin could likely be delayed until susceptibility results were available, without substantial increase in risk.[49] A single-center study reported no change in the frequency of fulminant sepsis or the duration of the sepsis episodes for a 2 year period with use of oxacillin compared with a 7 year period with vancomycin as the standard empiric gram-positive antibiotic.[50]

In addition to limited data supporting its effectiveness compared with antibiotics with narrower spectrums, the Centers for Disease Control and Prevention (CDC) has specifically targeted reducing excessive vancomycin use as a health care improvement goal.[51] In addition to the short-term consequences of vancomycin exposure, nephrotoxicity, and ototoxicity,[52,53] vancomycin use increases the risk of future sepsis in general and infections with vancomycin-resistant enterococci,[54] multidrug-resistant gram-negative bacilli,[55] vancomycin-intermediate and -resistant *S. aureus,* and invasive candidiasis in particular, for both the individual and the patient care unit.[56]

However, in centers where LOS due to methicillin-resistant *Staphylococcus aureus* (MRSA) is common, empiric vancomycin may be appropriate. A large retrospective study found that for infants with MRSA-associated bacteremia, empiric vancomycin therapy was associated with improved survival at 30 days.[5] Adjusting for confounding factors, adequate empiric antibiotic therapy with vancomycin doubled the odds of survival at 30 days (aOR = 2.06; 1.08, 3.82).[5]

Nafcillin/Oxacillin

The antistaphylococcal penicillins, nafcillin and oxacillin, are increasingly used as empiric therapy for LOS.[57] These antibiotics provide good activity against methicillin-sensitive *S. aureus* (MSSA), susceptible CoNS isolates, GBS, and other *Streptococcus* species, while having a narrower spectrum and less toxicity than vancomycin.

Recently, empiric use of oxacillin for LOS has been associated with an unexpected decrease in the incidence of LOS due to *S. aureus*.[58] This is thought to be due to decreased selective pressure on *S. aureus,* because the incidence of CoNS infections did increase with the change. Because CoNS are less pathogenic than *S. aureus*, this change resulted in three fewer deaths during the 2-year oxacillin period compared with the 2-year vancomycin period.[58] Several other centers have found that they were able to reduce vancomycin use dramatically without increases in mortality or measured morbidities. One center decreased their vancomycin use from 81% of antibiotic courses to 23% of antibiotic courses with no changes in the mortality rate.[59] A multicenter study of medication use in 220 NICUs found that nafcillin use increased by 158% over the 5 years of the study period.[60] Over that same period, mortality among the infants born weighing ≤1500 g did not change.[61]

The major therapeutic hole for these penicillins is MRSA. However, invasive MSSA infections are much more common than MRSA infections in infants, and beta-lactam antibiotics are superior to vancomycin for treatment of invasive MSSA.[44,62] Unless the incidence of MRSA is particularly high or there are very clear risk factors for MRSA, it seems appropriate to use the class of antibiotics that will be the most effective for the common organisms rather than using an antibiotic that, although it provides a more complete gram-positive spectrum of activity, is a less effective drug for most organisms. Although infants colonized with MRSA can have LOS caused by other types of organisms, due to the increased risk of invasive MRSA infection, colonized infants should probably be treated empirically with vancomycin when signs of LOS develop.[63]

Nafcillin and oxacillin likely have some activity against *Enterococcus* species and *L. monocytogenes*, but there are no approved criteria for testing for susceptibility of these antibiotic/organism combinations. Ampicillin or vancomycin should be used if these organisms are suspected. However, concern for these organisms should not have a significant impact on antibiotic selection for LOS. Infections due to *L. monocytogenes* are exceedingly rare after the first postnatal month.[64]

Cefazolin

Cefazolin, a first-generation cephalosporin, has the same general advantages and disadvantages as nafcillin/oxacillin, in that it has a narrower spectrum and less toxicity than vancomycin. There is not as much experience using cefazolin for LOS as there is with the antistaphylococcal penicillins, but it appears to have similar efficacy for the treatment of MSSA bacteremia in older patients.[65,66] Cefazolin has the additional theoretical benefit as an empiric agent for neonatal LOS of a spectrum that often includes *E. coli* and *Klebsiella* species in addition to gram-positive organisms.[67] Like all cephalosporins, cefazolin is not effective for the treatment of infections due to *Enterococcus* species or *L. monocytogenes*. Importantly, cefazolin is not effective for treatment of meningitis so should not be used unless meningitis has been ruled out. Studies in infants should be conducted before initiating widespread use of empiric cefazolin.

Cefotaxime

Cefotaxime is a third-generation cephalosporin that provides increased coverage against gram-negative bacteria while maintaining fair gram-positive activity.[18] Cefotaxime is the preferred treatment for cases of suspected or proven neonatal meningitis due to its superior central nervous system penetration and high rate of cerebrospinal fluid (CSF) sterilization.[12,68] In contrast to their high rates of resistance to ampicillin, most *E. coli* infections are susceptible to cefotaxime. The NRN found that only 3% of 94 early-onset *E. coli* infections were due to cephalosporin-resistant strains.[9] Similarly, a national surveillance study conducted in Germany found that 4% of 158 *E. coli* infections were resistant to cefotaxime.[25] Another surveillance study that included 5 years of neonatal bloodstream infections in England and Wales found that ≈3% of *E. coli* infections were resistant to cefotaxime.[69] Because of the broader spectrum of cefotaxime compared with ampicillin, this antibiotic is often used as a single agent, which has the advantage of reduced line entries and potentially lower toxicity.

However, cefotaxime is not effective against *Enterococcus* or *L. monocytogenes,* so ampicillin should be used in addition to cefotaxime if these organisms are suspected.[20] Additionally, third-generation cephalosporins are less effective than first-generation cephalosporins or antistaphylococcal penicillins against *S. aureus*.[70] Cefotaxime also does not exhibit synergy when combined with gentamicin, such that the addition of gentamicin to cefotaxime is less useful than when it is used alongside ampicillin or nafcillin.[18]

An additional concern with widespread cephalosporin use is the associated increase in resistant isolates, such that caution must be exercised before using cefotaxime as part of the standard empiric antibiotic strategy for infants. In settings where broad-spectrum antibiotic use is common, cephalosporin resistance rates among gram-negatives causing LOS can reach 50%.[71] Studies in adults have linked cephalosporin use to the selection of highly resistant gram-negative isolates and increased rates of infections due to *Pseudomonas aeruginosa* and extended-spectrum penicillinase producing enterobactericeae.[72] Additionally, cephalosporin use in infants unduly increases the risk of invasive candidiasis, which has significant associated morbidity and mortality and may be associated with an increased risk of all-cause mortality in hospitalized infants.[73,74] A study of infants with meconium aspiration syndrome found that exposure to cefotaxime was independently associated with an increased odds of death (aOR 2.1; 95% CI 1.4, 3.4).[75]

Due to these concerns with efficacy and safety, many experts only recommend the use of cefotaxime with suspected or proven neonatal meningitis, or as an alternative to gentamicin in instances of neonatal renal or auditory problems.[12]

Gentamicin

Similar to its role in EOS, gentamicin provides broad-spectrum gram-negative coverage with the additional potential benefit of synergy with other antibiotics for the treatment of some gram-positive infections.[18,23] Because gram-positive infections predominate after 3 days of age, the combination of ampicillin/gentamicin or nafcillin or oxacillin/gentamicin would be expected to provide a good balance of a relatively narrow spectrum that still provides effective coverage for the majority of expected pathogens.[59] Gentamicin is not typically used in combination with cefotaxime because cefotaxime alone provides good gram-negative coverage.

Pseudomonas Coverage

Approximately 2% to 5% of LOS cases are due to *P. aeruginosa*.[26,41] Because of this low incidence, empiric coverage of *P. aeruginosa* is not usually warranted. However, compared with other pathogens, *P. aeruginosa* is more likely to cause fulminant disease and has a much higher mortality than other pathogens.[76–78] An Australian surveillance study with an unusually high incidence of *Pseudomonas* LOS found that 52% of infants with *Pseudomonas* infection died and there was a significantly increased odds of mortality compared with other gram-negative bacilli (OR = 5.9; 95% CI 3.69, 9.47).[78] Consideration should be given to including empiric antibiotics that are effective against *P. aeruginosa* for infants with rapidly progressive clinical decompensation.

Although most cases are sporadic, *P. aeruginosa* has been known to cause outbreaks of disease in neonatal units in the past.[79] Compared with other organisms, the risk of infant-to-infant spread is much higher for *P. aeruginosa*. For this reason, empiric coverage of *P. aeruginosa* is warranted for neighbors of *Pseudomonas*-infected infants who develop signs of infection.[80] Ceftazidime, cefepime, piperacillin-tazobactam, and meropenem are the antibiotics most often used for empiric and definitive treatment of *P. aeruginosa*. Piperacillin-tazobactam and meropenem are also effective against anaerobic bacteria, so they may have greater detrimental effects on intestinal flora and risks of candidiasis and infections with resistant organisms.[81] When meningitis is a possibility, piperacillin-tazobactam may not be as effective as other antipseudomonal antibiotics because differential penetration of the two components across the blood–brain barrier may compromise achievement of a proper ratio of piperacillin to tazobactam concentrations in the CSF.[82] Fluoroquinolones are used in adults for treatment of *P. aeruginosa,* but should not generally be used in infants due to lack of safety data. The Food and Drug Administration recently upgraded the "black box" warning for fluoroquinolones due to findings that the risks of mitochondrial toxicity and other adverse events were more common than previously appreciated.[83]

Antifungals

Invasive candidiasis is a relatively uncommon cause of sepsis among infants but has a high mortality and leads to long-term neurodevelopmental impairment among survivors.[84] Empiric antifungal therapy should be considered for infants who do not show rapid improvement after initiation of empiric antibacterial agents. The risk of candidiasis is inversely related to gestational age and birth weight and is increased by exposure to third-generation cephalosporins and other broad-spectrum antibiotics and the presence of central venous catheters.[85] Fluconazole is a reasonable first-line antifungal if it has not been used for prophylaxis, in which case micafungin or amphotericin B deoxycholate should be considered instead.[86]

Early antifungal use has been shown to reduce mortality due to *Candida* LOS. A study that included 136 infants treated at NRN hospitals found that empiric antifungal treatment improved neurodevelopmental impairment–free survival for infants with candidiasis compared with those who only received definitive therapy. Fifty percent (19/38) of infants with invasive candidiasis who received empiric antifungal therapy had death or neurodevelopmental impairment compared with 64% (55/86) of those with delayed therapy (aOR 0.27; 95% CI 0.08–0.86).[87]

Antivirals

Neonatal herpes simplex virus (HSV) infections may lead to subtle or fulminant signs of sepsis in infants. Timing of presentation often depends on the manifestation of disease: disseminated disease usually presents around day 7 of age, skin–eye–mucous membrane disease around day 14 of age, and central nervous system disease around day 21 of age.[88] Delayed initiation of acyclovir to infants with HSV disease has been associated with increased mortality.[89] For infants who are ultimately diagnosed with HSV infection, empiric acyclovir therapy has been associated with improved survival compared with infants for whom acyclovir therapy is delayed until a definitive diagnosis is made (ORT 2.63; 95% CI 1.36–5.08).[89]

Conclusion

Most infants receiving empiric treatment actually do not have a bacterial infection. Uninfected infants receiving empiric treatment are exposed to the negative consequences of antibiotic use without corresponding benefit.[13,90] Recent studies have demonstrated that even short courses of empiric antibiotics lead to reductions in the biodiversity of intestinal microbes with a shift toward more pathogenic species like *Enterobacter*.[91] These alterations in biodiversity have been linked to increased risks of necrotizing enterocolitis, bacterial sepsis, invasive candidiasis, and death during infancy, as well as longer-term consequences that are still under study.[91] As we seek to improve care to achieve better short- and long-term outcomes, we must develop (1) better methods for identifying which infants truly have bacterial infections and (2) techniques that allow for accurate identification of the infecting organism rapidly enough that empiric therapy can promptly be replaced by definitive targeted therapy. While we await these capabilities, narrow-spectrum therapy with ampicillin and gentamicin for EOS or an antistaphylococcal penicillin and gentamicin for LOS is probably the best approach in most cases. Special risk factors may warrant broader empiric therapy, which should be narrowed as soon as culture results are available.

REFERENCES

1. Hornik CP, Fort P, Clark RH, et al. Early and late onset sepsis in very-low-birth-weight infants from a large group of neonatal intensive care units. *Early Hum Dev*. 2012;88(suppl 2):S69–S74.
2. Sivanandan S, Soraisham AS, Swarnam K. Choice and duration of antimicrobial therapy for neonatal sepsis and meningitis. *Int J Pediatr*. 2011;2011:712150.
3. Shane AL, Stoll BJ. Recent developments and current issues in the epidemiology, diagnosis, and management of bacterial and fungal neonatal sepsis. *Am J Perinatol*. 2013;30(2):131–141.
4. Berardi A, Buffagni AM, Rossi C, et al. Serial physical examinations, a simple and reliable tool for managing neonates at risk for early-onset sepsis. *World J Clin Pediatr*. 2016;5(4):358–364.
5. Thaden JT, Ericson JE, Cross H, et al. Survival benefit of empirical therapy for *Staphylococcus aureus* bloodstream infections in infants. *Pediatr Infect Dis J*. 2015;34:1175–1179.
6. Downie L, Armiento R, Subhi R, et al. Community-acquired neonatal and infant sepsis in developing countries: efficacy of WHO's currently recommended antibiotics–systematic review and meta-analysis. *Arch Dis Child*. 2013;98(2):146–154.
7. Bergin SP, Thaden J, Ericson JE, et al. Neonatal *Escherichia coli* bloodstream infections: clinical outcomes and impact of initial antibiotic therapy. *Pediatr Infect Dis J*. 2015;34(9):933–936.
8. Weston EJ, Pondo T, Lewis MM, et al. The burden of invasive early-onset neonatal sepsis in the United States, 2005-2008. *Pediatr Infect Dis J*. 2011;30(11):937–941.

9. Stoll BJ, Hansen NI, Sánchez PJ, et al. Early onset neonatal sepsis: the burden of group B Streptococcal and *E. coli* disease continues. *Pediatrics*. 2011;127(5):817–826.

10. Polin RA, Committee on Fetus and Newborn. Management of neonates with suspected or proven early-onset bacterial sepsis. *Pediatrics*. 2012;129(5):1006–1015.

11. Muller-Pebody B, Johnson AP, Heath PT, et al. Empirical treatment of neonatal sepsis: are the current guidelines adequate? *Arch Dis Child Fetal Neonatal Ed*. 2011;96(1):F4–F8.

12. Stockmann C, Spigarelli MG, Campbell SC, et al. Considerations in the pharmacologic treatment and prevention of neonatal sepsis. *Paediatr Drugs*. 2014;16(1):67–81.

13. Baltimore RS. Neonatal sepsis: epidemiology and management. *Paediatr Drugs*. 2003;5(11):723–740.

14. Hornik CP, Benjamin DK, Smith PB, et al. Electronic health records and pharmacokinetic modeling to assess the relationship between ampicillin exposure and seizure risk in neonates. *J Pediatr*. 2016;178:125–129.e121.

15. Verani JR, McGee L, Schrag SJ. Prevention of perinatal group B streptococcal disease–revised guidelines from CDC, 2010. *MMWR Recomm Rep*. 2010;59(RR–10):1–36.

16. Andrews JI, Diekema DJ, Hunter SK, et al. Group B streptococci causing neonatal bloodstream infection: antimicrobial susceptibility and serotyping results from SENTRY centers in the Western Hemisphere. *Am J Obstet Gynecol*. 2000;183(4):859–862.

17. Fluegge K, Supper S, Siedler A, et al. Antibiotic susceptibility in neonatal invasive isolates of *Streptococcus agalactiae* in a 2-year nationwide surveillance study in Germany. *Antimicrob Agents Chemother*. 2004;48(11):4444–4446.

18. Darmstadt GL, Batra M, Zaidi AK. Parenteral antibiotics for the treatment of serious neonatal bacterial infections in developing country settings. *Pediatr Infect Dis J*. 2009;28(1 suppl):S37–S42.

19. Kristich C, Rice L, Arias C. Enterococcal Infection - Treatment and Antibiotic Resistance. In: Gilmore M, Clewell D, Ike Y, et al, eds. *Enterococci: from Commensals to Leading Causes of Drug Resistant Infection*. Boston: Massachusetts Eye and Ear Infirmary; 2014.

20. Leazer R, Perkins AM, Shomaker K, et al. A meta-analysis of the rates of *Listeria monocytogenes* and *Enterococcus* in febrile infants. *Hosp Pediatr*. 2016;6(4):187–195.

21. Jiao Y, Zhang W, Ma J, et al. Early onset of neonatal listeriosis. *Pediatr Int*. 2011;53(6):1034–1037.

22. Mylonakis E, Paliou M, Hohmann EL, et al. Listeriosis during pregnancy: a case series and review of 222 cases. *Medicine (Baltimore)*. 2002;81(4):260–269.

23. Espaze EP, Reynaud AE. Antibiotic susceptibilities of *Listeria*: *in vitro* studies. *Infection*. 1988;16(suppl 2):S160–S164.

24. Spanggaard MH, Hønge BL, Schønheyder HC, et al. Short-term gentamicin therapy and risk of renal toxicity in patients with bacteraemia. *Scand J Infect Dis*. 2011;43(11–12):953–956.

25. Heideking M, Lander F, Hufnagel M, et al. Antibiotic susceptibility profiles of neonatal invasive isolates of Escherichia coli from a 2-year nationwide surveillance study in Germany, 2009-2010. *Eur J Clin Microbiol Infect Dis*. 2013;32(9):1221–1223.

26. Vergnano S, Menson E, Kennea N, et al. Neonatal infections in England: the NeonIN surveillance network. *Arch Dis Child Fetal Neonatal Ed*. 2011;96(1):F9–F14.

27. Friedman S, Shah V, Ohlsson A, et al. Neonatal *Escherichia coli* infections: concerns regarding resistance to current therapy. *Acta Paediatr*. 2000;89(6):686–689.

28. Bizzarro MJ, Dembry LM, Baltimore RS, et al. Changing patterns in neonatal *Escherichia coli* sepsis and ampicillin resistance in the era of intrapartum antibiotic prophylaxis. *Pediatrics*. 2008;121(4):689–696.

29. Alarcon A, Peña P, Salas S, et al. Neonatal early onset *Escherichia coli* sepsis: trends in incidence and antimicrobial resistance in the era of intrapartum antimicrobial prophylaxis. *Pediatr Infect Dis J*. 2004;23(4):295–299.

30. Hyde TB, Hilger TM, Reingold A, et al. Trends in incidence and antimicrobial resistance of early-onset sepsis: population-based surveillance in San Francisco and Atlanta. *Pediatrics*. 2002;110(4):690–695.

31. Terrone DA, Rinehart BK, Einstein MH, et al. Neonatal sepsis and death caused by resistant *Escherichia coli*: possible consequences of extended maternal ampicillin administration. *Am J Obstet Gynecol*. 1999;180(6 Pt 1):1345–1348.

32. Weissman SJ, Hansen NI, Zaterka-Baxter K, et al. Emergence of antibiotic resistance-associated clones among *Escherichia coli* recovered from newborns with early-onset sepsis and meningitis in the United States, 2008-2009. *J Pediatric Infect Dis Soc*. 2016;5(3):269–276.

33. Stoll BJ, Hansen N, Fanaroff AA, et al. Changes in pathogens causing early-onset sepsis in very-low-birth-weight infants. *N Engl J Med*. 2002;347(4):240–247.

34. Touw DJ, Westerman EM, Sprij AJ. Therapeutic drug monitoring of aminoglycosides in neonates. *Clin Pharmacokinet*. 2009;48(2):71–88.

35. Musiime GM, Seale AC, Moxon SG, et al. Risk of gentamicin toxicity in neonates treated for possible severe bacterial infection in low- and middle-income countries: systematic review. *Trop Med Int Health*. 2015;20(12):1593–1606.

36. Zimmerman E, Lahav A. Ototoxicity in preterm infants: effects of genetics, aminoglycosides, and loud environmental noise. *J Perinatol*. 2013;33(1):3–8.

37. Fuchs A, Zimmermann L, Bickle Graz M, et al. Gentamicin exposure and sensorineural hearing loss in preterm infants. *PLoS ONE*. 2016;11(7):e0158806.

38. Wortham JM, Hansen NI, Schrag SJ, et al. Chorioamnionitis and culture-confirmed, early-onset neonatal infections. *Pediatrics*. 2016;137(1):e20152323.

39. Hashavya S, Benenson S, Ergaz-Shaltiel Z, et al. The use of blood counts and blood cultures to screen neonates born to partially treated group B Streptococcus-carrier mothers for early-onset sepsis: is it justified? *Pediatr Infect Dis J*. 2011;30(10):840–843.

40. Testoni D, Hayashi M, Cohen-Wolkowiez M, et al. Late-onset bloodstream infections in hospitalized term infants. *Pediatr Infect Dis J*. 2014;33(9):920–923.

41. Boghossian NS, Page GP, Bell EF, et al. Late-onset sepsis in very low birth weight infants from singleton and multiple-gestation births. *J Pediatr*. 2013;162(6):1120–1124, 1124.

42. Arnold C, Clark R, Bosco J, et al. Variability in vancomycin use in newborn intensive care units determined from data in an electronic medical record. *Infect Control Hosp Epidemiol*. 2008;29(7):667–670.

43. Metsvaht T, Nellis G, Varendi H, et al. High variability in the dosing of commonly used antibiotics revealed by a Europe-wide point prevalence study: implications for research and dissemination. *BMC Pediatr*. 2015;15:41.

44. Ericson JE, Popoola VO, Smith PB, et al. Burden of invasive *Staphylococcus aureus* infections in hospitalized infants. *JAMA Pediatr*. 2015;169(12):1105–1111.

45. Källman J, Kihlström E, Sjöberg L, et al. Increase of staphylococci in neonatal septicaemia: a fourteen-year study. *Acta Paediatr*. 1997;86(5):533–538.

46. Kacica MA, Horgan MJ, Preston KE, et al. Relatedness of coagulase-negative staphylococci causing bacteremia in low-birthweight infants. *Infect Control Hosp Epidemiol*. 1994;15(10):658–662.

47. Rubin LG, Sánchez PJ, Siegel J, et al. Evaluation and treatment of neonates with suspected late-onset sepsis: a survey of neonatologists' practices. *Pediatrics*. 2002;110(4):e42.

48. Ericson JE, Thaden J, Cross HR, et al. No survival benefit with empirical vancomycin therapy for coagulase-negative staphylococcal bloodstream infections in infants. *Pediatr Infect Dis J*. 2015;34(4):371–375.

49. Blanchard AC, Quach C, Autmizguine J. Staphylococcal infections in infants: updates and current challenges. *Clin Perinatol*. 2015;42(1):119–132, ix.

50. Karlowicz MG, Buescher ES, Surka AE. Fulminant late-onset sepsis in a neonatal intensive care unit, 1988-1997, and the impact of avoiding empiric vancomycin therapy. *Pediatrics*. 2000;106(6):1387–1390.

51. Recommendations for preventing the spread of vancomycin resistance. Recommendations of the Hospital Infection Control Practices Advisory Committee (HICPAC). *MMWR Recomm Rep*. 1995;44(RR–12):1–13.

52. Vella-Brincat JW, Begg EJ, Robertshawe BJ, et al. Are gentamicin and/or vancomycin associated with ototoxicity in the neonate? A retrospective audit. *Neonatology*. 2011;100(2):186–193.

53. McKamy S, Hernandez E, Jahng M, et al. Incidence and risk factors influencing the development of vancomycin nephrotoxicity in children. *J Pediatr*. 2011;158(3):422–426.

54. Iosifidis E, Evdoridou I, Agakidou E, et al. Vancomycin-resistant *Enterococcus* outbreak in a neonatal intensive care unit: epidemiology, molecular analysis and risk factors. *Am J Infect Control*. 2013;41(10):857–861.

55. Ofek-Shlomai N, Benenson S, Ergaz Z, et al. Gastrointestinal colonization with ESBL-producing *Klebsiella* in preterm babies–is vancomycin to blame? *Eur J Clin Microbiol Infect Dis*. 2012;31(4):567–570.

56. Zaoutis TE, Prasad PA, Localio AR, et al. Risk factors and predictors for candidemia in pediatric intensive care unit patients: implications for prevention. *Clin Infect Dis*. 2010;51(5):e38–e45.

57. Chiu CH, Michelow IC, Cronin J, et al. Effectiveness of a guideline to reduce vancomycin use in the neonatal intensive care unit. *Pediatr Infect Dis J*. 2011;30(4):273–278.

58. Romanelli RM, Anchieta LM, Bueno E, et al. Empirical antimicrobial therapy for late-onset sepsis in a neonatal unit with high prevalence of coagulase-negative *Staphylococcus*. *J Pediatr (Rio J)*. 2016;92(5):472–478.

59. Holzmann-Pazgal G, Khan AM, Northrup TF, et al. Decreasing vancomycin utilization in a neonatal intensive care unit. *Am J Infect Control*. 2015;43(11):1255–1257.

60. Clark RH, Bloom BT, Spitzer AR, et al. Reported medication use in the neonatal intensive care unit: data from a large national data set. *Pediatrics*. 2006;117(6):1979–1987.

61. Stoll BJ, Hansen NI, Bell EF, et al. Trends in care practices, morbidity, and mortality of extremely preterm neonates, 1993-2012. *JAMA*. 2015;314(10):1039–1051.

62. Schweizer ML, Furuno JP, Harris AD, et al. Comparative effectiveness of nafcillin or cefazolin versus vancomycin in methicillin-susceptible *Staphylococcus aureus* bacteremia. *BMC Infect Dis*. 2011;11:279.

63. Popoola VO, Budd A, Wittig SM, et al. Methicillin-resistant *Staphylococcus aureus* transmission and infections in a neonatal intensive care unit despite active surveillance cultures and decolonization: challenges for infection prevention. *Infect Control Hosp Epidemiol*. 2014;35(4):412–418.

64. Okike IO, Awofisayo A, Adak B, et al. Empirical antibiotic cover for *Listeria monocytogenes* infection beyond the neonatal period: a time for change? *Arch Dis Child*. 2015;100(5):423–425.

65. Pollett S, Baxi SM, Rutherford GW, et al. Cefazolin versus nafcillin for methicillin-sensitive *Staphylococcus aureus* bloodstream infection in a California tertiary medical center. *Antimicrob Agents Chemother*. 2016;60(8):4684–4689.

66. Rao SN, Rhodes NJ, Lee BJ, et al. Treatment outcomes with cefazolin versus oxacillin for deep-seated methicillin-susceptible *Staphylococcus aureus* bloodstream infections. *Antimicrob Agents Chemother*. 2015;59(9):5232–5238.

67. Baxter Healthare Corporation. Cefazolin—cefazolin sodium injection, solution. https://dailymed.nlm.nih.gov/dailymed/drugInfo.cfm?setid=d91a8d13-99a0-4d87-88dc-71cbd37922b4. Accessed January 12, 2017.

68. Odio CM. Cefotaxime for treatment of neonatal sepsis and meningitis. *Diagn Microbiol Infect Dis*. 1995;22(1–2):111–117.

69. Blackburn RM, Verlander NQ, Heath PT, et al. The changing antibiotic susceptibility of bloodstream infections in the first month of life: informing antibiotic policies for early- and late-onset neonatal sepsis. *Epidemiol Infect*. 2014;142(4):803–811.

70. Kang N, Housman ST, Nicolau DP. Assessing the surrogate susceptibility of oxacillin and cefoxitin for commonly utilized parenteral agents against methicillin-susceptible *Staphylococcus aureus*: focus on ceftriaxone discordance between predictive susceptibility and *in vivo* exposures. *Pathogens*. 2015; 4(3):599–605.

71. Lona Reyes JC, Verdugo Robles M, Pérez Ramírez RO, et al. Etiology and antimicrobial resistance patterns in early and late neonatal sepsis in a Neonatal Intensive Care Unit. *Arch Argent Pediatr*. 2015;113(4):317–323.

72. Dancer SJ. The problem with cephalosporins. *J Antimicrob Chemother*. 2001;48(4):463–478.

73. Cotten CM, McDonald S, Stoll B, et al. The association of third-generation cephalosporin use and invasive candidiasis in extremely low birth-weight infants. *Pediatrics*. 2006;118(2):717–722.

74. Clark RH, Bloom BT, Spitzer AR, et al. Empiric use of ampicillin and cefotaxime, compared with ampicillin and gentamicin, for neonates at risk for sepsis is associated with an increased risk of neonatal death. *Pediatrics*. 2006;117(1):67–74.

75. Singh BS, Clark RH, Powers RJ, et al. Meconium aspiration syndrome remains a significant problem in the NICU: outcomes and treatment patterns in term neonates admitted for intensive care during a ten-year period. *J Perinatol*. 2009;29(7):497–503.

76. Tsai MH, Hsu JF, Chu SM, et al. Incidence, clinical characteristics and risk factors for adverse outcome in neonates with late-onset sepsis. *Pediatr Infect Dis J*. 2014;33(1):e7–e13.

77. Hammoud MS, Al-Taiar A, Thalib L, et al. Incidence, aetiology and resistance of late-onset neonatal sepsis: a five-year prospective study. *J Paediatr Child Health*. 2012;48(7):604–609.

78. Gordon A, Isaacs D. Late onset neonatal Gram-negative bacillary infection in Australia and New Zealand: 1992-2002. *Pediatr Infect Dis J*. 2006;25(1):25–29.

79. Jefferies JM, Cooper T, Yam T, et al. *Pseudomonas aeruginosa* outbreaks in the neonatal intensive care unit—a systematic review of risk factors and environmental sources. *J Med Microbiol*. 2012; 61(Pt 8):1052–1061.

80. Reichert F, Piening B, Geffers C, et al. Pathogen-specific clustering of nosocomial blood stream infections in very preterm infants. *Pediatrics*. 2016;137:(published online ahead of print).

81. Gibson MK, Wang B, Ahmadi S, et al. Developmental dynamics of the preterm infant gut microbiota and antibiotic resistome. *Nat Microbiol*. 2016;1:16024.

82. Leleu G, Kitzis MD, Vallois JM, et al. Different ratios of the piperacillin-tazobactam combination for treatment of experimental meningitis due to *Klebsiella pneumoniae* producing the TEM-3 extended-spectrum beta-lactamase. *Antimicrob Agents Chemother*. 1994;38(2):195–199.

83. Claris Lifesciences. Ciprofloxacin—ciprofloxacin injection, solution. https://dailymed.nlm.nih.gov/dailymed/drugInfo.cfm?setid=e82f52f2-ecf8-4c04-a206-f3253b265903. Accessed January 12, 2017.

84. Adams-Chapman I, Bann CM, Das A, et al. Neurodevelopmental outcome of extremely low birth weight infants with *Candida* infection. *J Pediatr*. 2013;163(4):961–967.

85. Kelly MS, Benjamin DK, Smith PB. The epidemiology and diagnosis of invasive candidiasis among premature infants. *Clin Perinatol*. 2015;42(1):105–117.

86. Botero-Calderon L, Benjamin DK, Cohen-Wolkowiez M. Advances in the treatment of invasive neonatal candidiasis. *Expert Opin Pharmacother*. 2015;16(7):1035–1048.

87. Greenberg RG, Benjamin DK, Gantz MG, et al. Empiric antifungal therapy and outcomes in extremely low birth weight infants with invasive candidiasis. *J Pediatr*. 2012;161(2):264–269.

88. Curfman AL, Glissmeyer EW, Ahmad FA, et al. Initial presentation of neonatal *Herpes simplex* virus infection. *J Pediatr*. 2016;172:121–126.

89. Shah SS, Aronson PL, Mohamad Z, et al. Delayed acyclovir therapy and death among neonates with *Herpes simplex* virus infection. *Pediatrics*. 2011;128(6):1153–1160.

90. Tzialla C, Borghesi A, Serra G, et al. Antimicrobial therapy in neonatal intensive care unit. *Ital J Pediatr*. 2015;41:27.

91. Greenwood C, Morrow AL, Lagomarcino AJ, et al. Early empiric antibiotic use in preterm infants is associated with lower bacterial diversity and higher relative abundance of *Enterobacter*. *J Pediatr*. 2014;165(1):23–29.

CHAPTER 3

When and How to Treat Neonatal CMV Infection

Kristin E.D. Weimer, MD, PhD, Sallie R. Permar, MD, PhD

- Congenital cytomegalovirus (CMV) is the leading infectious cause of hearing loss and neurologic deficits, affecting up to 1% of live births worldwide.
- Symptomatic congenital CMV infection should be treated with ganciclovir or valganciclovir for 6 months to reduce or ameliorate long-term neurologic deficits, including hearing loss and developmental delay.
- Studies suggest that some infants with asymptomatic congenital CMV infection may benefit from treatment.
- In premature infants, postnatal CMV infection can cause severe sepsis like disease and may contribute to long-term neurologic impairment and bronchopulmonary dysplasia.
- Premature infants with symptomatic postnatal CMV infection should be strongly considered for treatment.
- There is not enough evidence at this time to recommend routine treatment of asymptomatic premature infants with postnatal CMV infection.

Clinical Significance

Cytomegalovirus (CMV) is the most common infection in the newborn, affecting between 0.5% and 2.3% of live births worldwide.[1,2] The seroprevalence of CMV in adults ranges from 45% to 100%, depending on geographic location, socioeconomic status, and race.[3] Infants can acquire CMV infection in utero (congenital CMV), through maternal secretions at birth (perinatal), or after birth via breastfeeding (postnatal CMV). Historically, only congenital CMV was thought to cause clinically significant illness and lead to neurodevelopmental impairment in infants; however, new studies have shown that postnatal CMV infection in premature infants can cause severe disease and contribute to long-term sequelae. Although the infection types can be similar, the risk factors for transmission, severity of disease, long-term sequelae, and treatment recommendations differ based on route of infection (congenital vs. postnatal). We will therefore discuss these two modes of vertical viral transmission separately.

Congenital CMV Transmission and Outcomes

The highest risk of acquiring congenital CMV occurs in mothers with no prior immunity to CMV (primary infection, ≈40% transmission rate); however, transmission can occur with reactivation of a latent infection or maternal infection with a new strain of CMV (1%–2% transmission rate).[4,5] In fact, because of the high global prevalence of CMV seropositivity among women of childbearing age, the majority of congenital CMV infections occur in infants of women with prior immunity to CMV.[6]

Only 10% to 15% of infants with congenital CMV are symptomatic at birth. Symptoms range from mild to life-threatening multiorgan dysfunction and can include intrauterine growth restriction (IUGR), petechiae, jaundice, hepatosplenomegaly, microcephaly, chorioretinitis, and sensorineural hearing loss (SNHL).[7,8] Long-term sequelae include intellectual disability, seizures, chorioretinitis, optic nerve atrophy, psychomotor and speech delays, learning disabilities, and defects in dentition.[9] Of those infants who are asymptomatic at birth, 10% to 20% will develop neurologic impairment by 2 years of age, most commonly SNHL.[10–12] SNHL associated with CMV has a fluctuating and progressive course, with some children not developing symptoms until 6 years of age.[13,14] Infants with congenital CMV from a primary maternal infection are more likely to have severe sequelae.[7,8,15] Mortality in infants secondary to congenital CMV is 100 to 200 cases in the United States annually.[11] Overall, congenital CMV is the leading cause of developmental impairment and the leading nongenetic cause of SNHL in the developed world.[16,17]

Postnatal CMV Transmission and Outcomes

Infants acquire postnatal CMV through virus shed in maternal breast milk.[18,19] In the past, CMV was frequently transmitted to hospitalized infants through blood transfusions, but the use of CMV-seronegative or leukoreduced blood has essentially eliminated this mode of transmission.[20] Although harmless in full-term infants, postnatal CMV infection in very-low-birth-weight (VLBW, <1500 g birth weight) infants can result in a severe sepsis like illness characterized by pneumonitis, enteritis, hepatitis, and thrombocytopenia and may lead to long-term neurologic impairment.[21–23] In a meta-analysis of 17 studies, the risk of postnatal CMV infection in VLBW infants in the United States was approximately 6.5%, with 1.4% developing a sepsis like syndrome.[22] In most neonatal intensive care units (NICUs), the true prevalence is likely underestimated because CMV is not routinely tested for during sepsis evaluations.

It was initially thought that premature infants who survived a postnatal CMV infection, like full-term infants after postnatal infection, would have no long-term consequences. However, new studies suggest that this may not be the case. A prospective study that followed infants with and without a diagnosis of postnatal CMV initially showed that there were no differences in neurodevelopmental outcome between the two groups.[24] However, when the same population was followed longer, significant differences in neurodevelopment could be found beginning at 6 years of age.[21] In addition, a recent retrospective study on outcome data from over 300 NICUs found that VLBW infants with a diagnosis of postnatal CMV had an increased risk of the combined outcome of bronchopulmonary dysplasia (BPD) and death at 36 weeks corrected gestational age when compared with birth-weight–matched uninfected infants.[25] Other studies showed a variable association of postnatal CMV with BPD in premature infants.[26–30] A large, multicentered, prospective study is needed to fully determine the threat postnatal CMV poses to premature infants and determine how best to prevent virus transmission or disease in this population.

Treatment of Congenital CMV

Congenital CMV With Central Nervous System Involvement

Treatment of infants with congenital CMV infection and central nervous system (CNS) involvement is the most well-studied and least controversial population that will be discussed (Fig. 3.1). This population of infants has the highest risk for severe and permanent neurologic sequelae (up to 60%).[10,14,31,32]

The National Institute of Allergy and Infectious Diseases Collaborative Antiviral Study Group (CASG) led the majority of studies establishing a role for antiviral treatment of CMV in congenitally infected infants with CNS involvement. Ganciclovir, a nucleoside analogue, was first found to inhibit CMV replication in vitro and in animal models in the 1980s.[33] Subsequent phase I and II trials in the 1990s established safe dosing in infants and demonstrated some stabilization/improvement in hearing loss in symptomatic infants with congenital CMV infection.[34–36] The critical trial to

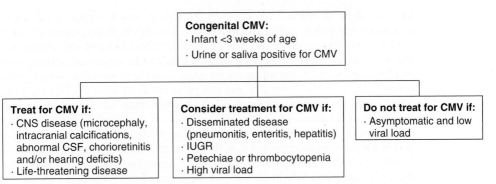

Figure 3.1 **Treatment Algorithm for Congenital CMV.** *IUGR,* intrauterine growth restriction.

evaluate ganciclovir efficacy against symptomatic congenital CMV enrolled 100 infants and took >8 years to complete.[37] Infants >32 weeks gestational age with confirmed congenital CMV infection with CNS involvement were randomized to receive either 6 weeks of intravenous (IV) ganciclovir (6 mg/kg every 12 hours) or no treatment. CNS involvement was defined as microcephaly, intracranial calcifications, abnormal cerebrospinal fluid, chorioretinitis, and/or hearing deficits. No placebo was given to the control group because of the ethical concerns of maintaining long-term IV access in this group. The primary endpoint was improved (or continued normal) brain stem-evoked response (BSER) in both ears between baseline and 6-month follow-up. Although the study was limited by poor follow-up (only 42 out of 100 participants completed both the baseline and follow-up BSER), treatment with ganciclovir was significantly better than no treatment.[37] None (0/25) of the ganciclovir-treated infants had worsening of their hearing compared with 41% (7/17) of the no-treatment group ($P < 0.01$), and 84% (21/25) had improvement or maintained normal hearing versus 59% (10/17) in the no-treatment group ($P < 0.06$). This significant improvement continued at follow-up at >1 year, but was less robust. To compare neurodevelopmental outcomes, Denver II developmental tests were performed at 6 weeks, 6 months, and 12 months. Infants treated with ganciclovir had significantly fewer developmental delays at 6 and 12 months than did untreated infants. Importantly, however, infants in the treatment group still had developmental delays compared with uninfected infants.[38] Although these results were promising, significant side effects were associated with IV ganciclovir treatment. Neutropenia was the most significant side effect, with 63% developing grade 3 or 4 toxicity versus 21% in the no-treatment group ($P < 0.01$) and ≈50% requiring a dose adjustment of ganciclovir.[37] There were also complications and risks associated with maintaining long-term IV access in this population (thrombus, infection, line replacement). An additional consideration is that ganciclovir can be carcinogenic and have gonadotoxicity in some animal models.[39–41]

Although ganciclovir was an effective treatment for congenital CMV, its widespread use was limited by the serious side effects and need for long-term IV access. Thus, the CASG evaluated the pharmacokinetics of the oral prodrug of ganciclovir, valganciclovir, and found it reached equivalent blood concentrations to ganciclovir at a dose of 16 mg/kg/dose twice a day.[42] There was also a reduced risk of neutropenia, with only 38% (9/24) developing grade 3 or 4 neutropenia and only 2 requiring a dose adjustment. In addition, the gonadotoxicity and carcinogenic effects of ganciclovir have not been seen with valganciclovir. Therefore, oral valganciclovir became the treatment of choice for congenital CMV infection.

Treatment of congenital CMV with ganciclovir or valganciclovir for 6 weeks eliminates or significantly reduces viral shedding; however, it usually returns to baseline shortly after cessation of therapy, and children can shed the virus for years.[35,40,43,44] Because many children can remain asymptomatic and may not develop SNHL or neurodevelopmental impairment until they are up to 6 years old, it was hypothesized that persistent viremia might contribute to pathogenesis and that a longer duration of therapy would improve outcomes. A randomized, placebo-controlled trial was done to address this question. Treatment with 6 weeks of valganciclovir was compared with 6 months of valganciclovir in infants with congenital CMV with CNS involvement (as defined in previous clinical trials). Hearing was similar between the two groups at 6 months, but was more likely to be improved or remain normal at 12 months in the 6-month treatment group compared with the 6-week treatment group (73% vs. 57%, $P = 0.01$), and this persisted at 24 months (77% vs. 64%, $P = 0.04$). Infants in the 6-month group also had significantly better neurodevelopmental outcomes, as determined using the Bayley Scales of Infant and Toddler Development, at 24 months. Interestingly, the incidence of neutropenia did not differ significantly between the two treatment groups. In the 4.5 months after valganciclovir was stopped in the 6-week treatment group, the rate of neutropenia was 27% in the 6-week treatment group and 21% in the 6-month treatment group.[45] The authors hypothesized that much of the neutropenia seen during CMV treatment can be attributed to congenital CMV infection rather than treatment. These studies effectively demonstrated that infants with congenital CMV with CNS involvement have improved hearing and neurodevelopmental outcomes with antiviral treatment with valganciclovir for 6 months compared with shorter or no treatment.

Limitations and Future Research

As with most drug therapies, safety and efficacy studies are limited in infants, particularly premature infants. The clinical trials establishing the pharmacokinetics, safety, and efficacy of ganciclovir and valganciclovir were all limited to infants >32 weeks gestation and >1200 g. There are several case studies of ganciclovir use in premature infants and one showing efficacy of ganciclovir followed by valganciclovir.[46-50] More studies are needed in premature infants, particularly extremely low-birth-weight infants (ELBW, <1000 g) to establish pharmacokinetics, safety, and efficacy. In addition, infants with congenital CMV with CNS disease who receive treatment should be followed long term to determine if their improvement persists as they age or if they would benefit from longer therapy, as has been observed for acyclovir treatment for congenital HSV infection.[51-54]

Summary

Infants with a diagnosis of congenital CMV that have CNS involvement should be treated with either ganciclovir (6 mg/kg IV every 12 hours) or valganciclovir (16 mg/kg PO every 12 hours) for a total of 6 months (Fig. 3.2). Treatment should begin within the first month of life, ideally <2 weeks. Valganciclovir should be preferentially used once the infant is safely tolerating oral intake. In infants <32 weeks gestation or <1200 g, dose adjustment may be needed based on side effects or viral load.

The major risk of treatment is neutropenia, which was most pronounced with ganciclovir and in the first 6 weeks of treatment with valganciclovir. Infants should be monitored with complete blood counts, serum transaminase levels, kidney function tests, and viral load measurements during therapy. An additional consideration is that ganciclovir can be carcinogenic and have gonadotoxicity in some animal models.[39-41] This has never been shown in human studies or for valganciclovir, but the potential risk should be discussed with families. Overall, although risks are associated with treatment, in this population, the benefits outweigh the risks.

Symptomatic Congenital CMV Without CNS Involvement and Asymptomatic Congenital CMV

Symptomatic Congenital CMV Without CNS Involvement

The randomized clinical trials addressing treatment of symptomatic congenital CMV were limited to those infants with CNS involvement at the time of diagnosis. In those infants with severe disease outside the CNS, like pneumonitis, there are case studies documenting successful treatment with ganciclovir.[55,56] However, many children only have mild, non–life-threatening symptoms at birth (i.e., jaundice, petechiae, transient thrombocytopenia). Although CNS involvement is a predictor of cognitive and motor development impairment, it is not predictive of the development of

Congenital CMV Treatment:		
Medication	**Duration**	**Monitoring**
• Ganciclovir 6 mg/kg/dose every 12 hours or • Valganciclovir 16 mg/kg/dose every 12 hours	• 6 months	Biweekly to monthly: • Complete blood count • Serum transaminase levels • Kidney function tests • CMV load (to assess for development of resistant virus and adherence)

Postnatal CMV Treatment:		
Medication	**Duration**	**Monitoring**
• Ganciclovir 6 mg/kg/dose every 12 hours or • Valganciclovir 16 mg/kg/dose every 12 hours • Preterm dosing awaiting pharmacokinetic (PK) trials	• Typically at least 3 weeks, depending on clinical improvement	Frequent (weekly): • Complete blood count • Serum transaminase levels • Kidney function tests Less frequent (biweekly to monthly) • CMV load

Figure 3.2   CMV Treatment Regimens and Monitoring.

SNHL.[31,57–59] In a prospective study of 180 children diagnosed with congenital CMV, the presence of IUGR or petechiae was predictive of SNHL.[58] In addition, another study of 127 children showed that petechiae and viremia were associated with SNHL.[60] These studies suggest that some infants with symptomatic congenital CMV infection, regardless of CNS involvement, are at high risk for developing SNHL and could be considered candidates for antiviral treatment.

Asymptomatic Congenital CMV Infection

Unlike symptomatic congenital CMV infection, there are no randomized controlled trials or large clinical studies to determine if treatment of asymptomatic congenital infections reduces the risk of late hearing loss and/or improves neurodevelopmental outcomes. Most published references recommend against treating those with asymptomatic infection and instead recommend close monitoring for neurodevelopmental delay and implementing early referral for ancillary services.[9,61–63] They cite no evidence of the benefit of treatment and the significant risks associated with treatment. However, the majority of these recommendations were published before the availability of valganciclovir as a treatment option.

As mentioned previously, 85% to 90% of infants with congenital CMV are asymptomatic at birth, but up to 20% of those will develop neurologic impairment, mostly commonly SNHL.[11,12,64] The two options for treatment include (1) treating all infants with congenital infection, regardless of symptoms, and (2) determining which infants with asymptomatic congenital CMV are at high risk for neurodevelopmental impairment and treat only those high-risk infants. The difficulty lies in determining which infants who are asymptomatic at birth will go on to develop SNHL. Ideally, an accurate predictor or biomarker could be established that will determine which infants will benefit most from therapy, thereby preventing unnecessary treatment of thousands of infants. However, such a predictor or biomarker does not currently exist.

The exact mechanism by which CMV causes SNHL is not clear; however, several studies suggest that direct viral cytopathology and viral-induced local inflammatory response play a role.[65,66] Pathology studies also show damage to vestibular endolymphatic systems in infected infants.[67] The progressive nature of the SNHL suggests that ongoing viral replication and damage may be responsible for part or all of the hearing loss seen. If this is true, treatment to reduce or eliminate CMV viral load should improve hearing outcomes, even in children who are asymptomatic and in particular those with high viral loads. This is similar to the theory that led to increasing the treatment duration of valganciclovir from 6 weeks to 6 months.

In fact, some studies have suggested that high plasma viral load is linked to the development of SNHL, regardless of whether the infant is symptomatic at birth.[58,60,68–70] The viral load linked to progression of SNHL in each study varied, but, in general, infants with viral loads of $<10^3$ copies/mL had no long-term complications, whereas those with viral loads $>10^5$ copies/mL were at increased risk for SNHL. These studies support the theory that high plasma viral load increases the risk for SNHL and that reducing viral load could prevent this complication. However, a plasma viral load cutoff needs to be validated in further studies and the positive and negative predictive values determined before plasma viral load risk assessment is recommended for routine clinical use.

In the only study comparing treatment versus no treatment in asymptomatic infants with congenital CMV infection, 12 infants were treated with ganciclovir 10 mg/kg for 21 days and 11 were observed off therapy.[71] The infants were followed for the next 4 to 10 years. Of the 18 children who completed follow-up, only 2 developed SNHL—both in the observation group ($P = 0.18$). Although these results suggest a possible benefit of treating asymptomatic congenital CMV, the study was significantly limited by the small sample size and low follow-up rates. This study also used a shorter treatment duration than is now recommended.

Limitations and Future Research

Although studies suggest a potential benefit of treatment, a large clinical trial is needed to determine if treatment improves neurodevelopmental outcomes in infants with congenital CMV infection without overt CNS disease at birth. Importantly, it remains to be determined whether treatment of asymptomatic congenital CMV infection diagnosed at birth can prevent the development of late hearing loss or improve neurodevelopmental outcome, and there is great need for a biomarker that could predict the risk of long-term deficits in congenitally infected infants. Clearly, more studies are needed to determine which infants are at risk for neurodevelopmental impairment or if all infants with congenital CMV, regardless of presentation, would benefit from treatment.

With the implementation of routine screening for CMV by some states and institutions, this will be an increasingly more relevant and important question to answer. Universal CMV testing at birth to define this population of infants provides researchers with the perfect opportunity to study the long-term consequences of asymptomatic or symptomatic congenital CMV infection without CNS involvement and if treatment improves outcomes.

Summary

Infants with symptomatic congenital CMV without CNS involvement should be considered for treatment if they have disseminated disease, IUGR, petechiae, or a high viral load (see Fig. 3.1). Physicians should consider treatment of asymptomatic CMV in infants with a high plasma viral load. The risks and potential benefits of valganciclovir should be discussed with the parents/caregivers. The treatment dose and duration should be the same as with symptomatic congenital CMV infection.

Treatment of Postnatal CMV Infection

Routine treatment of postnatal CMV infection in immunocompetent children, including term infants, is not recommended. CMV is a self-limited infection with no known short- or long-term complications in this population. However, as described earlier, premature VLBW infants infected postnatally with CMV can develop a severe sepsis like illness during an acute infection and may have an increased risk of developing BPD and neurodevelopmental impairment.[21–23,25,27]

Again, no large trials address treatment of premature infants with postnatal CMV infection. There are several small case studies of premature infants with severe postnatal CMV infection treated with ganciclovir who show significant clinical improvement with antiviral therapy.[20,46,47,49] In addition, in all of these studies, CMV load in plasma was eliminated or decreased by several logs. The majority of infants in these case studies had no apparent side effects from ganciclovir therapy[20,47,49]; however, in one report, therapy was discontinued after 28 days (and significant clinical improvement) in an ELBW infant secondary to neutropenia.[46]

The more difficult question is whether premature infants with asymptomatic postnatal CMV infection would benefit from treatment. In the retrospective studies by Kelly et al. and Mukhopadhyay et al. that showed an increased risk of BPD in infants with postnatal CMV infection, infants with postnatal CMV were tested at some point by their provider, presumably because they developed symptoms that could be consistent with CMV infection.[25,27] Therefore BPD might only be a complication in symptomatic postnatal CMV infection. However, the studies suggesting that postnatal CMV infection in VLBW infants may be associated with neurodevelopmental impairment were performed by screening all infants born to CMV-seropositive mothers at birth and following them prospectively.[21] These studies therefore represent both asymptomatic and symptomatic postnatal CMV-infected premature infants. Thus although some sequelae appear to affect only infants with symptomatic infection, others affect both groups.

Limitations and Future Research

The full impact of postnatal CMV infection on premature infants remains unclear. A large, multicentered, prospective trial is needed to define the full incidence of disease and determine the long-term sequelae. These vulnerable infants are already at high risk for morbidity and mortality, and decreasing the contribution of CMV to their neurodevelopmental and respiratory outcome could have a significant impact. Studies are also needed to assess the role of antiviral treatment in improving the outcome of symptomatic and asymptomatic postnatal CMV infection in premature infants.

Summary

Clinicians should strongly consider treating VLBW infants with severe acute disease after postnatal CMV acquisition. In these cases, treatment should consist of IV ganciclovir at a dose of 5 to 6 mg/kg IV every 12 hours for a minimum of 3 weeks, with the length of treatment depending on clinical course and viral load (see Fig. 3.2). In ELBW infants, drug levels should be monitored periodically, if possible, until adequate pharmacokinetic studies are available.[50]

There is insufficient evidence at this time to recommend treatment for asymptomatic VLBW infants with postnatal CMV infection. However, studies suggest these infants could develop long-term sequelae and the risks associated with treatment may be less than originally assumed prior to the availability of valganciclovir. Further studies are needed to quantitate the risk of long-term deficits due to postnatal CMV acquisition in premature infants and determine if these could be reduced with treatment for CMV in this vulnerable population. In addition, safe strategies should be devised for prevention of breast milk–associated CMV transmission in the NICU population, allowing the full benefits of breast milk feeding while also eliminating CMV as a contributor to negative health and developmental outcomes in premature infants.

REFERENCES

1. Kenneson A, Cannon MJ. Review and meta-analysis of the epidemiology of congenital cytomegalovirus (CMV) infection. *Rev Med Virol.* 2007;17:253–276.
2. Manicklal S, Emery VC, Lazzarotto T, et al. The "silent" global burden of congenital cytomegalovirus. *Clin Microbiol Rev.* 2013;26:86–102.

3. Cannon MJ, Schmid DS, Hyde TB. Review of cytomegalovirus seroprevalence and demographic characteristics associated with infection. *Rev Med Virol.* 2010;20:202–213.

4. Boppana SB, Rivera LB, Fowler KB, et al. Intrauterine transmission of cytomegalovirus to infants of women with preconceptional immunity. *N Engl J Med.* 2001;344:1366–1371.

5. Yow MD, Williamson DW, Leeds LJ, et al. Epidemiologic characteristics of cytomegalovirus infection in mothers and their infants. *Am J Obstet Gynecol.* 1988;158:1189–1195.

6. Wang C, Zhang X, Bialek S, et al. Attribution of congenital cytomegalovirus infection to primary versus non-primary maternal infection. *Clin Infect Dis.* 2011;52:e11–e13.

7. Malm G, Engman ML. Congenital cytomegalovirus infections. *Semin Fetal Neonatal Med.* 2007;12:154–159.

8. Pass RF, Fowler KB, Boppana SB, et al. Congenital cytomegalovirus infection following first trimester maternal infection: symptoms at birth and outcome. *J Clin Virol.* 2006;35:216–220.

9. Buonsenso D, Serranti D, Gargiullo L, et al. Congenital cytomegalovirus infection: current strategies and future perspectives. *Eur Rev Med Pharmacol Sci.* 2012;16:919–935.

10. Dollard SC, Grosse SD, Ross DS. New estimates of the prevalence of neurological and sensory sequelae and mortality associated with congenital cytomegalovirus infection. *Rev Med Virol.* 2007;17:355–363.

11. Ross SA, Boppana SB. Congenital cytomegalovirus infection: outcome and diagnosis. *Semin Pediatr Infect Dis.* 2005;16:44–49.

12. Stagno S, Whitley RJ. Herpesvirus infections of pregnancy. Part I: Cytomegalovirus and Epstein-Barr virus infections. *N Engl J Med.* 1985;313:1270–1274.

13. Dahle AJ, Fowler KB, Wright JD, et al. Longitudinal investigation of hearing disorders in children with congenital cytomegalovirus. *J Am Acad Audiol.* 2000;11:283–290.

14. Fowler KB, Dahle AJ, Boppana SB, et al. Newborn hearing screening: will children with hearing loss caused by congenital cytomegalovirus infection be missed? *J Pediatr.* 1999;135:60–64.

15. Fowler KB, Stagno S, Pass RF, et al. The outcome of congenital cytomegalovirus infection in relation to maternal antibody status. *N Engl J Med.* 1992;326:663–667.

16. Cannon MJ, Davis KF. Washing our hands of the congenital cytomegalovirus disease epidemic. *BMC Public Health.* 2005;5:70.

17. Smith RJ, Bale JF Jr, White KR. Sensorineural hearing loss in children. *Lancet.* 2005;365:879–890.

18. Capretti MG, Lanari M, Lazzarotto T, et al. Very low birth weight infants born to cytomegalovirus-seropositive mothers fed with their mother's milk: a prospective study. *J Pediatr.* 2009;154:842–848.

19. de Cates CR, Gray J, Roberton NR, et al. Acquisition of cytomegalovirus infection by premature neonates. *J Infect.* 1994;28:25–30.

20. Josephson CD, Caliendo AM, Easley KA, et al. Blood transfusion and breast milk transmission of cytomegalovirus in very-low-birth-weight infants: a prospective cohort study. *JAMA Pediatr.* 2014;168:1054–1062.

21. Brecht KF, Goelz R, Bevot A, et al. Postnatal human cytomegalovirus infection in preterm infants has long-term neuropsychological sequelae. *J Pediatr.* 2015;166:834–839 e1.

22. Lanzieri TM, Dollard SC, Josephson CD, et al. Breast milk-acquired cytomegalovirus infection and disease in VLBW and premature infants. *Pediatrics.* 2013;131:e1937–e1945.

23. Lombardi G, Garofoli F, Manzoni P, et al. Breast milk-acquired cytomegalovirus infection in very low birth weight infants. *J Matern Fetal Neonatal Med.* 2012;25(suppl 3):57–62.

24. Vollmer B, Seibold-Weiger K, Schmitz-Salue C, et al. Postnatally acquired cytomegalovirus infection via breast milk: effects on hearing and development in preterm infants. *Pediatr Infect Dis J.* 2004;23:322–327.

25. Kelly MS, Benjamin DK, Puopolo KM, et al. Postnatal cytomegalovirus infection and the risk for bronchopulmonary dysplasia. *JAMA Pediatr.* 2015;169:e153785.

26. Ehrenkranz RA, Walsh MC, Vohr BR, et al. Validation of the National Institutes of Health consensus definition of bronchopulmonary dysplasia. *Pediatrics.* 2005;116:1353–1360.

27. Mukhopadhyay S, Meyer SA, Permar SR, et al. Symptomatic postnatal cytomegalovirus testing among very-low-birth-weight infants: indications and outcomes. *Am J Perinatol.* 2016;33:894–902.

28. Neuberger P, Hamprecht K, Vochem M, et al. Case-control study of symptoms and neonatal outcome of human milk-transmitted cytomegalovirus infection in premature infants. *J Pediatr.* 2006;148:326–331.

29. Nijman J, de Vries LS, Koopman-Esseboom C, et al. Postnatally acquired cytomegalovirus infection in preterm infants: a prospective study on risk factors and cranial ultrasound findings. *Arch Dis Child Fetal Neonatal Ed.* 2012;97:F259–F263.

30. Sawyer MH, Edwards DK, Spector SA. Cytomegalovirus infection and bronchopulmonary dysplasia in premature infants. *Am J Dis Child.* 1987;141:303–305.

31. Pass RF, Stagno S, Myers GJ, et al. Outcome of symptomatic congenital cytomegalovirus infection: results of long-term longitudinal follow-up. *Pediatrics.* 1980;66:758–762.

32. Williams EJ, Gray J, Luck S, et al. First estimates of the potential cost and cost saving of protecting childhood hearing from damage caused by congenital CMV infection. *Arch Dis Child Fetal Neonatal Ed.* 2015;100:F501–F506.

33. Matthews T, Boehme R. Antiviral activity and mechanism of action of ganciclovir. *Rev Infect Dis.* 1988;10(suppl 3):S490–S494.

34. Trang JM, Kidd L, Gruber W, et al. Linear single-dose pharmacokinetics of ganciclovir in newborns with congenital cytomegalovirus infections. NIAID Collaborative Antiviral Study Group. *Clin Pharmacol Ther.* 1993;53:15–21.

35. Whitley RJ, Cloud G, Gruber W, et al. Ganciclovir treatment of symptomatic congenital cytomegalovirus infection: results of a phase II study. *J Infect Dis*. 1997;175:1080–1086.
36. Zhou XJ, Gruber W, Demmler G, et al. Population pharmacokinetics of ganciclovir in newborns with congenital cytomegalovirus infections. *Antimicrob Agents Chemother*. 1996;40:2202–2205.
37. Kimberlin DW, Lin CY, Sanchez PJ, et al. Effect of ganciclovir therapy on hearing in symptomatic congenital cytomegalovirus disease involving the central nervous system: a randomized, controlled trial. *J Pediatr*. 2003;143:16–25.
38. Oliver SE, Cloud GA, Sanchez PJ, et al. Neurodevelopmental outcomes following ganciclovir therapy in symptomatic congenital cytomegalovirus infections involving the central nervous system. *J Clin Virol*. 2009;46(suppl 4):S22–S26.
39. Faqi AS, Klug A, Merker HJ, et al. Ganciclovir induces reproductive hazards in male rats after short-term exposure. *Hum Exp Toxicol*. 1997;16:505–511.
40. Mareri A, Lasorella S, Iapadre G, et al. Anti-viral therapy for congenital cytomegalovirus infection: pharmacokinetics, efficacy and side effects. *J Matern Fetal Neonatal Med*. 2016;29:1657–1664.
41. Wutzler P. Thust R. Genetic risks of antiviral nucleoside analogues–a survey. *Antiviral Res*. 2001;49: 55–74.
42. Kimberlin DW, Acosta EP, Sanchez PJ, et al. Pharmacokinetic and pharmacodynamic assessment of oral valganciclovir in the treatment of symptomatic congenital cytomegalovirus disease. *J Infect Dis*. 2008;197:836–845.
43. Nigro G, Scholz H, Bartmann U. Ganciclovir therapy for symptomatic congenital cytomegalovirus infection in infants: a two-regimen experience. *J Pediatr*. 1994;124:318–322.
44. Syggelou A, Iacovidou N, Kloudas S, et al. Congenital cytomegalovirus infection. *Ann N Y Acad Sci*. 2010;1205:144–147.
45. Kimberlin DW, Jester PM, Sanchez PJ, et al. Valganciclovir for symptomatic congenital cytomegalovirus disease. *N Engl J Med*. 2015;372:933–943.
46. Fischer C, Meylan P, Bickle Graz M, et al. Severe postnatally acquired cytomegalovirus infection presenting with colitis, pneumonitis and sepsis like syndrome in an extremely low birthweight infant. *Neonatology*. 2010;97:339–345.
47. Mehler K, Oberthuer A, Lang-Roth R, et al. High rate of symptomatic cytomegalovirus infection in extremely low gestational age preterm infants of 22-24 weeks' gestation after transmission via breast milk. *Neonatology*. 2014;105:27–32.
48. Muller A, Eis-Hubinger AM, Brandhorst G, et al. Oral valganciclovir for symptomatic congenital cytomegalovirus infection in an extremely low birth weight infant. *J Perinatol*. 2008;28:74–76.
49. Okulu E, Akin IM, Atasay B, et al. Severe postnatal cytomegalovirus infection with multisystem involvement in an extremely low birth weight infant. *J Perinatol*. 2012;32:72–74.
50. Sunada M, Kinoshita D, Furukawa N, et al. Therapeutic drug monitoring of ganciclovir for postnatal cytomegalovirus infection in an extremely low birth weight infant: a case report. *BMC Pediatr*. 2016;16:141.
51. Kimberlin DW, Lin CY, Jacobs RF, et al. Natural history of neonatal herpes simplex virus infections in the acyclovir era. *Pediatrics*. 2001;108:223–229.
52. Kimberlin DW, Whitley RJ, Wan W, et al. Oral acyclovir suppression and neurodevelopment after neonatal herpes. *N Engl J Med*. 2011;365:1284–1292.
53. Tiffany KF, Benjamin DK Jr, Palasanthiran P, et al. Improved neurodevelopmental outcomes following long-term high-dose oral acyclovir therapy in infants with central nervous system and disseminated herpes simplex disease. *J Perinatol*. 2005;25:156–161.
54. Whitley R, Arvin A, Prober C, et al. A controlled trial comparing vidarabine with acyclovir in neonatal herpes simplex virus infection. *N Engl J Med*. 1991;324:444–449.
55. Hocker JR, Cook LN, Adams G, et al. Ganciclovir therapy of congenital cytomegalovirus pneumonia. *Pediatr Infect Dis J*. 1990;9:743–745.
56. Vallejo JG, Englund JA, Garcia-Prats JA, et al. Ganciclovir treatment of steroid-associated cytomegalovirus disease in a congenitally infected neonate. *Pediatr Infect Dis J*. 1994;13:239–241.
57. Noyola DE, Demmler GJ, Nelson CT, et al. Early predictors of neurodevelopmental outcome in symptomatic congenital cytomegalovirus infection. *J Pediatr*. 2001;138:325–331.
58. Rivera LB, Boppana SB, Fowler KB, et al. Predictors of hearing loss in children with symptomatic congenital cytomegalovirus infection. *Pediatrics*. 2002;110:762–767.
59. Weller TH, Hanshaw JB. Virologic and clinical observations on cytomegalic inclusion disease. *N Engl J Med*. 1962;266:1233–1244.
60. Bradford RD, Cloud G, Lakeman AD, et al. Detection of cytomegalovirus (CMV) DNA by polymerase chain reaction is associated with hearing loss in newborns with symptomatic congenital CMV infection involving the central nervous system. *J Infect Dis*. 2005;191:227–233.
61. Gandhi RS, Fernandez-Alvarez JR, Rabe H. Management of congenital cytomegalovirus infection: an evidence-based approach. *Acta Paediatr*. 2010;99:509–515.
62. James SH, Kimberlin DW. Advances in the prevention and treatment of congenital cytomegalovirus infection. *Curr Opin Pediatr*. 2016;28:81–85.
63. Smets K, De Coen K, Dhooge I, et al. Selecting neonates with congenital cytomegalovirus infection for ganciclovir therapy. *Eur J Pediatr*. 2006;165:885–890.
64. Fowler KB, Boppana SB. Congenital cytomegalovirus (CMV) infection and hearing deficit. *J Clin Virol*. 2006;35:226–231.
65. Fowler KB, McCollister FP, Dahle AJ, et al. Progressive and fluctuating sensorineural hearing loss in children with asymptomatic congenital cytomegalovirus infection. *J Pediatr*. 1997;130:624–630.

3

66. Strauss M. Human cytomegalovirus labyrinthitis. *Am J Otolaryngol.* 1990;11:292–298.
67. Davis LE, Johnsson LG, Kornfeld M. Cytomegalovirus labyrinthitis in an infant: morphological, virological, and immunofluorescent studies. *J Neuropathol Exp Neurol.* 1981;40:9–19.
68. Boppana SB, Fowler KB, Pass RF, et al. Congenital cytomegalovirus infection: association between virus burden in infancy and hearing loss. *J Pediatr.* 2005;146:817–823.
69. Lanari M, Lazzarotto T, Venturi V, et al. Neonatal cytomegalovirus blood load and risk of sequelae in symptomatic and asymptomatic congenitally infected newborns. *Pediatrics.* 2006;117:e76–e83.
70. Walter S, Atkinson C, Sharland M, et al. Congenital cytomegalovirus: association between dried blood spot viral load and hearing loss. *Arch Dis Child Fetal Neonatal Ed.* 2008;93:F280–F285.
71. Lackner A, Acham A, Alborno T, et al. Effect on hearing of ganciclovir therapy for asymptomatic congenital cytomegalovirus infection: four to 10 year follow up. *J Laryngol Otol.* 2009;123:391–396.

A

CHAPTER 4

Neonatal Herpes Simplex Virus Infection

Nazia Kabani, MD, BS, David W. Kimberlin, MD

4

- HSV is a virus that is capable of causing severe infection in a neonate, but fortunately with advances in medicine via research, it is treatable.
- There are three periods of acquisition of HSV: in utero, perinatal, and postnatal.
- HSV can be diagnosed via PCR of blood and CSF as well surface cultures and PCR.
- It is important to assess for disseminated HSV.
- HSV can be treated with IV acyclovir, and many neonates require oral suppression therapy.

Introduction

Of the viruses capable of infecting neonates, herpes simplex virus (HSV) is among the most severe, causing significant mortality and morbidity. Unlike many other viral pathogens, though, HSV is treatable using a commercially available antiviral drug: acyclovir. Neonatal HSV infection is primarily acquired in the peripartum period, which improves the likelihood that antiviral therapy can be beneficial, because viral damage is of a relatively short duration compared with injury to the developing fetal brain from viruses such as rubella, cytomegalovirus, and Zika virus, which are primarily acquired in utero. Studies conducted by the National Institute of Allergy and Infectious Diseases (NIAID) Collaborative Antiviral Study Group (CASG) over the course of four decades have advanced our knowledge of the favorable impact that antiviral therapy has on neonatal HSV disease outcomes, and many neonates now are effectively treated and experience no long-term sequelae of this potentially devastating infection.

Timing of Infection

Neonatal HSV is acquired in one of three distinct periods: in utero, perinatal, and postnatal. In a majority of cases (≈85%), the infants acquire the infection perinatally.[1] In approximately 10% of cases, neonates are infected postnatally, and in 5% the infection is acquired in utero.[1]

Risk Factors for Neonatal Infection

Risk factors that increase the likelihood of transmission from a mother with genital HSV shedding to her infant include:
1. Type of maternal infection (primary infection increases likelihood versus recurrent)[2-6]
2. Maternal antibody status (lower concentration of antibodies with primary infection)[6-9]
3. Prolonged duration of rupture of membranes[5]

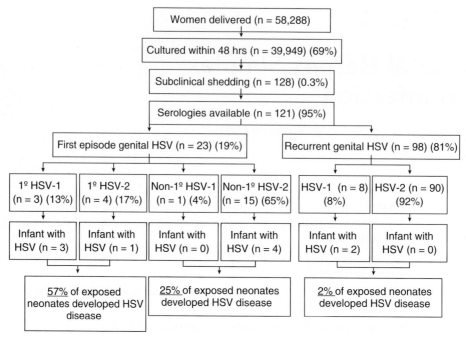

Figure 4.1   Risk of neonatal HSV disease as a function of type of maternal infection. (Adapted from Brown ZA, Wald A, Morrow RA, et al. Effect of serologic status and cesarean delivery on transmission rates of herpes simplex virus from mother to infant. *JAMA.* 2003;289:203–209.)

4. Integrity of mucocutaneous barriers (using fetal scalp probe, incisions, etc.)[6,10,11]
5. Mode of delivery (cesarean section versus vaginal delivery)[6]

    Neonates born to mothers with primary genital HSV infection near term, that is, a first episode of genital HSV infection, are at much greater risk of developing neonatal herpes than are neonates born to mothers with recurrent genital HSV infection. This increased risk is due to two factors.[2–6] First, the concentration of transplacentally acquired HSV-specific antibodies is lower in neonates born to women with primary infection.[8] In addition, these antibodies tend to be less reactive to the expressed peptides. Second, there is a larger burden of the virus being shed vaginally, and virus is shed for a longer period in the maternal genital tract of women with primary infection compared with women with recurrent HSV infection.[12] This was demonstrated in a landmark study of approximately 60,000 women in labor who did not have any symptoms of genital HSV infection at the time of delivery. Of these women, approximately 40,000 had a vaginal swab obtained within 48 hours of delivery for HSV detection (Fig. 4.1).[6] Of these ≈40,000, 121 (0.3%) women were identified as having asymptomatic shedding of HSV and had sera available for HSV serologic testing, thereby allowing for classification of first episodes versus recurrent maternal infections. The trial found that 57% of neonates born to mothers with primary infection developed neonatal HSV, 25% of neonates born to women with first-episode nonprimary infection developed neonatal HSV, and only 2% of neonates born to women with recurrent HSV developed neonatal HSV (see Fig. 4.1).[6] This same study also confirmed that cesarean delivery decreased transmission of HSV to the neonate when mothers are shedding in their genital tracts, affirming the results of a previous small study published in 1971.[5] Despite this degree of protection, though, the risk of HSV transmission is not eliminated by cesarean delivery.[13,15]

Clinical Manifestations of Neonatal Infection and Disease

Neonatal HSV infection is classified based upon the extent of involvement into one of three categories: disseminated disease; central nervous system (CNS) infection;

or skin, eyes, and mouth (SEM) infection. Disseminated disease involves multiple organs, including but not limited to lung, liver, adrenal glands, brain, and skin. CNS disease involves the brain and can have skin lesions as well. SEM disease is limited to just those areas. This classification is predictive of morbidity and mortality, with disseminated disease having the most significant mortality and CNS disease having the most significant morbidity.[16–22]

Disseminated infection can manifest as severe hepatitis, disseminated intravascular coagulopathy, pneumonitis, and possibly CNS involvement (seen in 60%–75% of cases).[17,21] The mean age at presentation is around 11 days. Interestingly, over 40% of disseminated HSV disease cases do not develop skin findings during the course of illness, which can complicate the diagnosis.[14,17,22,23]

Neonatal HSV CNS disease can present as seizures, lethargy, poor feeding, irritability and increased fussiness, tremors, temperature instability, and bulging fontanelle. The mean age of presentation is around 16 days.[17] Around 60% to 70% of neonates with CNS disease will have skin manifestations at some point in the disease course.[17,22] Mortality is usually due to devastating brain destruction and atrophy, causing neurologic and autonomic dysfunction.

SEM disease has the best overall outcome, with virtually no mortality and with morbidity associated solely with cutaneous recurrences but no neurologic sequelae. Additionally, neonates with SEM disease are most likely to have skin lesions, which facilitates diagnosis and allows prompt initiation of antiviral treatment before the disease progresses to involve other organs, including the CNS. Presenting signs and symptoms of SEM disease include skin vesicles, fever, lethargy, and conjunctivitis.[17] Mean age of presentation is around 12 days. If SEM disease is not treated, it will likely progress to CNS or disseminated disease.[14]

Diagnosis of Neonatal HSV Disease

Because the extent of involvement varies by disease classification, the diagnosis of neonatal HSV infections requires sampling of multiple sites:
1. Swabs of mouth, nasopharynx, conjunctivae, and rectum should be obtained for HSV surface cultures.
2. Specimens of skin vesicles should be obtained for culture and polymerase chain reaction (PCR).
3. Cerebrospinal fluid (CSF) should be obtained for HSV PCR.
4. Whole blood should be obtained for HSV PCR.
5. Alanine aminotransferase should be obtained as an indicator of hepatic involvement.[24]

In past decades, the presence of red blood cells in CSF was suggestive of HSV CNS infection, likely due to relatively advanced disease due to diagnostic limitations. However, with enhanced appreciation for neonatal HSV disease and the development of more advanced imaging and diagnostic capabilities, hemorrhagic HSV encephalitis is less common, and as a result most HSV CNS CSF indices do not have significant numbers of red blood cells. Performance of whole-blood PCR adds to the other diagnostic tools, but should not be used as the sole test for ruling in or ruling out neonatal HSV infection. Furthermore, viremia and DNAemia can occur in any of the three neonatal HSV disease classifications, so a positive whole blood PCR simply rules in neonatal HSV infection but does not assist in disease classification. Other rapid diagnostic techniques include direct fluorescent antibody staining of vesicle scrapings or enzyme immunoassay detection of HSV antigens, but these are less sensitive than PCR and culture and generally should not be used any longer. HSV isolates grown in culture or HSV DNA detected by PCR can be typed to determine whether it is HSV type 1 or HSV type 2. Chest radiographs and liver function tests can aid in the diagnosis of disseminated infection. Histologic testing is of low yield, as it has low sensitivity, and should not be used for diagnosis. Of note, all neonates with HSV disease, regardless of classification, need to have an ophthalmologic exam to look for ocular involvement. Infected neonates also should have neuroimaging studies (magnetic resonance imaging preferably, but computed tomography of the head or ultrasound are acceptable) performed to establish baseline brain anatomy.[24]

Treatment of Neonatal HSV Disease

Before antiviral therapies were available, disseminated HSV disease caused death by 1 year of age in 85% of those neonates affected. In neonates with CNS disease, the mortality rate was 50% (Table 4.1).[20] In a series of research studies conducted by the NIAID CASG between 1974 and 1997, parenteral vidarabine, lower-dose acyclovir (30 mg/kg/day), and higher-dose acyclovir (60 mg/kg/day) were evaluated sequentially.[18,20,25] In the first of these studies, 10 days of vidarabine decreased mortality compared with placebo at 1 year both for neonates with disseminated disease (down to 50% in the vidarabine group) and for those with CNS disease (down to 14% in the vidarabine group). After comparison of lower-dose acyclovir with vidarabine for 10 days, acyclovir became the primary treatment choice for neonatal HSV disease due to its favorable safety profile and its relative ease of administration (vidarabine required prolonged infusion times in large volumes of fluid). A subsequent study of higher-dose acyclovir for 21 days produced further reductions in 1-year mortality, to 29% for disseminated disease (Fig. 4.2) and 4% for CNS disease (Fig. 4.3).[16]

This series of studies determined that neonates with neonatal HSV disease should be treated with parenteral acyclovir at a dose of 60 mg/kg/day divided in three daily doses; the dosing interval may need to be increased in premature neonates, based on their creatinine clearance.[26] The recommended treatment duration now is 21 days for neonates with disseminated or CNS disease, whereas neonates with SEM disease should be treated for 14 days.[24] All neonates with CNS HSV disease should have a repeat lumbar puncture near the end of the 21-day course of acyclovir to document that the CSF PCR is negative; if the PCR remains positive, another week of parenteral acyclovir should be administered, and CSF analysis repeated in that

Table 4.1 MORTALITY AND MORBIDITY OUTCOMES AMONG 295 INFANTS WITH NEONATAL HSV INFECTION, EVALUATED BY THE NATIONAL INSTITUTES OF ALLERGY AND INFECTIOUS DISEASES COLLABORATIVE ANTIVIRAL STUDY GROUP BETWEEN 1974 AND 1997

Extent of Disease	Treatment			
	Placebo[20]	Vidarabine[18]	Acyclovir[18] 30 mg/kg/day	Acyclovir[16] 60 mg/kg/day
Disseminated Disease	n = 13	n = 28	n = 18	n = 34
Dead	11 (85%)	14 (50%)	11 (61%)	10 (29%)
Alive	2 (15%)	14 (50%)	7 (39%)	24 (71%)
Normal	1 (50%)	7 (50%)	3 (43%)	15 (63%)
Abnormal	1 (50%)	5 (36%)	2 (29%)	3 (13%)
Unknown	0 (0%)	2 (14%)	2 (29%)	6 (25%)
Central Nervous System Infection	n = 6	n = 36	n = 35	n = 23
Dead	3 (50%)	5 (14%)	5 (14%)	1 (4%)
Alive	3 (50%)	31 (86%)	30 (86%)	22 (96%)
Normal	1 (33%)	13 (42%)	8 (27%)	4 (18%)
Abnormal	2 (67%)	17 (55%)	20 (67%)	9 (41%)
Unknown	0 (0%)	1 (3%)	2 (7%)	9 (41%)
Skin, Eye, or Mouth Infection	n = 8	n = 31	n = 54	n = 9
Dead	0 (0%)	0 (0%)	0 (0%)	0 (0%)
Alive	8 (100%)	31 (100%)	54 (100%)	9 (100%)
Normal	5 (62%)	22 (71%)	45 (83%)	2 (22%)
Abnormal	3 (38%)	3 (10%)	1 (2%)	0 (0%)
Unknown	0 (0%)	6 (19%)	8 (15%)	7 (78%)

Adapted from Kimberlin DW. Advances in the treatment of neonatal herpes simplex infections. *Rev Med Virol.* 2001;11:157–163.

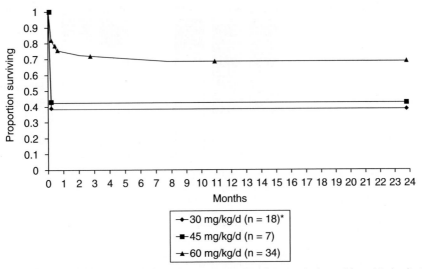

Figure 4.2 Mortality in patients with disseminated neonatal HSV disease. (Adapted from Kimberlin DW, Lin CY, Jacobs RF, et al. Safety and efficacy of high-dose intravenous acyclovir in the management of neonatal herpes simplex virus infections. *Pediatrics.* 2001;108:230–238.)

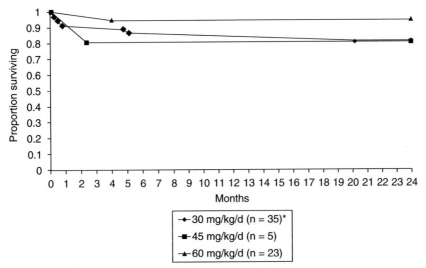

Figure 4.3 Mortality in patients with CNS neonatal HSV disease. (Adapted from Kimberlin DW, Lin CY, Jacobs RF, et al. Safety and efficacy of high-dose intravenous acyclovir in the management of neonatal herpes simplex virus infections. *Pediatrics.* 2001;108:230–238.)

manner until a negative CSF PCR is achieved.[17,27] In contrast, the value of serial whole-blood PCR determinations to gauge duration of therapy has not been established, and blood PCR should not be performed after the initial testing to establish whether neonatal HSV infection exists.

The primary toxicity of higher-dose parenteral acyclovir is neutropenia.[16] Absolute neutrophil counts (ANCs) should be monitored twice weekly throughout the course of parenteral therapy. If neutropenia of <500/μL develops, either the acyclovir can be held or granulocyte colony–stimulating factor can be administered.[16] Parenteral acyclovir dosing can be resumed when the ANC is >750/μL.

Oral acyclovir suppressive therapy for 6 months after acute parenteral treatment improves neurodevelopmental outcomes in neonates with CNS disease.[24] It is well known that HSV establishes latency in the sensory ganglia and occasionally reactivates

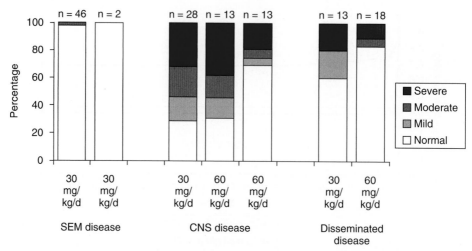

Figure 4.4 Morbidity among patients with known outcomes after 12 months of life. (Adapted from Kimberlin DW, Lin CY, Jacobs RF, et al. Safety and efficacy of high-dose intravenous acyclovir in the management of neonatal herpes simplex virus infections. *Pediatrics.* 2001;108:230–238 and Kimberlin DW, Whitley RJ, Wan W, et al; for the NIAID Collaborative Antiviral Study Group. Oral acyclovir suppression and neurodevelopment after neonatal herpes. *N Engl J Med.* 2011;365(14):1284–1292.)

and causes recurrence of disease. Reactivation may cause poor neurodevelopmental outcomes in neonates with CNS involvement. A recent study involving neonates with neonatal HSV with CNS involvement compared Bayley mental developmental scores at 1 year for neonates receiving suppressive therapy with acyclovir for 6 months versus neonates receiving placebo. The study found that the acyclovir group had a significantly higher mean Bayley score than the placebo group (88 vs. 68, *P* = 0.046).[28] It also demonstrated that that overall neurodevelopmental outcomes were better in the acyclovir group (Fig. 4.4). Suppressive acyclovir therapy also prevents skin recurrences in any classification of HSV disease.[28] Thus neonates should receive oral acyclovir at 300 mg/m^2/dose three times daily as suppressive therapy for 6 months after the initial parenteral treatment course. This dose should be adjusted for growth monthly, and ANCs should be monitored at 2 and 4 weeks after starting therapy and then monthly thereafter while oral acyclovir is administered.[24]

Outcomes of Neonatal HSV With Treatment

Improvements in morbidity after antiviral treatment is less dramatic than improvements in mortality for neonates with disseminated disease or CNS disease. Without treatment, 50% of neonates who survived disseminated HSV disease were developing normally at 1 year of age.[20] However, with use of higher-dose acyclovir for 21 days, the proportion of infants developing normally at 1 year of age after disseminated HSV disease has increased to 83%.[16] Similarly, for CNS HSV disease, 33% of patients develop normally at 1 year of age after 10 days of lower-dose acyclovir therapy, compared with 31% of children treated with higher-dose acyclovir for 21 days. With use of 6 months of oral acyclovir therapy, though, this percentage of infants with normal development at 1 year increases to 69%.[28] Morbidity of SEM disease also has dramatically improved since the introduction of antiviral treatment. In the pre-antiviral era, 38% of SEM patients were developing normally at 1 year of age, but with antiviral therapy this risk is eliminated (due to SEM disease not progressing to CNS or disseminated disease).[17]

Conclusion

Neonatal HSV disease is known to have devastating neurologic effects. Fortunately, over the past 4 decades, much has been learned regarding natural history, pathogenesis, diagnosis, and treatment of this severe infection. In the 21st century, neonatal HSV disease is treatable, and management recommendations have been standardized and implemented. As with any other area of medicine, though, information is fluid, and as more knowledge is obtained, more questions are formed. These questions in turn drive the next series of studies, with further promise of continued advances for years to come.

REFERENCES

1. Whitley RJ, Roizman B. Herpes simplex virus infections. *Lancet*. 2001;357:1513–1518.
2. Brown ZA, Benedetti J, Ashley R, et al. Neonatal herpes simplex virus infection in relation to asymptomatic maternal infection at the time of labor. *N Engl J Med*. 1991;324:1247–1252.
3. Brown ZA, Vontver LA, Benedetti J, et al. Effects on infants of a first episode of genital herpes during pregnancy. *N Engl J Med*. 1987;317:1246–1251.
4. Corey L, Wald A. Genital herpes. In: Holmes KK, Sparling PF, Mardh PA, et al, eds. *Sex Transm Dis*. 3rd ed. New York: McGraw-Hill; 1999:285–312.
5. Nahmias AJ, Josey WE, Naib ZM, et al. Perinatal risk associated with maternal genital herpes simplex virus infection. *Am J Obstet Gynecol*. 1971;110:825–837.
6. Brown ZA, Wald A, Morrow RA, et al. Effect of serologic status and cesarean delivery on transmission rates of herpes simplex virus from mother to infant. *JAMA*. 2003;289:203–209.
7. Yeager AS, Arvin AM. Reasons for the absence of a history of recurrent genital infections in mothers of neonates infected with herpes simplex virus. *Pediatrics*. 1984;73:188–193.
8. Prober CG, Sullender WM, Yasukawa LL, et al. Low risk of herpes simplex virus infections in neonates exposed to the virus at the time of vaginal delivery to mothers with recurrent genital herpes simplex virus infections. *N Engl J Med*. 1987;316:240–244.
9. Yeager AS, Arvin AM, Urbani LJ, et al. Relationship of antibody to outcome in neonatal herpes simplex virus infections. *Infect Immun*. 1980;29:532–538.
10. Parvey LS, Ch'ien LT. Neonatal herpes simplex virus infection introduced by fetal-monitor scalp electrodes. *Pediatrics*. 1980;65:1150–1153.
11. Kaye EM, Dooling EC. Neonatal herpes simplex meningoencephalitis associated with fetal monitor scalp electrodes. *Neurology*. 1981;31:1045–1047.
12. Whitley RJ. Herpes simplex viruses. In: Fields BN, Knipe DM, Howley PM, et al, eds. *Fields Virology*. 3rd ed. Philadelphia: Lippincott—Raven Publishers; 1996:2297–2342.
13. Anonymous. ACOG practice bulletin. Management of herpes in pregnancy. Number 8 October 1999. Clinical management guidelines for obstetrician-gynecologists. *Int J Gynaecol Obstet*. 2000;68:165–173.
14. Whitley RJ, Corey L, Arvin A, et al. Changing presentation of herpes simplex virus infection in neonates. *J Infect Dis*. 1988;158:109–116.
15. Peng J, Krause PJ, Kresch M. Neonatal herpes simplex virus infection after cesarean section with intact amniotic membranes. *J Perinatol*. 1996;16:397–399.
16. Kimberlin DW, Lin CY, Jacobs RF, et al. Safety and efficacy of high-dose intravenous acyclovir in the management of neonatal herpes simplex virus infections. *Pediatrics*. 2001;108:230–238.
17. Kimberlin DW, Lin CY, Jacobs RF, et al. Natural history of neonatal herpes simplex virus infections in the acyclovir era. *Pediatrics*. 2001;108:223–229.
18. Whitley R, Arvin A, Prober C, et al. A controlled trial comparing vidarabine with acyclovir in neonatal herpes simplex virus infection. *N Engl J Med*. 1991;324:444–449.
19. Whitley R, Arvin A, Prober C, et al. Predictors of morbidity and mortality in neonates with herpes simplex virus infections. *N Engl J Med*. 1991;324:450–454.
20. Whitley RJ, Nahmias AJ, Soong SJ, et al. Vidarabine therapy of neonatal herpes simplex virus infection. *Pediatrics*. 1980;66:495–501.
21. Whitley RJ. Herpes simplex virus infections. In: Remington JS, Klein JO, eds. *Infectious Diseases of the Fetus and Newborn Infants*. 3rd ed. Philadelphia: W.B. Saunders Company; 1990:282–305.
22. Sullivan-Bolyai JZ, Hull HF, Wilson C, et al. Presentation of neonatal herpes simplex virus infections: implications for a change in therapeutic strategy. *Pediatr Infect Dis*. 1986;5:309–314.
23. Arvin AM, Yeager AS, Bruhn FW, et al. Neonatal herpes simplex infection in the absence of muco-cutaneous lesions. *J Pediatr*. 1982;100:715–721.
24. American Academy of Pediatrics. Herpes simplex. In: Brady TD, Jackson MA, Long SS, et al., eds. *Red Book: 2015 Report of the Committee on Infectious Diseases*. 30th ed. Elk Grove Village, IL: American Academy of Pediatrics; 2015:432–443.
25. Whitley RJ, Yeager A, Kartus P, et al. Neonatal herpes simplex virus infection: follow-up evaluation of vidarabine therapy. *Pediatrics*. 1983;72:778–785.
26. Englund JA, Fletcher CV, Balfour HH Jr. Acyclovir therapy in neonates. *J Pediatr*. 1991;119:129–135.
27. Kimberlin DW, Lakeman FD, Arvin AM, et al. Application of the polymerase chain reaction to the diagnosis and management of neonatal herpes simplex virus disease. *J Infect Dis*. 1996;174:1162–1167.
28. Kimberlin DW, Whitley RJ, Wan W, et al; for the NIAID Collaborative Antiviral Study Group. Oral acyclovir suppression and neurodevelopment after neonatal herpes. *N Engl J Med*. 2011;365(14):1284–1292.
29. Kimberlin DW. Advances in the treatment of neonatal herpes simplex infections. *Rev Med Virol*. 2001;11:157–163.

4

CHAPTER 5

Antibiotic Stewardship

Tamara I. Herrera, MD, Charles Michael Cotten, MD, MHS

- Antibiotics are lifesaving and improve outcomes in neonatal clinical care.
- Increasing evidence in animal and human models links antibiotic exposure with alterations in the microbiome, the developing immune system, and subsequent effects on health.
- Empiric antibiotic use is linked to emergence of infections caused by multidrug-resistant organisms and to increased risk of necrotizing enterocolitis and mortality.
- The primary goal of antibiotic stewardship programs in NICUs is to reduce morbidity and save lives by appropriate use of antibiotics in the treatment of proven and suspected neonatal infections. A secondary goal is to reduce health care costs.
- Implementation of multidisciplinary stewardship strategies has led to a reduction in antibiotic resistance, length of hospitalization, adverse events, and rates of clinical failure.

Introduction

Neonatal sepsis remains a serious complication, especially among very low birth weight infants (VLBW, <1500 g at birth), with mortality inversely related to gestational age.[1-3] Obstetric and pediatric caregivers have focused efforts on reducing the risk of early-onset sepsis (EOS) caused by *group B Streptococcus* (GBS), with early onset defined as culture-positive infection in the first 72 hours of life.[4,5] Implementation of universal screening and intrapartum antibiotic prophylaxis (IAP) to prevent vertical transmission of GBS infection in women with risk factors has resulted in a significant decline in the incidence of GBS EOS in infants.[6,7] However, most recently the incidence of EOS has stabilized.[8] With the current approach, >30% of mothers delivering infants in the United States are exposed to IAP, and not all cases of GBS sepsis are prevented.[9] In addition to EOS, late-onset sepsis (LOS), that is, blood or spinal fluid culture–positive infections that occur after the first 3 postnatal days, is associated with increased mortality and morbidity in infants hospitalized in neonatal intensive care units (NICUs). Although the overall frequency of LOS is decreasing, the incidence is still relatively high, and risk increases with decreasing gestational age.[10-12]

The intrapartum GBS prevention guidelines have resulted in a decrease in EOS; however, a considerable number of initially asymptomatic infants continue to be evaluated for sepsis and receive empiric antibiotics based on risk factors. At least in part, this is because the clinical presentation of infections in the neonatal period can be subtle.[13] Although prophylactic maternal and empiric neonatal antibiotic use has saved lives, the increase in antibiotic exposure carries risk. Increasing evidence links antibiotic exposure in the neonatal period with short- and long-term health outcomes, including (1) emergence of multiresistant infections, (2) LOS, (3) necrotizing enterocolitis (NEC), (4) invasive candidiasis, and (5) death. IAP exposure is associated with ampicillin-resistant *Escherichia coli* sepsis[1,14] and other antibiotic-resistant pathogens causing infections in infants.[15]

Genes conferring antibiotic resistance are present in the intestinal microbiome of term and preterm infants in a NICU environment as well as the intestine of healthy infants.[16–18] Animal studies have identified antibiotic-induced microbiome disturbance and downstream effects on the developing immune system that suggest mechanisms underlying the link between antibiotic exposure in the neonatal period and adverse outcomes.[19–22] The emergence of resistant pathogens and recent evidence linking antibiotic practice variations with health outcomes has led to initiation of antibiotic stewardship programs. Antibiotic stewardship is a current global focus, with ongoing efforts by many nations, including the U.S. Centers for Disease Control (CDC) (https://www.cdc.gov/getsmart/healthcare/), the Australian Commission on Safety and Quality in Healthcare (https://www.safetyandquality.gov.au/our-work/healthcare-associated-infection/antimicrobial-stewardship/), the United Kingdom Guidance for antimicrobial stewardship in hospitals (England) ARHAI Antimicrobial Stewardship (http://www.dh.gov.uk/prod_consum_dh/groups/dh_digitalassets/documents/digitalasset/dh_131181.pdf), and South Africa (http://www.fidssa.co.za/SAASP).

The aims of this review are to (1) describe the importance and current rationale of antibiotic use in the NICU, (2) review the extent and variation in antibiotic practice in NICUs, (3) discuss the emergence of resistant organisms in neonatal infections, (4) present evidence identifying the links between antimicrobial exposure and short- and long-term clinical outcomes, and (5) discuss the importance and impact of antibiotic stewardship.

Discussions of more global stewardship efforts is beyond the scope of this review. We acknowledge that the content of this review is largely focused on stewardship efforts in the United States, based on the diagnostic approaches, antimicrobial choices available, and the most frequent causative pathogens. In other parts of the world, pathogens are different, antibiotic resistance rates may be higher than the United States, and available diagnostic tests and therapeutic options are different.[23,24]

Rationale for Empiric Use of Antibiotics in Infants: What Is Causing the Infections?

Empiric antibiotic therapy should be directed against the most frequent bacteria causing neonatal sepsis (Table 5.1). However, identification of neonatal sepsis is challenging, as infants with infections may be asymptomatic, clinical signs may be difficult to distinguish from other noninfectious conditions, and available diagnostic tests are not often informative in deciding which infant will have a verifiable infection.[5] As a result, clinicians frequently use antibiotics empirically in high-risk infants or those presenting with subtle or significant signs before culture results are available.[25,26]

Table 5.1 MOST FREQUENT ORGANISMS ASSOCIATED WITH EOS AND LOS (UNITED STATES AND ENGLAND)

Early-Onset Sepsis	Late-Onset Sepsis
Group B *Streptococcus* 43%–50%	Coagulase-negative *Staphylococcus* 42%
Escherichia coli 18%–29%	*Staphylococcus aureus* 10%
Listeria monocytogenes 6%	Enterococci 9%
Viridans group *Streptococcus* 5%	Group B *Streptococcus* 5%
Group A *Streptococcus* 2%	*Escherichia coli* 8%
Enterococci 2%–3%	*Klebsiella* spp. 5%
Nontypeable *Haemophilus influenzae* 3%	*Enterobacter* spp. 5%
Staphylococcus aureus 2%	*Pseudomonas* spp. 3%
	Candida spp. 5%

Epidemiology data on EOS extracted from Stoll et al[4] and Vergnano et al[30].
Epidemiology data on LOS extracted from Shane and Stoll.[34]

Avoiding delays in treating true infections results in overtreatment. Antibiotics—particularly ampicillin, gentamicin, vancomycin, and cefotaxime—continue to be the most commonly prescribed drugs in NICUs.[27] A review of 1600 infants who received antibiotic therapy during their NICU stay showed that only 5% of antibiotic use was for culture-proven infections.[28]

EOS is attributed to maternal intrapartum transmission of pathogens.[4,29] EOS remains a serious disease with an incidence between 0.77 and 0.98 per 1000 live births and a mortality of approximately 10%. Premature infants have a much higher incidence of EOS than do term infants (up to 5%) and have an increased mortality.[4,8] GBS remains the most frequently isolated pathogen in EOS among term infants in the United States and other developed countries, whereas *E. coli* has been identified as the most common cause among VLBW infants.[3,4,8,30] Bacteria less commonly associated with EOS include other streptococci (most commonly viridans group streptococci), *Listeria monocytogenes, Enterococcus* spp., gram-negative enteric bacilli such as nontypeable *Haemophilus influenza*, and *Staphylococcus aureus*.[3,8,31] Missed opportunities for prevention of GBS disease exist, as only 76% of known GBS-colonized mothers and 66% with unknown GBS colonization and a risk factor in the United States, and as little as 19% in the United Kingdom, receive appropriate IAP.

Infants staying weeks in the NICU are at risk for LOS.[10] Premature infants are at highest risk of LOS due to immature skin and mucosal barriers, a multitude of invasive procedures, and an immature immune system that relies largely on innate immunity and neutrophil function for defense against infection.[3,32–35] LOS is likely due to nosocomial or horizontal acquisition of pathogens, and the incidence of LOS varies inversely with birth weight and gestational age.[11] More than 10 years ago, a large cohort study from the National Institute of Child Health and Human Development Neonatal Research Network revealed that the majority of VLBW infants develop at least one episode of proven infection during their hospital stay.[12] More recent data from three multicenter cohorts demonstrate that the incidence of LOS among extremely premature infants has decreased significantly from approximately 20% to 10%, although the distribution of bacterial pathogens is similar.[36–38] The most common pathogens associated with LOS are listed in Table 5.1. Although gram-negative infection and invasive candidiasis are less common, the case mortality rate is two to three times higher than with gram-positive infections.[11,34,39]

EOS and LOS are associated with an increased risk of bronchopulmonary dysplasia (BPD), white matter injury, intraventricular hemorrhage, retinopathy of prematurity, growth abnormalities, and neurodevelopmental delay.[40–42] Term and near-term infants who had infections are also more likely to have long-term neurologic sequalae.[43,44]

Variations in Antimicrobial Practice: What Is the Range of Practice Among Neonatologists?

Antibiotic prescribing practice for infants varies widely across centers.[45–47] An overall 40-fold variation in antibiotic use was observed across 127 California NICUs from 2.4% to 97% of patient-days.[48] Variation in antibiotic prescribing practice was independent of the burden of culture-proven sepsis, NEC, surgical volume, and mortality among centers. Overuse of antibiotics in NICUs may be a result of institutional practices regarding thresholds for sepsis screening and empiric treatment rather than case-by-case or individual physician decision making. In a cohort of 331 late preterm infants, antibiotic use was more common among those admitted to a NICU at a university teaching hospital compared with community hospitals.[49]

Variation in dosing and therapeutic drug monitoring protocols between NICUs has also been reported, suggesting that either subtherapeutic or toxic antibiotic doses may be common.[50] Whereas antibiotic overdosing may increase toxicity and compromise the safety of the neonatal population, underdosing may lead to low concentration of the drug, particularly at sites of heavy microbial concentrations such as mucosal surfaces and biofilms surrounding central lines, increasing the likelihood of ineffective treatment and development of resistant microbes.[15] Evaluation of antibiotic use and misuse is therefore important, because antibiotic-resistant infections are on the rise.[51,52] When medications have been studied, variations in pharmacokinetics related to gestational and postnatal age have been identified, providing a basis for optimization of dosing and monitoring to achieve therapeutic targets in the majority of infants while minimizing adverse events.[53–55]

Empiric Broad-Spectrum and Prolonged Antibiotic Use and NICU Outcomes

Appropriate use of antibiotics is crucial to improve outcomes and save lives for culture-proven infection. However, antibiotics are frequently prescribed in infants with sterile cultures in the first postnatal days based on a constellation of antepartum risk factors or a perceived clinical suspicion of infection. Concerns remain about the benefits of antibiotic therapy for microbiologically unproven suspected sepsis, particularly in extremely premature infants. In an observational study that included four NICUs, the most common reasons for inappropriate days of use of antibiotics were failure to discontinue treatment within 72 hours after initiation, failure to adjust coverage based on microbiology results, and prolonged prophylaxis after chest tube placement.[56]

Infants unnecessarily exposed to antibiotics are placed at risk for serious complications, even death, with no clinical benefit. Among a large cohort of VLBW infants admitted to NICU's in the Canadian Neonatal Network, exposure to antibiotic therapy in those without culture-proven sepsis or NEC was associated with an increased risk in mortality and morbidity, including stage 3 or higher retinopathy of prematurity (ROP).[57] In a study including 906 VLBW infants, antibiotic therapy for >48 hours during the first week after birth was associated with subsequent BPD and development of resistant gram-negative bacteria in routine endotracheal cultures.[58] In another cohort of VLBW infants who received antibiotics during the first 2 postnatal weeks, investigators observed that each additional antibiotic day was associated with increased risk of BPD by approximately 13% and with increased severity of the disease.[59] Longer courses (≥5 days) of empiric antibiotics in the first postnatal days was associated with increased risk of NEC or death in extremely low birth weight (ELBW) infants with sterile cultures[45,59] and increased length of stay.

Antibiotic utilization practices in the NICU influence the epidemiology of infections in infants, as early use of empiric broad-spectrum antibiotics selects for resistant bacteria. Extended-spectrum beta lactamase–producing (ESBL) gram-negative bacteria and other multiresistant organisms have emerged globally, at least in part as a consequence of misuse and prolonged empiric antibiotic therapy.[60–62] An analysis of two NICUs initially assigned to either a narrow-spectrum antibiotic regimen (penicillin or flucloxacillin/tobramycin) or a broad-spectrum regimen (ampicillin/cefotaxime) and exchanged after 6 months revealed that the relative risk for colonization with resistant strains was 18 times higher for the amoxicillin/cefotaxime group, with *Enterobacter cloacae* being the predominant isolated pathogen.[63] Because of emerging antibiotic-resistant gram-negative strains, the use of piperacillin-tazobactam and meropenem has increased, as they provide better coverage.[27] Of note, the spread of resistant pathogens increases risk of serious infections among the entire NICU population.[64] Exposure to broad-spectrum antibiotics, particularly third-generation cephalosporins, in ELBW infants has also been associated with invasive fungal infection and increased risk of subsequent poor neurodevelopmental outcome.[65,66]

Antibiotic Resistance: Emerging Problem for Neonatal Infections

Colonization of infants hospitalized in NICUs by antibiotic-resistant bacteria affects not only the colonized infants, who can develop infection, but also other hospitalized infants for whom colonization serves as a reservoir.[15] Risks associated with antibiotic-resistant infections include increased virulence of these pathogens, difficulties in diagnosing and initiating prompt and appropriate therapy, and limited treatment options. Although the benefits of appropriately indicated antibiotic therapy are well defined, widespread and prolonged use of antibiotics, as well as using antibiotics at less than therapeutic doses, has contributed to the increased emergence of resistant strains.[67]

The World Health Organization reported in 2014 that the proportion of *E. coli, Klebsiella pneumoniae,* and *S. aureus* resistant to commonly used antimicrobial agents exceeded 50% in many settings.[68] Broad-spectrum empiric antibiotic therapy, particularly with third-generation cephalosporins, does not always provide coverage for these resistant pathogens and may increase emergence of further resistance in the NICU.[69]

As a result of implementation of IAP to prevent early-onset GBS disease, GBS isolates with increasing minimum inhibitory concentrations to penicillin, ampicillin, and cefazolin; alterations in a penicillin-binding protein (PBP2X); and in vitro resistance to clindamycin or erythromycin have been reported. Fortunately, the incidence of antibiotic-resistant early-onset GBS disease is very low and remains stable.[70]

Vancomycin remains an adequate treatment option for most late-onset neonatal infections caused by gram-positive bacteria, particularly coagulase-negative staphylococci (CoNS) and methicillin-resistant *S. aureus* (MRSA),[71] but increasing resistance of MRSA species to vancomycin, oxacillin, and linezolid has been reported.[72,73] Decreased glycopeptide susceptibility has also been observed among strains of CoNS, including *S. epidermidis, S. warneri,* and *S. haemolyticus.*[74] The emergence of vancomycin-intermediate *S. aureus* (VISA) and heterogeneous vancomycin-intermediate *S. aureus* (hVISA) over the past decade as a result of varied mutations has posed new challenges for clinicians treating infants with these infections.[75]

Widespread use of vancomycin may also lead to development and transmission of vancomycin-resistant enterococci (VRE). VRE has been associated with higher mortality than vancomycin-susceptible *Enterococcus* strains.[76,77] Antibiotic options for VRE infections are limited to bacteriostatic agents such as linezolid, with limited clinical experience and pharmacokinetic data in the neonatal population.[78]

The recent rapid spread of multiresistant gram-negative bacteria is much more threatening. ESBL-producing gram-negative pathogens have emerged, particularly *Klebsiella pneumoniae* and *E. coli* with resistance to third-generation cephalosporins, as well as *Klebsiella* strains resistant to carbapenems and other gram-negative organisms resistant to piperacillin-tazobactam and aminoglycosides.[23,79-82]

With the looming threat of emergent resistance, empiric antibiotic therapy for sepsis should have the narrowest spectrum possible while still providing coverage for the local epidemiology of each NICU. Better hand washing and infection control practices, avoiding broad-spectrum antibiotics and prolonged or unnecessary treatments for suspected infections, synthesis of more potent antibiotics, and prospective surveillance of antibiotic use by a multidisciplinary team are of paramount importance to mitigate the emergence of antimicrobial-resistant infections.[69,83]

Antibiotic Practice and Stewardship Efforts in NICUs

Starting Antibiotics: Who to Treat?

A challenge for antibiotic stewardship in the NICU is that presentation of sepsis in the neonatal population can be subtle and nonspecific and often overlaps with other noninfectious morbidities. As a result, neonatologists have a low threshold to obtain cultures and start empiric antibiotic therapy.[84] The CDC 2002 and 2010 revised guidelines for GBS prevention provided algorithms for the evaluation of infants at risk for EOS.[70,85] However, a large proportion of uninfected infants continue to receive antibiotic treatment.[13,28] Efforts to improve accuracy of identifying infants who should receive empiric antibiotic treatment include the development of an online multivariate tool to quantify risk of EOS among term and near-term infants. This tool incorporates objective data available at the time of birth, accounting for maternal intrapartum antibiotic treatment and subsequent modification of neonatal risk, population prevalence of EOS, maternal clinical signs and GBS colonization status, and neonatal clinical signs. Use of this model can aid clinicians in deciding neonatal management and could possibly safely reduce antibiotic treatment in 80,000 to 240,000 U.S. infants each year.[86–88]

Blood culture remains the gold standard for the diagnosis of neonatal sepsis. However, four common scenarios are the subject of debate and result in treatment of unproven sepsis: (1) premature infants with signs indistinguishable from sepsis, (2) term infants with transient tachypnea of the newborn (TTN), (3) infants born to mothers with chorioamnionitis, and (4) blood cultures contaminated with CoNS.

Premature infants with respiratory distress syndrome (RDS) are commonly exposed to antibiotic treatment despite sterile cultures, as clinical and radiologic findings of early-onset pneumonia are indistinguishable from those of RDS. Recommendations on the management of VLBW infants with RDS at risk of EOS are limited, and markers for the diagnosis of sepsis have little utility in the presence of RDS.[89,90] Term infants with TTN are more likely to receive antibiotic therapy based on the fear of a missed infection; however, several investigators have proposed a more conservative approach for these infants with no concomitant specific infectious risk factors to reduce antibiotic exposure with no negative impact on the clinical outcome.[91–93]

Another concern is the management of infants born to mothers with chorioamnionitis. Recent reports indicate that the risk of EOS among these infants is strongly associated with gestational age. The low incidence of EOS (<1%) among well-appearing infants born at term to mothers with chorioamnionitis has called into question current guidelines recommending systematic antibiotic treatment of these infants while awaiting cultures.[94–96] In contrast, the risk of EOS among premature infants exposed to chorioamnionitis is substantial, as the incidence approaches 16%, and thus antibiotic treatment for this group remains justified.[97] Further data are emerging in use of the EOS risk calculator as a mechanism to reduce the numbers of infants empirically treated for EOS.[98]

CoNS is the most common cause of LOS in NICUs. Difficulties exist in differentiating true CoNS infection from culture contamination, as this organism is a common skin commensal.[99] A false-positive blood culture can lead to increased laboratory costs and unnecessary prolonged treatment with vancomycin.[100] Studies have shown that obtaining two peripheral blood cultures may reduce the number of infants diagnosed with CoNS infection and therefore reduce unnecessary antibiotic use.[101–103] Species identification and selected strain genotyping of CoNS may also aid in the interpretation of blood culture results.[104,105]

Biomarkers for Neonatal Infection: Are They Useful?

Although different strategies have been proposed based on the combination of multiple hematologic findings, early complete blood cell (CBC) count adds little diagnostic information in the evaluation of asymptomatic or symptomatic infants with suspected sepsis.[106] In a study including the largest series of CBC counts in infants with EOS admitted to different NICUs, low white blood cell (WBC) counts were associated with infection. However, the low sensitivity of CBC count-derived indices showed poor diagnostic utility to rule out infection reliably in these infants.[107] Similarly, although high and low WBC counts were associated with LOS with the highest specificity for counts <1000/mm and >50,000/mm, no CBC count index showed adequate sensitivity to rule out LOS reliably.[108]

Recent studies suggest that serial values of C-reactive protein (CRP) and immature:total neutrophil ratio (I:T ratio) provide some degree of predictive value for the diagnosis of neonatal sepsis. However, they need to be interpreted in conjunction with other clinical and laboratory parameters, as they are not sufficiently powerful to guide management of neonatal sepsis.[107,109–111] In a cohort study, two serial normal I:T ratios and a negative blood culture in the first 24 hours of life had a negative predictive value of 100%, suggesting that antibiotics can be safely discontinued at

24 hours in these infants.[112] Newer biomarkers, including cytokines and cell surface markers, are promising in the sorting out of high-risk infants to empirically treat while awaiting blood culture results due to their negative predictive value.[111,113–116]

Recent reports suggest that gene expression patterns may distinguish infected from uninfected infants in the early neonatal period.[117,118] Further studies are needed to determine the diagnostic utility in clinical practice of these molecular-level biomarkers, but in the short term these investigations will contribute to the understanding of mechanisms and variations of the neonatal immune response.

Initial Therapy for Suspected Early- and Late-Onset Sepsis: What to Use?

Ampicillin and gentamicin should remain the empiric antimicrobial treatment of choice for suspected EOS, as this combination targets the most prevalent pathogens with low rates of resistance.[4,119–121] Broadening empiric antibiotic treatment to increase the spectrum of gram-negative coverage or the penetration of the drug to certain tissues may be tempting, but evidence suggests that it is unsafe and ineffective.[122] A multicenter cohort study of 128,914 infants showed that the empiric combined use of ampicillin/cefotaxime during the first 3 postnatal days was associated with increased risk of death before discharge compared with the use of ampicillin/gentamicin for all gestational ages.[123]

Cephalosporins should be used cautiously in infants for LOS, as there is an association with increased risk for invasive candidiasis,[65,124] adverse events,[125,126] and development of resistance.[127,128] Third-generation cephalosporins may best be reserved for infants with suspected or proven gram-negative meningitis or significant renal insufficiency contraindicating the use of aminoglycosides.[129]

Carbapenems may be a feasible option to treat infections caused by ESBL strains, but clinical experience in infants is limited, and adverse events, most importantly the increased risk of seizures, must be taken into account.[54,130–132] A cohort study including 267 infants with positive *E. coli* cultures showed that absence of an antimicrobial agent against the infecting *E. coli* strain in the initial empiric treatment was not associated with increased 30-day mortality, suggesting that initiating treatment with aminoglycosides and later adding more potent, broader antibiotics may be safe.[133]

Vancomycin is commonly used for empiric therapy of LOS due to the prevalence of CoNS and concerns for emerging β-lactamase–resistant strains, including MRSA. A multicenter survey among neonatologists revealed that at least 75% prescribe a vancomycin-containing regimen for suspected LOS in VLBW infants.[134] However, empiric vancomycin started before culture results are available is not recommended because of the very low frequency of fulminant sepsis caused by CoNS,[135] the associated increase in the emergence of vancomycin-resistant strains,[136] and the lack of evidence suggesting improved morbidity and mortality outcomes.[137,138] In 1995, the CDC recommended hospitals develop guidelines for the appropriate use of vancomycin as part of stewardship efforts.[139] Implementation of vancomycin-reduction guidelines in NICUs with low prevalence of MRSA infections showed that initiation of empiric therapy with nafcillin or oxacillin combined with gentamicin was associated with a reduction in vancomycin exposure without compromising short-term patient safety.[137] A retrospective study comparing cloxacillin with vancomycin for empiric treatment of LOS reported no significant differences in duration of CoNS bacteremia, suggesting that reserving vancomycin for confirmed cases of CoNS infection resistant to oxacillin was safe and effective.[140] Clinicians can be somewhat reassured regarding using antibiotics other than vancomycin for empiric treatment of suspected LOS when methicillin-susceptible *S. aureus* or CoNS is the causative organism, as retrospective cohort analysis indicates that being on vancomycin when the culture is obtained and these organisms are identified offers no survival advantage.[138] Alternatively, when MRSA is the causative organism, being on vancomycin was protective, suggesting that local microbiograms and epidemiology provide important guidance of local selection of empiric antibiotics.[141] Therefore appropriate empiric therapy for LOS includes the combination of a semisynthetic penicillin such as oxacillin or nafcillin with an aminoglycoside while waiting for cultures, whereas vancomycin should be reserved for the following cases: (1) NICUs with high prevalence of MRSA, (2) infants known to be MRSA colonized, (3) proven infection with MRSA or oxacillin-resistant CoNS, (4) clinical deterioration despite antibiotic therapy, and (5) critically ill infants with presumed sepsis.[84,129,137,142]

Reevaluating Antibiotic Therapy: How Long to Treat?

When microbiology results and susceptibility profiles are available, the initial antibiotic regimen should be reviewed to determine whether antibiotics should be continued, modified, or discontinued. Susceptibility profiles provide the opportunity to change antimicrobial agents to a narrow-spectrum, less toxic, or more effective regimen. As most blood cultures become positive within 48 hours when bacteremia is significant and any growth beyond this time more likely corresponds to a contaminant, a timely review at this point may reduce antibiotic use.[143,144] Over 60% of the antibiotics used were used after 48 hours of empirical treatment, and 26% occurring beyond 5 days. Infants with suspected clinical sepsis and pneumonia accounted for much of the antibiotic exposure beyond 5 days.[28] Unjustified prolonged antibiotic therapy has been attributed to institutional decisions rather than severity of illness, so changing and informing the rationale underlying antibiotic prescription are urgently needed.[145]

Antibiotics should be continued past 48 hours in infants with positive cultures. When an infant is critically ill and clinical signs of infection persist beyond 48 hours, the possibility of false-negative culture results also may justify continuation of treatment.[146] Conversely, discontinuation of empiric antibiotics by 48 to 72 hours in infants with sterile blood cultures and without clinical signs of infection has been reported to be safe.[46] More recent data regarding time to positive results using automated blood culture systems support reducing antibiotic duration to 24 to 36 hours in infants who remain clinically well and have negative cultures.[147,148] One concern is that IAP may mask true neonatal infection by reducing the likelihood that a pathogen will be recovered in a blood culture; however, there is reassuring evidence that pathogens grow in infected infants even when intrapartum antibiotics are used.[70,147]

Antibiotic use in well-appearing infants born to mothers with chorioamnion-itis who received adequate intrapartum antibiotic therapy has been the subject of debate. In 2012 the American Academy of Pediatrics' Committee on the Fetus and Newborn (COFN) issued guidelines on the management of sepsis recommending that antibiotics be discontinued after 48 hours in asymptomatic infants exposed to chorioamnionitis with normal laboratory findings and negative blood cultures, while continuing therapy in those infants with abnormal laboratory findings despite sterile cultures if intrapartum antibiotics were administered.[5,149] As a result of these practices, Kiser et al. found that a large number of infants exposed to chorioamnionitis and with sterile blood cultures received prolonged antibiotic therapy and were subject to additional invasive procedures and prolonged hospital stay solely on the basis of abnormal laboratory findings.[96] In 2014 an expert commentary on the COFN recommendations supported discontinuation of antibiotic therapy at 48 hours of life in well-appearing term infants born to mothers with chorioamnionitis and with sterile blood cultures and at 72 hours in infants with abnormal laboratory findings or in those born prematurely.[150] In a case series of 698 well-appearing infants ≥34 weeks gestation born to mothers with chorioamnionitis who were managed initially with empiric antibiotics pending blood culture results according to guidelines, only 1 (0.14%) had culture-positive EOS.[151] Implementation of a strategy based on risk factors and the infant's clinical appearance rather than the obstetric diagnosis of chorioamnionitis would have reduced the proportion of infants undergoing laboratory tests and antibiotic therapy to 12% without underdiagnosing EOS. Isolated abnormal laboratory results should not justify continuation of empiric antibiotics for more than 48 hours in these infants.[87,97,150]

In the case of LOS, antibiotic treatment should be continued for at least 48 hours before cessation is considered, due to the increased proportion of late-onset infections caused by *Staphylococcus* and the increased median time to positivity of cultures for those organisms (18 hours or more compared with <12 hours for GBS and *E. coli*, the major pathogens associated with EOS).[148]

Table 5.2 ONE APPROACH TO TERM AND LATE-PRETERM INFANTS RECEIVING EMPIRICAL ANTIBIOTICS FOR EOS WITH STERILE CULTURES AT 48 HOURS[146]

Clinical Situation	Duration of Antibiotic Therapy
Clinical signs of infection persisting over 24 hours	7 days
Normal laboratory screening that was drawn for risk factors in a well-appearing infant	48 hours
Abnormal initial CBC drawn for risk factors in an infant with transient clinical signs (less than 8 hours)	Obtain CRP at 24 and 48 hours. If normal and infant continues well, stop antibiotics at 48 hours.

Data from Cotten CM, Smith PB: Duration of empirical antibiotic therapy for infants suspected of early-onset sepsis. *Curr Opin Pediatr* 25:167–171, 2013.

Clinicians will continue to be concerned about infants with signs of infection that resolve in the first 24 to 48 hours and whether or not it is safe to stop antibiotics that had been empirically initiated. Some are likely to rely on laboratory values for admittedly imperfect guidance. One potential set of guidelines for clinicians who are using screening laboratory results to guide decisions to continue antibiotics or not is presented in Table 5.2.

Reducing Infection Risk

Antibiotic stewardship begins with prevention of infections. In the last decade, large consortia incorporating hundreds of intensive care units have reported decreasing rates of sepsis in the NICU.[10,36–38] Obstetric interventions are necessary to reduce preterm deliveries, as the burden of infections and volume of antibiotic use is the highest among premature infants.[129] In addition to working with obstetricians to identify safe and effective strategies to prevent preterm birth, caregivers of newborns must work with obstetrics colleagues on antenatal antibiotic strategies and guidelines because antibiotic use in neonates may be strongly influenced by prenatal antibiotic exposures.[84]

Within the NICU, adherence to infection-prevention strategies is of paramount importance. A decrease in true infections is likely accompanied by fewer suspected infections and therefore less antibiotic use. Hand hygiene remains the most effective method for reducing hospital-acquired infections. Other efforts are focused on care in placement and maintenance of central catheters to reduce central line–associated bloodstream infections, appropriate suctioning practices, and positioning of the infant to reduce tracheal colonization of ventilated infants and adequate care of the skin of extremely premature infants.[152–154] Universal use of gloves and masks for patient contact in the intensive care setting has not been demonstrated to reduce transmission of resistant-pathogens compared with usual care.[155,156]

Although antibiotic stewardship continues to be a priority, antibiotic use remains high among the neonatal population, but as noted earlier, the incidence of infection is decreasing. The Pediatrix medical group has demonstrated in their 100,000 babies campaign that a decrease in use of third-generation cephalosporins and an increase in use of fluconazole prophylaxis are associated with reduction in invasive candidiasis.[38,157,158]

Examples of Targeted Antibiotic Stewardship

Management of suspected pneumonia, as it accounts for a significant proportion of prolonged antibiotic use in the NICU due to difficulties in distinguishing from other noninfectious conditions such as RDS and TTN, has been a target for antibiotic stewardship efforts.[28,89,93] The diagnosis of pneumonia in hospitalized infants is difficult, because the target population often has evolving or proven BPD, and clinical signs may be attributed to a new infection or the underlying chronic lung disease. Once the diagnosis of pneumonia is made, Engle et al. suggested that 4 days of antibiotic therapy compared with 7 days may be sufficient in term and near-term infants who are asymptomatic by 48 hours of therapy.[159] Those suggestions, however, are unproven, and most infants with a respiratory decompensation will not have an infectious cause. Further data are needed to determine the optimal treatment duration for premature infants with a health care–acquired pneumonia. Moreover, validating diagnostic criteria, as well as screening of respiratory viral panels, could reduce overtreatment of suspected pneumonia.[160,161]

Infectious complications play an important role in surgical conditions, such as abdominal wall defects. Perioperative antibiotic prophylaxis for infants varies widely among centers, but there is evidence that prolonged courses (over 48 hours) do not prevent surgical site infections and may increase the risk of infections by multiresistant pathogens.[162–164] Although the optimal duration remains to be determined, standardizing perioperative prophylaxis offers an additional antimicrobial stewardship target.[144]

Results of implementing the Kaiser Permanente EOS risk calculator were recently published. In analysis of over 200,000 infants, use of this multivariable risk prediction model among near-term and term infants reduced the proportion of infants undergoing sepsis evaluation from 14% to 5% and those receiving empiric antibiotic treatment in the first 24 hours of life from 5% to 2.6%, as well as antibiotic days from 16 to 8.5 days per 100 births. Initiation of treatment of infants with EOS presenting with more severe clinical illness was not delayed, and sepsis-associated clinical outcome or readmissions for EOS after discharge were not increased.[98]

National Attention for Antibiotic Stewardship

Get Smart for Healthcare is a CDC campaign launched in 2009 focused on improving antibiotic prescribing practices in inpatient and outpatient health care facilities through implementation of stewardship programs to optimize clinical outcomes and ultimately save lives while reducing the burden of antibiotic resistance, adverse events, and health care costs. Multiple providers, including infectious disease specialists, neonatologists, clinical pharmacists, clinical microbiologists, nurses, hospital administrators, and policymakers, are essential for the success of these stewardship programs. To date, 39% of all hospitals in the United States have stewardship programs, with the national goal being 100% by 2020 (http://www.cdc.gov/getsmart/healthcare). Strategies implemented in stewardship programs vary widely based on the needs of each hospital, as well as the availability of resources and expertise (Table 5.3). Establishment of stewardship programs should start with one recommended action: Implementing too many interventions simultaneously is not recommended. Education is essential to provide a foundation of knowledge that enhances the acceptance of stewardship strategies. However, the effectiveness of education alone is limited, and development of evidence-based clinical guidelines that include local microbiology and resistance patterns is needed.[165] Antibiotic "timeout" is a strategy that promotes reviewing indications for antibiotic continuation 48 hours after initiation, when more diagnostic information is available.[166] A key element is antibiotic de-escalation, in which review of microbiology results 48 to 72 hours after initiation permits empiric antibiotic treatment to be discontinued, reduced in number, or narrowed in spectrum.[167] A study showed that nearly 60% of infants continue to receive broad-spectrum empiric therapy despite culture results allowing de-escalation.[168] To achieve potential synergism and broader coverage, empiric regimens targeted at gram-negative organisms often consist of a combination of antimicrobial agents. Available evidence does not support such "double coverage" for treatment of gram-negative infections, as it does not result in improved outcome compared with monotherapy and may lead to antibiotic resistance, adverse events, and increased costs.[169,170] Prospective audit of antibiotic use with real-time feedback to the prescriber, formulary restriction, and preauthorization strategies can result in reduced inappropriate use of antibiotics and cost.[165] Computer-based surveillance can greatly facilitate good stewardship by tracking antimicrobial use and generating electronic alerts for redundant drug combinations, prolonged duration of therapy, antimicrobial-resistant patterns, and adverse events.[165] Periodic assessments of the actions targeted to reduce antibiotic misuse, monitor clinical

Table 5.3   STEWARDSHIP PROGRAMS AND PRINCIPLES FOR ANTIBIOTIC USE IN NICUs

Education	Provide a foundation of knowledge to enhance acceptance of stewardship strategies.
Coordinated multidisciplinary approach of the stewardship program	Infectious disease specialist, neonatologist, clinical pharmacist, clinical microbiologist, nursing leadership, hospital administrators, and policymakers are essential for decision making and success of the program.
Leadership commitment	Appointing a single leader responsible for program outcomes has demonstrated to be effective.
Prescription approval of antibiotics	Preauthorization requirements by an antibiotic expert can lead to significant reductions in antimicrobial use and cost.
Rational empiric initiation of antibiotics	Initiate antibiotics when bacterial infections are likely. Indication for all courses of antibiotics must be readily identifiable.
Facility-specific treatment recommendations	Optimize antibiotic selection and duration for common indications, especially for specific syndromes and surgical prophylaxis. Develop consensus guidelines for the NICU.
Dosing optimization	Use pharmacodynamics and pharmacokinetic principles to optimize antimicrobial dosing.
Therapeutic monitoring	Reduce adverse events and administration errors.
Adjust coverage based on susceptibility and resistance patterns	Reduce the proportion of antimicrobial-resistant organisms in the hospital and community.
Establish duration of antibiotic therapy	Determine treatment duration based on the disease process, and discontinue when bacterial infection has not been identified.
Antibiotic "timeouts"	Review the need to continue antibiotics at 48 hours with new diagnostic information with other members of the treating team.
Avoid combination of antimicrobial agents	There are insufficient data to recommend empiric combination therapy.
Antibiotic de-escalation	Reassess therapy based on microbiology results and discontinue, reduce in number, or narrow in spectrum empiric antibiotics.
Parenteral to oral conversion of antibiotics	Switch to oral agents when the condition of the patient allows to reduce length of stay, the need for intravenous access, and costs.
Interactions with other drugs	Detection and prevention of interaction between antibiotics and other drugs.
Prospective audit and feedback of antibiotic use	Direct interaction and feedback to the prescriber or other external experts can reduce inappropriate use of antibiotics.
Computer-based surveillance	Monitoring antimicrobial prescription, resistance patterns, and adverse events can facilitate stewardship strategies. Generate automated alerts for redundant drug combinations and prolonged duration of therapy.

Adapted from CDC Get Smart for Healthcare. Core Elements of Hospital Antibiotic Stewardship Programs. http://www.cdc.gov/getsmart/healthcare/implementation/core-elements.html

outcomes, and accumulate data regarding dosing in the intensive care nursery population will inform ongoing local and national infection and antibiotic stewardship efforts.

Summary

Although EOS and LOS in infants have decreased in the last two decades, sepsis remains a significant cause of morbidity and mortality in the neonatal population. Antibiotics are an unavoidable fact of life for thousands of infants. However, most of these infants are not infected. Evidence from animal studies linking antibiotic exposure in the neonatal period with variations in the evolving microbiome and subsequent effects on health is emerging, and antibiotic overuse and misuse can lead to emergence of resistant pathogens. Judicious use of antibiotics appears to be a critical step to reducing risk of death and complications, especially in preterm infants. Increasing knowledge of antibiotic pharmacokinetics and selective use of antibiotics through evidence-based protocols will help clinicians in the management of neonatal infections. The combination of ampicillin and an aminoglycoside is the most suitable choice for initial empiric therapy for suspected EOS. Empiric therapy for suspected LOS should include oxacillin and an aminoglycoside in NICUs where MRSA is not endemic. Vancomycin should be reserved for infants at risk for MRSA infections. Use of third-generation cephalosporins should be discouraged when meningitis is not suspected. Ongoing efforts to reduce infection risk and stewardship programs and general guidelines for antibiotic use managed by a multidisciplinary team are essential to optimize outcomes for our vulnerable neonatal patients.

REFERENCES

1. Stoll BJ, Hansen N, Fanaroff AA, et al. Changes in pathogens causing early-onset sepsis in very-low-birth-weight infants. *N Engl J Med*. 2002;347:240–247.
2. Stoll BJ, Hansen NI, Higgins RD, et al. Very low birth weight preterm infants with early onset neonatal sepsis: the predominance of gram-negative infections continues in the National Institute of Child Health and Human Development Neonatal Research Network, 2002-2003. *Pediatr Infect Dis J*. 2005;24:635–639.
3. Camacho-Gonzalez A, Spearman PW, Stoll BJ. Neonatal infectious diseases: evaluation of neonatal sepsis. *Pediatr Clin North Am*. 2013;60:367–389.
4. Stoll BJ, Hansen NI, Sanchez PJ, et al. Early onset neonatal sepsis: the burden of group B *Streptococcal* and *E. coli* disease continues. *Pediatrics*. 2011;127:817–826.
5. Polin RA, Committee on Fetus and Newborn. Management of neonates with suspected or proven early-onset bacterial sepsis. *Pediatrics*. 2012;129:1006–1015.
6. Committee on Infectious Diseases, Committee on Fetus and Newborn, Baker CJ, et al. Policy statement-recommendations for the prevention of perinatal group B streptococcal (GBS) disease. *Pediatrics*. 2011;128:611–616.
7. Schrag SJ, Zywicki S, Farley MM, et al. Group B streptococcal disease in the era of intrapartum antibiotic prophylaxis. *N Engl J Med*. 2000;342:15–20.
8. Schrag SJ, Farley MM, Petit S, et al. Epidemiology of invasive early-onset neonatal sepsis, 2005 to 2014. *Pediatrics*. 2016;138:e20162013.
9. Van Dyke MK, Phares CR, Lynfield R, et al. Evaluation of universal antenatal screening for group B *Streptococcus*. *N Engl J Med*. 2009;360:2626–2636.
10. Stoll BJ, Hansen NI, Bell EF, et al. Trends in care practices, morbidity, and mortality of extremely preterm neonates, 1993-2012. *JAMA*. 2015;314:1039–1051.
11. Stoll BJ, Hansen N, Fanaroff AA, et al. Late-onset sepsis in very low birth weight neonates: the experience of the NICHD Neonatal Research Network. *Pediatrics*. 2002;110:285–291.
12. Stoll BJ, Hansen NI, Adams-Chapman I, et al. Neurodevelopmental and growth impairment among extremely low-birth-weight infants with neonatal infection. *JAMA*. 2004;292:2357–2365.
13. Mukhopadhyay S, Eichenwald EC, Puopolo KM. Neonatal early-onset sepsis evaluations among well-appearing infants: projected impact of changes in CDC GBS guidelines. *J Perinatol*. 2013;33: 198–205.
14. Tsai CH, Chen YY, Wang KG, et al. Characteristics of early-onset neonatal sepsis caused by *Escherichia coli*. *Taiwan J Obstet Gynecol*. 2012;51:26–30.
15. Patel SJ, Saiman L. Antibiotic resistance in neonatal intensive care unit pathogens: mechanisms, clinical impact, and prevention including antibiotic stewardship. *Clin Perinatol*. 2010;37:547–563.
16. Fouhy F, Ogilvie LA, Jones BV, et al. Identification of aminoglycoside and beta-lactam resistance genes from within an infant gut functional metagenomic library. *PLoS ONE*. 2014;9:e108016.
17. Brooks B, Firek BA, Miller CS, et al. Microbes in the neonatal intensive care unit resemble those found in the gut of premature infants. *Microbiome*. 2014;2:1.
18. Moore AM, Ahmadi S, Patel S, et al. Gut resistome development in healthy twin pairs in the first year of life. *Microbiome*. 2015;3:27.
19. Zeissig S, Blumberg RS. Life at the beginning: perturbation of the microbiota by antibiotics in early life and its role in health and disease. *Nat Immunol*. 2014;15:307–310.
20. Schokker D, Zhang J, Zhang LL, et al. Early-life environmental variation affects intestinal microbiota and immune development in new-born piglets. *PLoS ONE*. 2014;9:e100040.
21. Candon S, Perez-Arroyo A, Marquet C, et al. Antibiotics in early life alter the gut microbiome and increase disease incidence in a spontaneous mouse model of autoimmune insulin-dependent diabetes. *PLoS ONE*. 2015;10:e0125448.
22. Deshmukh HS, Liu Y, Menkiti OR, et al. The microbiota regulates neutrophil homeostasis and host resistance to *Escherichia coli* K1 sepsis in neonatal mice. *Nat Med*. 2014;20:524–530.
23. Investigators of the Delhi Neonatal Infection Study (DeNIS) collaboration. Characterisation and antimicrobial resistance of sepsis pathogens in neonates born in tertiary care centres in Delhi, India: a cohort study. *Lancet Glob Health*. 2016;4:e752–e760.
24. Lu Q, Zhou M, Tu Y, et al. Pathogen and antimicrobial resistance profiles of culture-proven neonatal sepsis in Southwest China, 1990–2014. *J Paediatr Child Health*. 2016;52:939–943.
25. Gerdes JS. Diagnosis and management of bacterial infections in the neonate. *Pediatr Clin North Am*. 2004;51:939–959.
26. Fanaroff AA, Korones SB, Wright LL, et al. Incidence, presenting features, risk factors and significance of late onset septicemia in very low birth weight infants. The National Institute of Child Health and Human Development Neonatal Research Network. *Pediatr Infect Dis J*. 1998;17:593–598.
27. Clark RH, Bloom BT, Spitzer AR, et al. Reported medication use in the neonatal intensive care unit: data from a large national data set. *Pediatrics*. 2006;117:1979–1987.

28. Cantey JB, Wozniak PS, Sanchez PJ. Prospective surveillance of antibiotic use in the neonatal intensive care unit: results from the SCOUT study. *Pediatr Infect Dis J.* 2015;34:267–272.
29. Hornik CP, Fort P, Clark RH, et al. Early and late onset sepsis in very-low-birth-weight infants from a large group of neonatal intensive care units. *Early Hum Dev.* 2012;88:S69–S74.
30. Vergnano S, Menson E, Kennea N, et al. Neonatal infections in England: the NeonIN surveillance network. *Arch Dis Child Fetal Neonatal Ed.* 2011;96:F9–F14.
31. Simonsen KA, Anderson-Berry AL, Delair SF, et al. Early-onset neonatal sepsis. *Clin Microbiol Rev.* 2014;27:21–47.
32. Wynn JL, Wong HR. Pathophysiology and treatment of septic shock in neonates. *Clin Perinatol.* 2010;37:439–479.
33. Cuenca AG, Wynn JL, Moldawer LL, et al. Role of innate immunity in neonatal infection. *Am J Perinatol.* 2013;30:105–112.
34. Shane AL, Stoll BJ. Neonatal sepsis: progress towards improved outcomes. *J Infect.* 2014;68(suppl 1):S24–S32.
35. Chu A, Hageman JR, Schreiber M, et al. Antimicrobial therapy and late onset sepsis. *NeoReviews.* 2012;13:e94–e102.
36. Greenberg R, et al. for the Eunice Kennedy Shriver National Institute of Child Health and Human Development Neonatal Research Network: Late-Onset Sepsis in Extremely Premature Infants: 2000-2011. *Pediatr Infect Dis J.* 2017.
37. Horbar JD, Edwards EM, Greenberg LT, et al. Variation in performance of neonatal intensive care units in the United States. *JAMA Pediatrics.* 2017;e164396.
38. Ellsbury DL, Clark RH, Ursprung R, et al. A multifaceted approach to improving outcomes in the NICU: The Pediatrix 100 000 Babies Campaign. *Pediatrics.* 2016;137:e20150389.
39. Downey LC, Smith PB, Benjamin DK Jr. Risk factors and prevention of late-onset sepsis in premature infants. *Early Hum Dev.* 2010;86(suppl 1):7–12.
40. Glass HC, Bonifacio SL, Chau V, et al. Recurrent postnatal infections are associated with progressive white matter injury in premature infants. *Pediatrics.* 2008;122:299–305.
41. Adams-Chapman I. Long-term impact of infection on the preterm neonate. *Semin Perinatol.* 2012;36:462–470.
42. Procianoy RS, Silveira RC. Association between high cytokine levels with white matter injury in preterm infants with sepsis. *Pediatr Crit Care Med.* 2012;13:183–187.
43. Levent F, Baker CJ, Rench MA, et al. Early outcomes of group B streptococcal meningitis in the 21st century. *Pediatr Infect Dis J.* 2010;29:1009–1012.
44. Libster R, Edwards KM, Levent F, et al. Long-term outcomes of group B streptococcal meningitis. *Pediatrics.* 2012;130:e8–e15.
45. Cotten CM, Taylor S, Stoll B, et al. Prolonged duration of initial empirical antibiotic treatment is associated with increased rates of necrotizing enterocolitis and death for extremely low birth weight infants. *Pediatrics.* 2009;123:58–66.
46. Cordero L, Ayers LW. Duration of empiric antibiotics for suspected early-onset sepsis in extremely low birth weight infants. *Infect Control Hosp Epidemiol.* 2003;24:662–666.
47. Liem TB, Krediet TG, Fleer A, et al. Variation in antibiotic use in neonatal intensive care units in the Netherlands. *J Antimicrob Chemother.* 2010;65:1270–1275.
48. Schulman J, Dimand RJ, Lee HC, et al. Neonatal intensive care unit antibiotic use. *Pediatrics.* 2015;135:826.
49. Aliaga S, Boggess K, Ivester TS, et al. Influence of neonatal practice variation on outcomes of late preterm birth. *Am J Perinatol.* 2014;31:659–666.
50. Kadambari S, Heath PT, Sharland M, et al. Variation in gentamicin and vancomycin dosage and monitoring in UK neonatal units. *J Antimicrob Chemother.* 2011;66:2647–2650.
51. Bizzarro MJ, Gallagher PG. Antibiotic-resistant organisms in the neonatal intensive care unit. *Semin Perinatol.* 2007;31:26–32.
52. Institute of Medicine (US) Forum on Microbial Threats. Antibiotic Resistance. *Implications for Global Health and Novel Intervention Strategies: Workshop Summary.* Washington (DC): National Academies Press (US); 2010. doi:10.17226/12925. Available from: https://www.ncbi.nlm.nih.gov/books/NBK54255/.
53. Tremoulet A, Le J, Poindexter B, et al. Characterization of the population pharmacokinetics of ampicillin in neonates using an opportunistic study design. *Antimicrob Agents Chemother.* 2014;58:3013–3020.
54. Smith PB, Cohen-Wolkowiez M, Castro LM, et al. Population pharmacokinetics of meropenem in plasma and cerebrospinal fluid of infants with suspected or complicated intra-abdominal infections. *Pediatr Infect Dis J.* 2011;30:844–849.
55. Piper L, Smith PB, Hornik CP, et al. Fluconazole loading dose pharmacokinetics and safety in infants. *Pediatr Infect Dis J.* 2011;30:375–378.
56. Patel SJ, Oshodi A, Prasad P, et al. Antibiotic use in neonatal intensive care units and adherence with Centers for Disease Control and Prevention 12 step campaign to prevent antimicrobial resistance. *Pediatr Infect Dis J.* 2009;28:1047–1051.
57. Ting JY, Synnes A, Roberts A, et al. Association between antibiotic use and neonatal mortality and morbidities in very low-birth-weight infants without culture-proven sepsis or necrotizing enterocolitis. *JAMA Pediatr.* 2016;170:1181–1187.
58. Novitsky A, Tuttle D, Locke RG, et al. Prolonged early antibiotic use and bronchopulmonary dysplasia in very low birth weight infants. *Am J Perinatol.* 2015;32:43–48.

59. Cantey JB, Huffman LW, Subramanian A, et al. Antibiotic exposure and risk for death or broncho-pulmonary dysplasia in very low birth weight infants. *J Pediatr.* 2017;181:289–293.
60. Sehgal R, Gaind R, Chellani H, et al. Extended-spectrum beta lactamase-producing gram-negative bacteria: clinical profile and outcome in a neonatal intensive care unit. *Ann Trop Paediatr.* 2007;27:45–54.
61. Linkin DR, Fishman NO, Patel JB, et al. Risk factors for extended-spectrum beta-lactamase-producing Enterobacteriaceae in a neonatal intensive care unit. *Infect Control Hosp Epidemiol.* 2004;25:781–783.
62. Touati A, Achour W, Cherif A, et al. Outbreak of *Acinetobacter baumannii* in a neonatal intensive care unit: antimicrobial susceptibility and genotyping analysis. *Ann Epidemiol.* 2009;19:372–378.
63. de Man P, Verhoeven BA, Verbrugh HA, et al. An antibiotic policy to prevent emergence of resistant bacilli. *Lancet.* 2000;355:973–978.
64. Solomon SL, Oliver KB. Antibiotic resistance threats in the United States: stepping back from the brink. *Am Fam Physician.* 2014;89:938–941.
65. Cotten CM, McDonald S, Stoll B, et al. The association of third-generation cephalosporin use and invasive candidiasis in extremely low birth-weight infants. *Pediatrics.* 2006;118:717–722.
66. Benjamin DK Jr, Stoll BJ, Fanaroff AA, et al. Neonatal candidiasis among extremely low birth weight infants: risk factors, mortality rates, and neurodevelopmental outcomes at 18 to 22 months. *Pediatrics.* 2006;117:84–92.
67. Tzialla C, Borghesi A, Pozzi M, et al. Neonatal infections due to multi-resistant strains: epidemiology, current treatment, emerging therapeutic approaches and prevention. *Clin Chim Acta.* 2015;451:71–77.
68. World Health Organization. Antimicrobial resistance: global report on surveillance; 2014. Geneva, Switzerland. Available from http://apps.who.int/iris/bitstream/10665/112642/1/9789241564748_eng.pdf?ua=1.
69. Cantey JB, Milstone AM. Bloodstream infections: epidemiology and resistance. *Clin Perinatol.* 2015;42:1–16, vii.
70. Verani JR, McGee L, Schrag SJ, et al. Prevention of perinatal group B streptococcal disease–revised guidelines from CDC, 2010. *MMWR Recomm Rep.* 2010;59:1–36.
71. Gray JW, Patel M. Management of antibiotic-resistant infection in the newborn. *Arch Dis Child Educ Pract Ed.* 2011;96:122–127.
72. Steinkraus G, White R, Friedrich L. Vancomycin MIC creep in non-vancomycin-intermediate *Staphylococcus aureus* (VISA), vancomycin-susceptible clinical methicillin-resistant *S. aureus* (MRSA) blood isolates from 2001-05. *J Antimicrob Chemother.* 2007;60:788–794.
73. Bal AM, Gould IM. Antibiotic resistance in *Staphylococcus aureus* and its relevance in therapy. *Expert Opin Pharmacother.* 2005;6:2257–2269.
74. Center KJ, Reboli AC, Hubler R, et al. Decreased vancomycin susceptibility of coagulase-negative staphylococci in a neonatal intensive care unit: evidence of spread of *Staphylococcus warneri.* *J Clin Microbiol.* 2003;41:4660–4665.
75. Howden BP, Davies JK, Johnson PD, et al. Reduced vancomycin susceptibility in *Staphylococcus aureus*, including vancomycin-intermediate and heterogeneous vancomycin-intermediate strains: resistance mechanisms, laboratory detection, and clinical implications. *Clin Microbiol Rev.* 2010;23:99–139.
76. Iosifidis E, Evdoridou I, Agakidou E, et al. Vancomycin-resistant *Enterococcus* outbreak in a neonatal intensive care unit: epidemiology, molecular analysis and risk factors. *Am J Infect Control.* 2013;41:857–861.
77. Duchon J, Graham Iii P, Della-Latta P, et al. Epidemiology of enterococci in a neonatal intensive care unit. *Infect Control Hosp Epidemiol.* 2008;29:374–376.
78. Garazzino S, Tovo PA. Clinical experience with linezolid in infants and children. *J Antimicrob Chemother.* 2011;66(suppl 4):iv23–iv41.
79. Pitout JD, Laupland KB. Extended-spectrum beta-lactamase-producing *Enterobacteriaceae*: an emerging public-health concern. *Lancet Infect Dis.* 2008;8:159–166.
80. Patel SJ, Saiman L. Antibiotic Resistance in Neonatal Intensive Care Unit Pathogens: Mechanisms, Clinical Impact, and Prevention Including Antibiotic Stewardship. *Clin Perinatol.* 2010;37:547–563.
81. Gupta A, Della-Latta P, Todd B, et al. Outbreak of extended-spectrum beta-lactamase-producing *Klebsiella pneumoniae* in a neonatal intensive care unit linked to artificial nails. *Infect Control Hosp Epidemiol.* 2004;25:210–215.
82. Stapleton PJ, Murphy M, McCallion N, et al. Outbreaks of extended spectrum beta-lactamase-producing *Enterobacteriaceae* in neonatal intensive care units: a systematic review. *Arch Dis Child Fetal Neonatal Ed.* 2016;101:F72–F78.
83. Neu HC. The crisis in antibiotic resistance. *Science.* 1992;257:1064–1073.
84. Cantey JB, Patel SJ. Antimicrobial stewardship in the NICU. *Infect Dis Clin North Am.* 2014;28:247–261.
85. Schrag S, Gorwitz R, Fultz-Butts K, et al. Prevention of perinatal group B streptococcal disease. Revised guidelines from CDC. *MMWR Recomm Rep.* 2002;51:1–22.
86. Puopolo KM, Draper D, Wi S, et al. Estimating the probability of neonatal early-onset infection on the basis of maternal risk factors. *Pediatrics.* 2011;128:e1155–e1163.
87. Escobar GJ, Puopolo KM, Wi S, et al. Stratification of risk of early-onset sepsis in newborns >/= 34 weeks' gestation. *Pediatrics.* 2014;133:30–36.
88. Kaiser Permanente Division of Research. Probability of Neonatal Early-Onset Sepsis Based on Maternal Risk factors and the Infant's Clinical Presentation; 2017. Available from https://neonatalsepsiscalculator.kaiserpermanente.org.

89. Shani L, Weitzman D, Melamed R, et al. Risk factors for early sepsis in very low birth weight neonates with respiratory distress syndrome. *Acta Paediatr*. 2008;97:12–15.

90. Kallman J, Ekholm L, Eriksson M, et al. Contribution of interleukin-6 in distinguishing between mild respiratory disease and neonatal sepsis in the newborn infant. *Acta Paediatr*. 1999;88:880–884.

91. Salama H, Abughalwa M, Taha S, et al. Transient tachypnea of the newborn: Is empiric antimicrobial therapy needed? *J Neonatal Perinatal Med*. 2013;6:237–241.

92. Li J, Wu J, Du L, et al. Different antibiotic strategies in transient tachypnea of the newborn: an ambispective cohort study. *Eur J Pediatr*. 2015;174:1217–1223.

93. Weintraub AS, Cadet CT, Perez R, et al. Antibiotic use in newborns with transient tachypnea of the newborn. *Neonatology*. 2013;103:235–240.

94. Taylor JA, Opel DJ. Choriophobia: a 1-act play. *Pediatrics*. 2012;130:342–346.

95. Linder N, Fridman E, Makhoul A, et al. Management of term newborns following maternal intrapartum fever. *J Matern Fetal Neonatal Med*. 2013;26:207–210.

96. Kiser C, Nawab U, McKenna K, et al. Role of guidelines on length of therapy in chorioamnionitis and neonatal sepsis. *Pediatrics*. 2014;133:992–998.

97. Benitz WE, Wynn JL, Polin RA. Reappraisal of guidelines for management of neonates with suspected early-onset sepsis. *J Pediatr*. 2015;166:1070–1074.

98. Kuzniewicz MW, Puopolo KM, Fischer A, et al. A quantitative, risk-based approach to the management of neonatal early-onset sepsis. *JAMA Pediatr*. 2017;171:365–371.

99. Venkatesh MP, Placencia F, Weisman LE. Coagulase-negative staphylococcal infections in the neonate and child: an update. *Semin Pediatr Infect Dis*. 2006;17:120–127.

100. Van Hal SJ, Frostis V, Miyakis S, et al. Prevalence and significance of coagulase-negative staphylococci isolated from blood cultures in a tertiary hospital. *Scand J Infect Dis*. 2008;40:551–554.

101. Struthers S, Underhill H, Albersheim S, et al. A comparison of two versus one blood culture in the diagnosis and treatment of coagulase-negative staphylococcus in the neonatal intensive care unit. *J Perinatol*. 2002;22:547–549.

102. Healy CM, Baker CJ, Palazzi DL, et al. Distinguishing true coagulase-negative *Staphylococcus* infections from contaminants in the neonatal intensive care unit. *J Perinatol*. 2013;33:52–58.

103. Beekmann SE, Diekema DJ, Doern GV. Determining the clinical significance of coagulase-negative staphylococci isolated from blood cultures. *Infect Control Hosp Epidemiol*. 2005;26:559–566.

104. Kim SD, McDonald LC, Jarvis WR, et al. Determining the significance of coagulase-negative staphylococci isolated from blood cultures at a community hospital: a role for species and strain identification. *Infect Control Hosp Epidemiol*. 2000;21:213–217.

105. Seybold U, Reichardt C, Halvosa JS, et al. Clonal diversity in episodes with multiple coagulase-negative *Staphylococcus* bloodstream isolates suggesting frequent contamination. *Infection*. 2009;37: 256–260.

106. Benitz WE. Adjunct laboratory tests in the diagnosis of early-onset neonatal sepsis. *Clin Perinatol*. 2010;37:421–438.

107. Hornik CP, Benjamin DK, Becker KC, et al. Use of the complete blood cell count in early-onset neonatal sepsis. *Pediatr Infect Dis J*. 2012;31:799–802.

108. Hornik CP, Benjamin DK, Becker KC, et al. Use of the complete blood cell count in late-onset neonatal sepsis. *Pediatr Infect Dis J*. 2012;31:803–807.

109. Philip AG, Mills PC. Use of C-reactive protein in minimizing antibiotic exposure: experience with infants initially admitted to a well-baby nursery. *Pediatrics*. 2000;106:E4.

110. Hengst JM. The role of C-reactive protein in the evaluation and management of infants with suspected sepsis. *Adv Neonatal Care*. 2003;3:3–13.

111. Shah BA, Padbury JF. Neonatal sepsis: an old problem with new insights. *Virulence*. 2014;5:170–178.

112. Murphy K, Weiner J. Use of leukocyte counts in evaluation of early-onset neonatal sepsis. *Pediatr Infect Dis J*. 2012;31:16–19.

113. Ozkan H, Koksal N, Cetinkaya M, et al. Serum mannose-binding lectin (MBL) gene polymorphism and low MBL levels are associated with neonatal sepsis and pneumonia. *J Perinatol*. 2012;32:210–217.

114. Resch B, Gusenleitner W, Muller WD. Procalcitonin and interleukin-6 in the diagnosis of early-onset sepsis of the neonate. *Acta Paediatr*. 2003;92:243–245.

115. Ng PC, Ang IL, Chiu RW, et al. Host-response biomarkers for diagnosis of late-onset septicemia and necrotizing enterocolitis in preterm infants. *J Clin Invest*. 2010;120:2989–3000.

116. Genel F, Atlihan F, Gulez N, et al. Evaluation of adhesion molecules CD64, CD11b and CD62L in neutrophils and monocytes of peripheral blood for early diagnosis of neonatal infection. *World J Pediatr*. 2012;8:72–75.

117. Cernada M, Serna E, Bauerl C, et al. Genome-wide expression profiles in very low birth weight infants with neonatal sepsis. *Pediatrics*. 2014;133:e1203–e1211.

118. Wynn JL, Guthrie SO, Wong HR, et al. Postnatal age is a critical determinant of the neonatal host response to sepsis. *Mol Med*. 2015;21:496–504.

119. Muller-Pebody B, Johnson AP, Heath PT, et al. Empirical treatment of neonatal sepsis: are the current guidelines adequate? *Arch Dis Child Fetal Neonatal Ed*. 2011;96:F4–F8.

120. Maayan-Metzger A, Barzilai A, Keller N, et al. Are the "good old" antibiotics still appropriate for early-onset neonatal sepsis? A 10 year survey. *Isr Med Assoc J*. 2009;11:138–142.

121. Manan MM, Ibrahim NA, Aziz NA, et al. Empirical use of antibiotic therapy in the prevention of early onset sepsis in neonates: a pilot study. *Arch Med Sci*. 2016;12:603–613.

122. Falciglia G, Hageman JR, Schreiber M, et al. Antibiotic therapy and early onset sepsis. *NeoReviews*. 2012;13:e86.

5

123. Clark RH, Bloom BT, Spitzer AR, et al. Empiric use of ampicillin and cefotaxime, compared with ampicillin and gentamicin, for neonates at risk for sepsis is associated with an increased risk of neonatal death. *Pediatrics*. 2006;117:67–74.

124. Benjamin DK Jr, DeLong ER, Steinbach WJ, et al. Empirical therapy for neonatal candidemia in very low birth weight infants. *Pediatrics*. 2003;112:543–547.

125. Martin E, Fanconi S, Kalin P, et al. Ceftriaxone–bilirubin-albumin interactions in the neonate: an *in vivo* study. *Eur J Pediatr*. 1993;152:530–534.

126. Arnold CJ, Ericson J, Cho N, et al. Cefepime and ceftazidime safety in hospitalized infants. *Pediatr Infect Dis J*. 2015;34:964–968.

127. Martelius T, Jalava J, Karki T, et al. Nosocomial bloodstream infections caused by *Escherichia coli* and *Klebsiella pneumoniae* resistant to third-generation cephalosporins, Finland, 1999-2013: Trends, patient characteristics and mortality. *Infect Dis (Lond)*. 2016;48:229–234.

128. Patel SJ, Green N, Clock SA, et al. Gram-negative bacilli in infants hospitalized in the neonatal intensive care unit. *J Pediatric Infect Dis Soc*. 2016.

129. Cantey JB. Optimizing the use of antibacterial agents in the neonatal period. *Paediatr Drugs*. 2016;18:109–122.

130. Ambroise M. Emerging trends in antibiotic use in neonates: new or not-so-new drugs for new bugs. *Newborn Infant Nurs Rev*. 2009;9:48–52.

131. Hornik CP, Herring AH, Benjamin DK Jr, et al. Adverse events associated with meropenem versus imipenem/cilastatin therapy in a large retrospective cohort of hospitalized infants. *Pediatr Infect Dis J*. 2013;32:748–753.

132. Cohen-Wolkowiez M, Poindexter B, Bidegain M, et al. Safety and effectiveness of meropenem in infants with suspected or complicated intra-abdominal infections. *Clin Infect Dis*. 2012;55:1495–1502.

133. Bergin SP, Thaden JT, Ericson JE, et al. Neonatal *Escherichia coli* bloodstream infections: clinical outcomes and impact of initial antibiotic therapy. *Pediatr Infect Dis J*. 2015;34:933–936.

134. Rubin LG, Sanchez PJ, Siegel J, et al. Evaluation and treatment of neonates with suspected late-onset sepsis: a survey of neonatologists' practices. *Pediatrics*. 2002;110:e42.

135. Karlowicz MG, Buescher ES, Surka AE. Fulminant late-onset sepsis in a neonatal intensive care unit, 1988-1997, and the impact of avoiding empiric vancomycin therapy. *Pediatrics*. 2000;106: 1387–1390.

136. Isaacs D. Rationing antibiotic use in neonatal units. *Arch Dis Child Fetal Neonatal Ed*. 2000;82:F1–F2.

137. Chiu CH, Michelow IC, Cronin J, et al. Effectiveness of a guideline to reduce vancomycin use in the neonatal intensive care unit. *Pediatr Infect Dis J*. 2011;30:273–278.

138. Ericson JE, Thaden J, Cross HR, et al. No survival benefit with empirical vancomycin therapy for coagulase-negative staphylococcal bloodstream infections in infants. *Pediatr Infect Dis J*. 2015;34: 371–375.

139. Recommendations for preventing the spread of vancomycin resistance. Recommendations of the Hospital Infection Control Practices Advisory Committee (HICPAC). *MMWR Recomm Rep*. 1995;44: 1–13.

140. Lawrence SL, Roth V, Slinger R, et al. Cloxacillin versus vancomycin for presumed late-onset sepsis in the Neonatal Intensive Care Unit and the impact upon outcome of coagulase negative staphylococcal bacteremia: a retrospective cohort study. *BMC Pediatr*. 2005;5:49.

141. Thaden JT, Ericson JE, Cross H, et al. Survival benefit of empirical therapy for *Staphylococcus aureus* bloodstream infections in infants. *Pediatr Infect Dis J*. 2015;34:1175–1179.

142. Holzmann-Pazgal G, Khan AM, Northrup TF, et al. Decreasing vancomycin utilization in a neonatal intensive care unit. *Am J Infect Control*. 2015;43:1255–1257.

143. Kumar Y, Qunibi M, Neal TJ, et al. Time to positivity of neonatal blood cultures. *Arch Dis Child Fetal Neonatal Ed*. 2001;85:F182–F186.

144. Patel SJ, Saiman L. Principles and strategies of antimicrobial stewardship in the neonatal intensive care unit. *Semin Perinatol*. 2012;36:431–436.

145. Cantey JB, Sanchez PJ. Prolonged antibiotic therapy for "culture-negative" sepsis in preterm infants: it's time to stop! *J Pediatr*. 2011;159:707–708.

146. Cotten CM, Smith PB. Duration of empirical antibiotic therapy for infants suspected of early-onset sepsis. *Curr Opin Pediatr*. 2013;25:167–171.

147. Garcia-Prats JA, Cooper TR, Schneider VF, et al. Rapid detection of microorganisms in blood cultures of newborn infants utilizing an automated blood culture system. *Pediatrics*. 2000;105:523–527.

148. Jardine L, Davies MW, Faoagali J. Incubation time required for neonatal blood cultures to become positive. *J Paediatr Child Health*. 2006;42:797–802.

149. Brady MT, Polin RA. Prevention and management of infants with suspected or proven neonatal sepsis. *Pediatrics*. 2013;132:166–168.

150. Polin RA, Watterberg K, Benitz W, et al. The conundrum of early-onset sepsis. *Pediatrics*. 2014;133: 1122–1123.

151. Shakib J, Buchi K, Smith E, et al. Management of newborns born to mothers with chorioamnionitis: is it time for a kinder, gentler approach? *Acad Pediatr*. 2015;15:340–344.

152. Polin RA, Denson S, Brady MT, et al. Strategies for prevention of health care-associated infections in the NICU. *Pediatrics*. 2012;129:e1085–e1093.

153. Kilbride HW, Wirtschafter DD, Powers RJ, et al. Implementation of evidence-based potentially better practices to decrease nosocomial infections. *Pediatrics*. 2003;111:e519–e533.

154. Andersen C, Hart J, Vemgal P, et al. Prospective evaluation of a multi-factorial prevention strategy on the impact of nosocomial infection in very-low-birthweight infants. *J Hosp Infect*. 2005;61:162–167.

155. Huskins WC, Huckabee CM, O'Grady NP, et al. Intervention to reduce transmission of resistant bacteria in intensive care. *N Engl J Med*. 2011;364:1407–1418.
156. Harris AD, Pineles L, Belton B, et al. Universal glove and gown use and acquisition of antibiotic-resistant bacteria in the ICU: a randomized trial. *JAMA*. 2013;310:1571–1580.
157. Chang YJ, Choi IR, Shin WS, et al. The control of invasive *Candida* infection in very low birth weight infants by reduction in the use of 3rd generation cephalosporin. *Korean J Pediatr*. 2013;56:68–74.
158. Aliaga S, Clark RH, Laughon M, et al. Changes in the incidence of candidiasis in neonatal intensive care units. *Pediatrics*. 2014;133:236–242.
159. Engle WD, Jackson GL, Sendelbach D, et al. Neonatal pneumonia: comparison of 4 vs 7 days of antibiotic therapy in term and near-term infants. *J Perinatol*. 2000;20:421–426.
160. Langley JM, Bradley JS. Defining pneumonia in critically ill infants and children. *Pediatr Crit Care Med*. 2005;6:S9–S13.
161. Kidszun A, Hansmann A, Winter J, et al. Detection of respiratory viral infections in neonates treated for suspicion of nosocomial bacterial sepsis: a feasibility study. *Pediatr Infect Dis J*. 2014;33:102–104.
162. Alvarez P, Fuentes C, Garcia N, et al. Evaluation of the duration of the antibiotic prophylaxis in paediatric postoperative heart surgery patients. *Pediatr Cardiol*. 2012;33:735–738.
163. Amadeo B, Zarb P, Muller A, et al. European Surveillance of Antibiotic Consumption (ESAC) point prevalence survey 2008: paediatric antimicrobial prescribing in 32 hospitals of 21 European countries. *J Antimicrob Chemother*. 2010;65:2247–2252.
164. Alphonso N, Anagnostopoulos PV, Scarpace S, et al. Perioperative antibiotic prophylaxis in paediatric cardiac surgery. *Cardiol Young*. 2007;17:12–25.
165. Dellit TH, Owens RC, McGowan JE Jr, et al. Infectious Diseases Society of America and the Society for Healthcare Epidemiology of America guidelines for developing an institutional program to enhance antimicrobial stewardship. *Clin Infect Dis*. 2007;44:159–177.
166. Graber CJ, Jones MM, Glassman PA, et al. Taking an antibiotic time-out: utilization and usability of a self-stewardship time-out program for renewal of vancomycin and piperacillin-tazobactam. *Hosp Pharm*. 2015;50:1011–1024.
167. Masterton RG. Antibiotic de-escalation. *Crit Care Clin*. 2011;27:149–162.
168. Cantey JB, Lopez-Medina E, Nguyen S, et al. Empiric antibiotics for serious bacterial infection in young infants: opportunities for stewardship. *Pediatr Emerg Care*. 2015;31:568–571.
169. Johnson SJ, Ernst EJ, Moores KG. Is double coverage of gram-negative organisms necessary? *Am J Health Syst Pharm*. 2011;68:119–124.
170. Boyd N, Nailor MD. Combination antibiotic therapy for empiric and definitive treatment of gram-negative infections: insights from the Society of Infectious Diseases Pharmacists. *Pharmacotherapy*. 2011;31:1073–1084.

CHAPTER 6

Candida Prophylaxis

Mihai Puia Dumitrescu, MD, MPH, Daniel K. Benjamin Jr., MD, MPH, PhD

- Invasive candidiasis (IC) is associated with high morbidity and mortality in infants.
- Fluconazole is the most common drug used for Candida prophylaxis in infants and reduces the incidence of IC.
- Fluconazole dosing of 6 mg/kg twice weekly is recommended for prophylaxis in infants.
- Fluconazole prophylaxis is not associated with significant short- and long-term toxicity or increased incidence of fluconazole-resistant Candida isolates in the intensive care nursery.
- Fluconazole prophylaxis should be limited to high-risk infants admitted to intensive care nurseries with a moderate to high incidence of IC.

Epidemiology

Invasive candidiasis (IC) is a major cause of morbidity and mortality in hospitalized infants. *Candida* species represent a group of opportunistic pathogens naturally present, primarily as saprophytes, on the skin and oral and gastrointestinal mucosa, but whose presence can become pathologic due to factors related to the organism, the host, or both. Candidemia is one of the most common health care–associated bloodstream infections in U.S. hospitals and is the fourth most common cause of nosocomial bloodstream infections in the United States.[1]

Incidence and Mortality

Extreme prematurity is strongly associated with risk of developing IC.[2,3] The risk of IC for infants <750 g is higher compared with infants with birth weights 750 to 1000 g, 13% versus 6%, respectively.[4] Among infants with a birth weight of 1001 to 1500 g, the incidence of IC is 1% or less.[3,5] The incidence of IC in infants has decreased in the United States over the last decade.[6] Data from a study of 130,523 infants admitted to 128 neonatal intensive care units (NICUs) participating in the National Nosocomial Infections Surveillance System showed that the incidence of IC in infants with a birth weight <1000 g decreased from 6.6% in 1995 to 1999 to 5.1% in 2000 to 2004.[3] In a study of 709,325 infants from 322 NICUs from 1997 to 2010, the annual incidence of IC decreased from 3.6 per 1000 infants to 1.4 per 1000 infants, with the greatest decrease among infants with a birth weight of 750 g (83 to 24 per 1000 infants) and infants with a birth weight of 750 to 999 g (24 to 12 per 1000 infants).[6]

IC is associated with high mortality: 34% in very low birth weight infants (VLBW) (<1500 g birth weight)[4,7] versus 16% to 28% in older children.[8,9] For extremely low birth weight (ELBW, <1000 g birth weight) infants, mortality is >30%, and up to 70% of survivors have long-term neurodevelopmental impairment.[2,10]

Candida Species in Infants

Candida albicans causes >50% of cases of IC in infants.[3,11–14] The second-most frequent species isolated in this population is *C. parapsilosis,* which accounts for approximately one third of IC cases, followed by *C. glabrata.*[15] *C. albicans* is the most pathogenic of the *Candida* species, with mortality twofold to threefold higher than *C. parapsilosis.*[7] *C. glabrata* and *C. krusei,* recognized for their resistance to azoles, represent only 2% and 1% of all cases, respectively.[3] *C. krusei* is inherently resistant to fluconazole, and *C. glabrata* is resistant to fluconazole in >50% of cases.[16]

Risk Factors

Risk factors for IC in infants include factors that promote colonization of mucosal surfaces, interrupt anatomic barriers to organism invasion, or otherwise weaken the immune response.[17] In addition to prematurity, risk factors for IC in infants include admission to a high-incidence medical center,[4] broad-spectrum antibiotic therapy (specifically including third-generation cephalosporins or carbapenems),[2,18] and *Candida* colonization.[19,20] Other risk factors have been described but have much less influence on the incidence within a unit.[2,11,21]

Prophylaxis

Prevention of IC in infants plays an important role in the management of high-risk patients. Providers should minimize infant exposure to broad-spectrum antibiotics (e.g., carbapenems and cephalosporins) and remove central venous catheters as quickly as possible.[21,22] Given poor diagnostic methods and inaccuracy of clinician predictions of infections, clinicians should initiate empiric antifungal therapy in infants at high risk of IC.[23,24]

Antifungals are used for prophylaxis to decrease the risk of IC.[23] The use of medication for prophylaxis is either selective, for high-risk groups of infants,[25–27] or broad on admission to the NICU.[28] Fluconazole prophylaxis for IC has been evaluated in a number of trials in premature infants.

Fluconazole

Fluconazole is a triazole approved by the U.S. Food and Drug Administration (FDA) for treatment of cryptococcosis and *Candida* infections, and is the most used antifungal in the neonatal period.[29] Fluconazole is approved by the FDA for prophylaxis of IC in patients undergoing bone marrow transplantation, but is not approved for use in infants. However, in clinical practice, it is frequently used for prophylaxis against IC in premature infants.[30–32]

Evidence for Efficacy of Fluconazole

Fluconazole is effective as prophylaxis for IC (Table 6.1). In a single-center, randomized trial 103 infants <1500 g birth weight were given fluconazole (6 mg/kg/day every 3 days for the first week then daily) or placebo for 28 days. Rectal colonization by *Candida* species was detected in 8/53 (15%) of the fluconazole-treated infants and 23/50 (46%) of the placebo-treated infants ($P = 0.0005$).[33] A single-center, randomized trial of 100 ELBW infants demonstrated a significant reduction in both fungal colonization and IC using 3 mg/kg of intravenous fluconazole.[34] The infants were treated for the first 6 weeks of life, and dosing interval varied by postnatal age from 24 hours to 72 hours. In this cohort, IC developed in 10 of 50 (20%) of the infants in the placebo group and 0 of 50 (0%) of those in the fluconazole group ($P = 0.008$).[34] A few years later, this same center performed a prospective, randomized, double-blind

Table 6.1   RANDOMIZED PLACEBO-CONTROLLED TRIALS OF FLUCONAZOLE PROPHYLAXIS IN INFANTS

Enrollment Period	Enrolled Infants (N)	Population	Incidence of IC (%)	Mortality (%)
1998–1999[33]	fluconazole: 53	<1500 g	4	9
	placebo: 50		4	20
1998–2000[34]	fluconazole: 50	<1000 g	0	8
	placebo: 50		20	20
2004–2005[32]	fluconazole: 220	<1500 g	3	8
	placebo: 106		13	9
2008–2011[35]	fluconazole: 188	<750 g	3	14
	placebo: 173		9	14

6

clinical trial in ELBW infants comparing 3 mg/kg dosed twice weekly (group A) with the previous regimen (group B).[30] They observed that twice-weekly dosing of prophylactic fluconazole to be as effective in decreasing IC as the more frequent dosing regimen. IC developed in 2 of 41 (5%) of group A and 1 of 40 (3%) of group B infants ($P=0.68$).[30] Use of less frequent dosing decreases cost and patient exposure to fluconazole.[30]

In a multicenter, randomized, double-blind, placebo-controlled trial of fluconazole at eight tertiary centers, investigators assigned 322 VLBW infants to receive 6 mg/kg fluconazole, 3 mg/kg fluconazole, or placebo.[32] Doses were given every 72 hours for the first 2 weeks, then every 48 hours. Infants 1001 to 1500 g were treated for 4 weeks, and infants <1000 g were treated for 6 weeks. The incidence of IC was 3 of 112 (2.7%) in the 6-mg group, 4 of 104 (3.8%) in the 3-mg group, and 14 of 106 (13.2%) in the placebo group ($P = 0.005$ for the 6 mg/kg group and $P = 0.02$ for the 3 mg/kg group versus the placebo group).[32]

In another randomized, blinded, placebo-controlled trial of 362 infants <750 g birth weight, fluconazole prophylaxis decreased the incidence of definite or probable IC from 16 of 173 (9%) in the placebo group to 6 of 188 (3%) in the fluconazole group ($P = 0.02$). However, the study's primary endpoint, death or IC, was not statistically different between the fluconazole and placebo groups (30 of 188 [16%] versus 36 of 173 [21%], respectively; $P = 0.24$).[35] In this study, fluconazole prophylaxis was not associated with an improved rate of neurodevelopmental impairment at 18 to 22 weeks corrected age (37 of 118 [31%] in the fluconazole group versus 29 of 107 [27%] in the placebo group; $P = 0.60$).[35]

Dosage for Fluconazole Prophylaxis

Until recently, fluconazole dosing in infants was based upon limited pharmacokinetics data.[36] Fluconazole has excellent properties as an agent for prophylaxis, but pharmacodynamic exposure targets for infants for the prevention of candidiasis are not well described. Preventative strategies should consider plasma concentrations, predicted tissue concentrations at sites of potential colonization, and the minimal inhibitory concentration (MIC) of colonizing *Candida* species.[37] Clinical trials of fluconazole prophylaxis in premature infants have found that both 3 mg/kg and 6 mg/kg dosing are effective at preventing IC in centers with a moderate to high burden.[34]

The typical MICs of *Candida* species in infants range from 0.25 to 4 µg/mL.[30,32–34] Dosing of fluconazole that maintains the proportion of time with concentration above the MIC (T>MIC) of >40% may prevent emergence of more resistant *Candida* isolates.[38] A 3 mg/kg twice-weekly regimen would be expected to prevent the growth of *Candida* species with an MIC of ≤2 µg/mL; the 6 mg/kg twice-weekly regimen would be needed if the targeted MIC range of *Candida* species is ≤4 µg/mL.[37] Neonatal units should consider their specific *Candida* MICs from surveillance and in vitro susceptibility testing of fungal isolates when considering dosing for prevention.[37]

Antifungal Prophylaxis and Development of Resistance

The potential for selection of resistant *Candida* isolates is a concern surrounding implementation of widespread antifungal prophylaxis. Mechanisms of azole resistance include alteration in fungal cell drug influx, drug efflux, or the target enzyme, lanosterol demethylase. Factors associated with development of resistance include intermittent dosing intervals, the amount of drug, the length of treatment, and the immune status of the patients.[37,39]

Antifungal resistance is observed in adult patients with neutropenia after prophylaxis with fluconazole.[39–42] In infants, increased prevalence of colonization and infections with fluconazole-resistant non-*albicans* strains are reported in some studies[34,43–45] but not in others.[3,46–49] In a multicenter, randomized, placebo-controlled trial of fluconazole prophylaxis in 361 infants <750 g birth weight receiving either fluconazole 6 mg/kg or placebo twice a week for 42 days, the MIC of colonizing *Candida* isolates increased in the fluconazole group, but most isolates remained in the susceptible range.[50]

Number Needed to Treat (NNT)

Fluconazole prophylaxis should be limited to high-risk patients. The NNT for fluconazole prophylaxis represents the number of infants who would need to receive prophylaxis to prevent one additional case of IC. Although the relative reduction in IC incidence with fluconazole prophylaxis is approximately 80% in most trials, it is unclear if the benefits of routine prophylaxis will be clinically meaningful in low-incidence settings.[24] For example, if the baseline incidence of IC without prophylaxis is 30%, assuming an 80% relative reduction to 6% with prophylaxis, the NNT is 4. If the baseline incidence is 5%, the NNT is 25, and if the baseline incidence is 1%, the NNT is 125.

Conclusions

IC infections are a major cause of morbidity and mortality in infants. Over the last decade, the incidence of IC has decreased in the United States.[6] Appropriate use of antifungals in infants is important for both prevention and treatment of infection. The high mortality and high rates of neurodevelopmental impairment among surviving infants suggest that improved treatment strategies are needed.[2] Randomized controlled trials have demonstrated safety and efficacy of fluconazole prophylaxis for the prevention of IC in premature infants. Fluconazole prophylaxis should be considered in premature infants in NICUs with moderate to high risk (at least 5%) of IC at a dose of 6 mg/kg twice weekly.

REFERENCES

1. Wisplinghoff H, Bischoff T, Tallent SM, et al. Nosocomial bloodstream infections in US hospitals: analysis of 24,179 cases from a prospective nationwide surveillance study. *Clin Infect Dis.* 2004;39: 309–317.
2. Benjamin DK Jr, Stoll BJ, Fanaroff AA, et al. Neonatal candidiasis among extremely low birth weight infants: risk factors, mortality rates, and neurodevelopmental outcomes at 18 to 22 months. *Pediatrics.* 2006;117:84–92.
3. Fridkin SK, Kaufman D, Edwards JR, et al. Changing incidence of *Candida* bloodstream infections among NICU patients in the United States: 1995–2004. *Pediatrics.* 2006;117:1680–1687.
4. Benjamin DK Jr, Stoll BJ, Gantz MG, et al. Neonatal candidiasis: epidemiology, risk factors, and clinical judgment. *Pediatrics.* 2010;126:e865–e873.
5. Manzoni P, Arisio R, Mostert M, et al. Prophylactic fluconazole is effective in preventing fungal colonization and fungal systemic infections in preterm neonates: a single-center, 6-year, retrospective cohort study. *Pediatrics.* 2006;117:e22–e32.
6. Aliaga S, Clark RH, Laughon M, et al. Changes in the incidence of candidiasis in neonatal intensive care units. *Pediatrics.* 2014;133:236–242.
7. Stoll BJ, Hansen N, Fanaroff AA, et al. Late-onset sepsis in very low birth weight neonates: the experience of the NICHD Neonatal Research Network. *Pediatrics.* 2002;110:285–291.

8. Singhi SC, Reddy TC, Chakrabarti A. Candidemia in a pediatric intensive care unit. *Pediatr Crit Care Med*. 2004;5:369–374.

9. Young GA, Bosly A, Gibbs DL, et al. A double-blind comparison of fluconazole and nystatin in the prevention of candidiasis in patients with leukaemia. Antifungal Prophylaxis Study Group. *Eur J Cancer*. 1999;35:1208–1213.

10. Adams-Chapman I, Bann CM, Das A, et al. Neurodevelopmental outcome of extremely low birth weight infants with Candida infection. *J Pediatr*. 2013;163:961–967.e3.

11. Saiman L, Ludington E, Pfaller M, et al. Risk factors for candidemia in Neonatal Intensive Care Unit patients. The National Epidemiology of Mycosis Survey study group. *Pediatr Infect Dis J*. 2000;19: 319–324.

12. Feja KN, Wu F, Roberts K, et al. Risk factors for candidemia in critically ill infants: a matched case-control study. *J Pediatr*. 2005;147:156–161.

13. Barton M, O'Brien K, Robinson JL, et al. Invasive candidiasis in low birth weight preterm infants: risk factors, clinical course and outcome in a prospective multicenter study of cases and their matched controls. *BMC Infect Dis*. 2014;14:327.

14. Chitnis AS, Magill SS, Edwards JR, et al. Trends in *Candida* central line-associated bloodstream infections among NICUs, 1999–2009. *Pediatrics*. 2012;130:e46–e52.

15. Pammi M, Holland L, Butler G, et al. *Candida parapsilosis* is a significant neonatal pathogen: a systematic review and meta-analysis. *Pediatr Infect Dis J*. 2013;32:e206–e216.

16. Pfaller MA, Messer SA, Boyken L, et al. Variation in susceptibility of bloodstream isolates of *Candida glabrata* to fluconazole according to patient age and geographic location. *J Clin Microbiol*. 2003;41: 2176–2179.

17. Chapman RL, Faix RG. Invasive neonatal candidiasis: an overview. *Semin Perinatol*. 2003;27:352–356.

18. Benjamin DK Jr, DeLong ER, Steinbach WJ, et al. Empirical therapy for neonatal candidemia in very low birth weight infants. *Pediatrics*. 2003;112:543–547.

19. Manzoni P, Farina D, Leonessa M, et al. Risk factors for progression to invasive fungal infection in preterm neonates with fungal colonization. *Pediatrics*. 2006;118:2359–2364.

20. Saiman L, Ludington E, Dawson JD, et al. Risk factors for *Candida* species colonization of neonatal intensive care unit patients. *Pediatr Infect Dis J*. 2001;20:1119–1124.

21. Kaufman D. Strategies for prevention of neonatal invasive candidiasis. *Semin Perinatol*. 2003;27:414–424.

22. Zaoutis TE, Prasad PA, Localio AR, et al. Risk factors and predictors for candidemia in pediatric intensive care unit patients: implications for prevention. *Clin Infect Dis*. 2010;51:e38–e45.

23. Smith JA, Kauffman CA. Recognition and prevention of nosocomial invasive fungal infections in the intensive care unit. *Crit Care Med*. 2010;38:S380–S387.

24. Ericson JE, Benjamin DK Jr. Fluconazole prophylaxis for prevention of invasive candidiasis in infants. *Curr Opin Pediatr*. 2014;26:151–156.

25. Eggimann P, Garbino J, Pittet D. Management of *Candida* species infections in critically ill patients. *Lancet Infect Dis*. 2003;3:772–785.

26. Shorr AF, Chung K, Jackson WL, et al. Fluconazole prophylaxis in critically ill surgical patients: a meta-analysis. *Crit Care Med*. 2005;33:1928–1935, quiz 36.

27. Rex JH, Sobel JD. Prophylactic antifungal therapy in the intensive care unit. *Clin Infect Dis*. 2001; 32:1191–1200.

28. Pelz RK, Hendrix CW, Swoboda SM, et al. Double-blind placebo-controlled trial of fluconazole to prevent candidal infections in critically ill surgical patients. *Ann Surg*. 2001;233:542–548.

29. Hsieh EM, Hornik CP, Clark RH, et al. Medication use in the neonatal intensive care unit. *Am J Perinatol*. 2014;31:811–821.

30. Kaufman D, Boyle R, Hazen KC, et al. Twice weekly fluconazole prophylaxis for prevention of invasive *Candida* infection in high-risk infants of <1000 grams birth weight. *J Pediatr*. 2005;147:172–179.

31. Kaufman DA, Manzoni P. Strategies to prevent invasive candidal infection in extremely preterm infants. *Clin Perinatol*. 2010;37:611–628.

32. Manzoni P, Stolfi I, Pugni L, et al. A multicenter, randomized trial of prophylactic fluconazole in preterm neonates. *N Engl J Med*. 2007;356:2483–2495.

33. Kicklighter SD, Springer SC, Cox T, et al. Fluconazole for prophylaxis against candidal rectal colonization in the very low birth weight infant. *Pediatrics*. 2001;107:293–298.

34. Kaufman D, Boyle R, Hazen KC, et al. Fluconazole prophylaxis against fungal colonization and infection in preterm infants. *N Engl J Med*. 2001;345:1660–1666.

35. Benjamin DK Jr, Hudak ML, Duara S, et al. Effect of fluconazole prophylaxis on candidiasis and mortality in premature infants: a randomized clinical trial. *JAMA*. 2014;311:1742–1749.

36. Saxen H, Hoppu K, Pohjavuori M. Pharmacokinetics of fluconazole in very low birth weight infants during the first two weeks of life. *Clin Pharmacol Ther*. 1993;54:269–277.

37. Wade KC, Benjamin DK Jr, Kaufman DA, et al. Fluconazole dosing for the prevention or treatment of invasive candidiasis in young infants. *Pediatr Infect Dis J*. 2009;28:717–723.

38. Andes D, Forrest A, Lepak A, et al. Impact of antimicrobial dosing regimen on evolution of drug resistance *in vivo*: fluconazole and *Candida albicans*. *Antimicrob Agents Chemother*. 2006;50:2374–2383.

39. Loeffler J, Stevens DA. Antifungal drug resistance. *Clin Infect Dis*. 2003;36:S31–S41.

40. Ullmann AJ, Akova M, Herbrecht R, et al. ESCMID* guideline for the diagnosis and management of Candida diseases 2012: adults with haematological malignancies and after haematopoietic stem cell transplantation (HCT). *Clin Microbiol Infect*. 2012;18(suppl 7):53–67.

41. Mulu A, Kassu A, Anagaw B, et al. Frequent detection of "azole" resistant *Candida* species among late presenting AIDS patients in northwest Ethiopia. *BMC Infect Dis*. 2013;13:82.

6

42. White TC, Marr KA, Bowden RA. Clinical, cellular, and molecular factors that contribute to antifungal drug resistance. *Clin Microbiol Rev.* 1998;11:382–402.
43. Sarvikivi E, Lyytikainen O, Soll DR, et al. Emergence of fluconazole resistance in a *Candida parapsilosis* strain that caused infections in a neonatal intensive care unit. *J Clin Microbiol.* 2005;43:2729–2735.
44. Martin A, Pappas A, Lulic-Botica M, et al. Impact of 'targeted' fluconazole prophylaxis for preterm neonates: efficacy of a highly selective approach? *J Perinatol.* 2012;32:21–26.
45. Ballot DE, Bosman N, Nana T, et al. Background changing patterns of neonatal fungal sepsis in a developing country. *J Trop Pediatr.* 2013;59:460–464.
46. Hope WW, Castagnola E, Groll AH, et al. ESCMID* guideline for the diagnosis and management of *Candida* diseases 2012: prevention and management of invasive infections in neonates and children caused by Candida spp. *Clin Microbiol Infect.* 2012;18(suppl 7):38–52.
47. Kaufman DA. "Getting to Zero": preventing invasive *Candida* infections and eliminating infection-related mortality and morbidity in extremely preterm infants. *Early Hum Dev.* 2012;88(suppl 2):S45–S49.
48. Manzoni P, Leonessa M, Galletto P, et al. Routine use of fluconazole prophylaxis in a neonatal intensive care unit does not select natively fluconazole-resistant *Candida* subspecies. *Pediatr Infect Dis J.* 2008;27:731–737.
49. Austin N, McGuire W. Prophylactic systemic antifungal agents to prevent mortality and morbidity in very low birth weight infants. *Cochrane Database Syst Rev.* 2013;CD003850.
50. Autmizguine J, Smith PB, Prather K, et al. Effect of Fluconazole Prophylaxis on Fluconazole *Candida* Susceptibility in Premature Infants. In: *Society of Pediatric Research.* San Francisco, CA: 2017.

CHAPTER 7

Diagnosis, Risk Factors, Outcomes, and Evaluation of Invasive *Candida* Infections

David Kaufman, MD, Hillary Liken, MD, Namrita J. Odackal, DO

- Major risk factors for invasive *Candida* infections include extreme prematurity, a compromised gastrointestinal function or barrier, and exposure to broad spectrum antibiotics, acid suppression medications, or high dose postnatal steroids.
- The highest risk patients are infants less than 1000 grams at birth or 28 weeks gestation due to their high mortality and risk of neurodevelopmental impairments from infection. Preventative measures including targeted antifungal prophylaxis have lowered the incidence in this group from 5-10% to 0-2%.
- *Candida* pathogenesis involves exposure, adherence, and colonization, followed by infection and commonly organ involvement. All infected infants need screening for end-organ dissemination.
- Cultures are critical to diagnosis and should include blood, urine and cerebrospinal fluid at the time of presentation. Additionally, peritoneal cultures should be obtained in any infant with necrotizing enterocolitis or bowel perforation requiring laparotomy or drainage.
- Congenital cutaneous candidiasis is an invasive infection that requires prompt recognition and evaluation as well as systemic treatment for 14 days. Dermatologic findings of congenital cutaneous candidiasis commonly involve skin desquamation, maculopapular and/or erythematous rashes.
- Survival is improved with central venous catheter removal for candidemia. Infection related outcomes are also improved with prompt antifungal dosing for all infected patients and empiric therapy in high-risk patients.

How Are ICI Infections Defined?

Invasive *Candida* infections (ICI) are generally defined as the presence of *Candida* species in a body fluid or tissue sample that should normally be sterile.[1] Such ICI include bloodstream infections (BSIs), urinary tract infections (UTIs), peritonitis, meningitis, cutaneous candidiasis, and any infection of an otherwise sterile tissue, such as bones and joints. These invasive infections are frequently identified and defined based on a positive culture of blood, urine, cerebrospinal fluid (CSF), peritoneal fluid, or tissue. For congenital cutaneous candidiasis, diagnosis requires a diffuse rash with identification of *Candida* or yeast from the skin, placenta, or umbilical cord.[2] Consensus definitions distinguishing colonization, infection, and dissemination, linking them to important clinical outcomes, have emerged.

When ICIs develop, they can be classified as early-onset (<72 hours after birth) or late-onset (≥72 hours after birth), similar to other neonatal infections. The exception is cutaneous candidiasis, which is sometimes further specified as congenital cutaneous candidiasis (CCC) when it occurs in the first week after birth.[2,3]

These ICIs can disseminate directly or hematogenously throughout the body, even in spite of antifungal therapy. This can lead to end-organ abscesses and damage to the heart, eyes, liver, kidneys, lungs, brain, or spleen.[4]

How Does *Candida* Cause Invasive Infections? (Fig. 7.1)

Candida species represent a group of opportunistic pathogens that are naturally present, primarily as saprophytes, on the skin and oral and gastrointestinal (GI) mucosa, but whose presence can become pathologic due to factors related to the organism, the host, or both (Fig. 7.1). This is the case in infants, who have an underdeveloped immune system with little to no adaptive and minimal innate immunity. Additionally, critical barriers to organisms (e.g., the skin and respiratory tract) are breached with intravenous catheters and/or endotracheal tubes. As an opportunistic organism, *Candida* species can also lead to infections if the host is exposed to a large number of organisms and/or when *Candida* can proliferate easily. Proliferation is favorable under certain conditions, such as when antibiotics eradicate competitive flora or H_2-blockers decrease stomach acidity.

What Are Predisposing Factors for ICI in the NICU?

ICIs are of special concern in premature infants, with early gestational age being the highest risk factor. Understanding why this population is susceptible, as well as other potential risk factors, is helpful in identifying patients most at risk for infection and potential candidates for preventative measures (Figs. 7.1 and 7.2).

Prematurity

One of the main risk factors for infants acquiring ICI is prematurity. The more premature the infant, the more underdeveloped the immune system and the barrier defenses and the greater the likelihood of procedures, antibiotic exposures, and use of other medications that all contribute to colonization and ICI.

Colonization (Fig. 7.1 and Table 7.1)

Local colonization of the skin or mucosal surfaces can lead to ICI, with *Candida* penetrating epidermal barriers to infect underlying tissue or directly invading the bloodstream and spreading hematogenously. Very low birth weight (VLBW; <1500 g at birth) infants are more susceptible to colonization with *Candida* and are also at a higher risk of progression to an invasive infection.[5] Colonization rates are inversely correlated with gestational age and birth weight. In the first weeks after birth, >50% of extremely low birth weight (ELBW; <1000 g at birth) and 25% to 50% of VLBW infants are colonized, compared with 5% to 10% of full-term infants.[1] Colonization during the first two weeks of life occurs primarily on the skin and in

Table 7.1 *CANDIDA COLONIZATION FACTORS*

Candida Species	*C. Albicans*	*C. Parapsilosis*
Risk Factors for Colonization	Early-onset neutropenia Use of cephalosporins Use of CVC or IV lipids	Early-onset neutropenia Use of cephalosporins H_2 blockers
High-Risk Colonization of Progression to ICI	Colonization of three or more body sites or devices Central venous catheter colonization Endotracheal tube colonization Urine colonization	
Protective Factors	Cesarean section	

CVC, central venous catheter; *IV*, intravenous; *ICI*, invasive *Candida* infection.

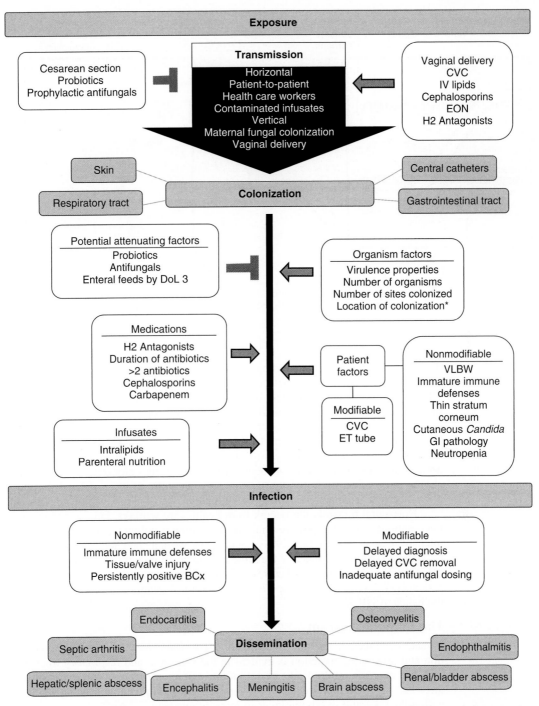

Figure 7.1 Pathogenesis of invasive *Candida* infections: Exposure, colonization, infection, and dissemination. Arrows indicate factors increasing risk, some of which are modifiable, and the "blocking" symbol represents factors that decrease or prevent the risk of ICI. *BCx*, Blood culture; *CVC*, central venous catheter; *EON*, early-onset neutropenia; *ET*, endotracheal tube; *IV*, intravenous; *VLBW*, very low birth weight. *High-risk colonization sites, including CVC, ET, urine.

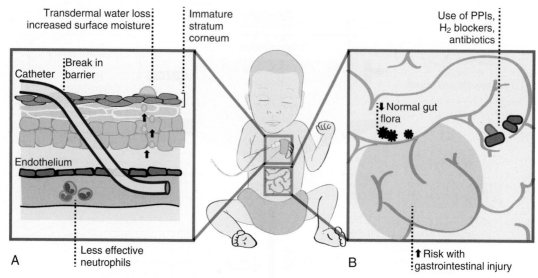

Figure 7.2 Risk factors for invasive *Candida* infections. (A) Effects of immature skin, neutrophil function and central venous catheter. (B) Gastrointestinal tract predisposing factors. *PPI,* Proton-pump inhibitor.

the gastrointestinal tract, including the rectum and oropharynx, followed a week or two later by respiratory tract colonization in high-risk patients.[6] Progression to infection occurs in approximately one of four colonized infants, influenced by both the number and location of colonized sites.[7] Colonization of three or more sites and/ or at a high-risk site (urine, catheter tips, drains, and surgical devices) is more likely to be associated with progression to ICI.[8–12]

Colonization can occur by way of vertical transmission from the mother or horizontal transmission from nosocomial sources. Early colonization (≤1 week of age) is more often attributed to maternal sources, with an increased risk for early colonization in premature infants born vaginally.[13,14]

Horizontal transmission occurs from health care workers, family, and medical interventions. In a prospective trial studying fungal colonization in six neonatal intensive care units (NICUs), 29% of health care workers had hand cultures positive for *Candida* species, with nearly the same percentage of infants (23%) having mucosal colonization. Although *C. albicans* was the more common fungal isolate in all NICU patients (14% vs. 7%), *C. parapsilosis* was the most common species isolated from the hands of NICU staff.[13]

The Immune System

Immaturity of the immune system's primary or physical barriers in controlling colonization and preventing infection is evident in the skin, gut, and respiratory tract (Fig. 7.2). For example, at 26 weeks gestation the stratum corneum is composed of only three cell layers and produces a thin keratin layer, compared with being 15 layers with a thick keratin overlying layer in term infants (Fig. 7.2A).[15]

Neutrophils are one of the most important components in the innate immune system's initial response to *Candida* infections, both through direct phagocytosis and through neutrophil extracellular trap formation (NET). Premature infants have neutrophils that may be less effective at seeking out sites of infection, phagocytosing pathogens, and producing NETs.[16] In addition, preterm infants have a multitude of decreased immune cellular functions and protein production.

The Gut Microbiome

Like the immune system, the gut microbiota and the microorganisms that comprise it play an important role in suppressing *Candida* colonization and preventing invasive infection. The intestinal microbiota of preterm infants are different and less diverse in composition than that of term infants.[17] Athymic neonatal mice colonized with *C. albicans* had a significant reduction in systemic infection when they were also colonized with probiotic species (*Lactobacillus acidophilus, L. reuteri, L. casei GG* [LGG], or *Bifidobacterium animalis*).[18] Premature infants given daily probiotics (*L. reuters* and *L. rhamnosus,* respectively) had significantly lower *Candida* stool colonization than the control preterm infants, and daily LGG with lactoferrin decreased ICIs without changing *Candida* colonization.[19,20]

Medications

Certain medications, including antibiotics, H_2 antagonists, and postnatal corticosteroids, increase the risk of ICI (Fig. 7.2B). Longer antibiotic duration, needing two or more antibiotics, third- and fourth-generation cephalosporin, and carbapenem antibiotics are associated with increased risk of ICI.[21–23] Dexamethasone and high-dose hydrocortisone (>1 mg/kg/day) are associated with increased risk.[24,25] In one study, ELBW infants exposed to hydrocortisone alone at 1 mg/kg/day with a weaning schedule had an incidence of ICI of 9% verus 10% in the control groups.[26]

Lines, Tubes, and Feedings

Use of central venous catheters (Fig. 7.2A) and endotracheal tubes increases the risk of ICI in infants.[11,22,23] Infants who receive larger amounts of expressed milk from their mothers generally have fewer infections, but a decrease in ICI has not been demonstrated. These studies have not controlled if milk was fresh or frozen. Freezing then thawing human milk is associated with reduction of protective components such as maternal white blood cells, lactoferrin, IgA, and lysozyme. Studies of pasteurized donor human milk have not demonstrated a decrease in infections of any type.[27] Prospective epidemiologic studies have found that infants who are not able to or do not receive enteral feedings by 3 days after birth are more likely to develop candidiasis, which may be related to the patient or the feeding practices.[28]

Gastrointestinal Pathology and Abdominal Surgery

GI pathology (Fig. 7.2B) is associated with an increased risk for candidemia in patients with tracheoesophageal fistula, gastroschisis, omphalocele, Hirschsprung disease, intestinal atresias, or necrotizing enterocolitis (NEC).[29,30]

Candida Pathogenesis

Biofilm Formation (Fig. 7.3A)

C. albicans, C. parapsilosis, and other *Candida* species are able to form biofilms, which can promote invasion and resist killing by antifungal therapy. The biofilms of *C. albicans* are made up of multiple morphologies, including yeast, hyphae, pseudohyphae, and germ tubes, whereas those formed by *C. parapsilosis* are made up of only two cell types: hyphae and yeast. These biofilms have the ability to adhere to medical devices and prevent the penetration of antifungals.[31] This explains in part the need to remove central venous catheters to clear candidemia and improve outcomes.[28]

Evading Host Immune System (Fig. 7.3B)

C. albicans has mechanisms that try to evade the normal human immune response, making it especially dangerous to premature infants who are immunocompromised. *C. albicans* can conceal its surface structures from the host immune system, and phagocytes have difficulty recognizing *C. albicans* because its hyphae contain surface proteins that mimic complement receptors. The fungus also degrades cell-surface complement C3b, reducing immune recognition. Even if *Candida* is recognized, its hyphae may interfere with lysosomal fusion as well as killing the macrophage attempting to destroy it by puncturing it via filament elongation.[32]

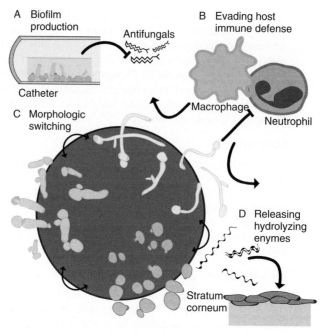

Figure 7.3 *Candida* virulence factors. (A) Biofilm formation, (B) evading host immune system, (C) morphologic switching, and (D) hydrolyzing enzymes.

Morphologic Switching (Fig. 7.3C)

Morphologic switching reflects the ability of *C. albicans* to take on both yeast and filamentous forms. Additionally, as a filamentous fungus, it can be present as both hyphae and pseudohyphae. Changes between these forms are normally triggered by environmental factors, such as pH, temperature, and presence of amino acids. Animal studies have found that infection with wild-type strains, capable of both yeast and filamentous forms, had the greatest mortality when compared with infection with either the filamentous-only or the yeast-only forms.[33] The yeast form facilitates cell and tissue invasion. Once inside human cells, pseudohyphae formation increases destruction and evades the host's immune response.[33] Another study found that although both hyphal forms of *C. albicans* are virulent, pseudohyphal forms are more easily cleared from tissue and had attenuated virulence compared with hyphal forms.[34]

Hydrolyzing Enzymes (Fig. 7.3D)

C. albicans produces hydrolyzing enzymes that include proteases, phospholipases, and lipases, which enable *C. albicans* to digest epithelial cells and invade host tissue. The phospholipase enzymes are important in penetrating host cells. Just as the *Int1* gene helped define mechanisms of adhesion, the study of genes such as *C. albicans* phospholipase B (*caPLB1*) have demonstrated their important role in the penetration of host cells.[35] Secreted aspartic proteases (SAPs) are another group of enzymes that enable *Candida* to progress from colonization to invasive infection. SAPs break down different proteins, including keratin and collagen, making them advantageous in invading host tissues.[36] SAPs are produced by most *Candida* species, except for *C. glabrata*, with *C. albicans* producing the highest amounts.

Which Organisms Cause ICI in the NICU?

The majority of invasive *Candida* infections in the NICU are due to the species *C. albicans*, which causes around 50% to 60% of cases of ICI in infants.[23,29,30,37–39] The second-most frequent species is *C. parapsilosis*, which accounts for approximately one third of cases followed to a lesser degree by *C. glabrata*.[40] Infections due to

C. tropicalis, C. lusitania, C. krusei, C. guillermondii, and other species occur less frequently. *C. albicans* is the most pathogenic of the *Candida* species, with mortality two to three times higher compared with *C. parapsilosis* and other non-*albicans* candidemia.[41] This pathogenicity is attributed to the virulence factors of *C. albicans* described earlier, including morphologic switching and factors that help it evade host immune defenses.[33]

What Is the Incidence of ICI in the NICU?

There is variation between rates of ICI in different NICUs as well as the incidence reported in the literature. Considerable variation exists between rates and risk for ICI based on patient demographics; largely gestational age or birth weight cutoffs for resuscitation of extremely premature infants; and practices related to feeding, medication, and antibiotic usage of individual NICUs.[21,29,42] NICUs that do not resuscitate infants <25 weeks, for example, would have a lower rate of ICI in infants <1000 g compared with centers caring for 23- and 24-week-gestation infants. The number of inborn or outborn patients with NEC, gastroschisis, and other complex GI diseases influences rates.[29] Lastly, infection control practices and use of antifungal prophylaxis are major factors affecting the incidence of ICI. Antifungal prophylaxis is associated with an incidence of 0% to 2% even at the lowest gestational ages and highest-risk patients.[12,37,43,44]

The literature also has limitations in describing incidence. Few studies include all types of ICI as defined earlier and are largely limited to the incidence of *Candida* BSIs and/or meningitis. In the absence of antifungal prophylaxis, the incidence of ICI (not including CCC) in ELBW infants is around 10%[22] and exceeds 20% in those <25 weeks gestation.[22] *Candida* UTIs occur in 3% to 4% of ELBW infants.[12,22,45] Meningitis and peritonitis (often complicating focal bowel perforation and stage III NEC) may be seen in an additional 1% to 2% of ELBWs.[46]

Examining candidemia alone, the largest report is from 128 US NICUs using the National Nosocomial Infections Surveillance system data from 1995 to 2004 (N = 130,523 infants).[39] Despite limitations resulting from data accrual during an era when antifungal prophylaxis and other preventative measures were being introduced, it found that for ELBW infants, the median NICU-specific infection rate was 7.5%, but 25% of NICUs had rates of 13.5% or higher. The pooled mean candidemia rates for infants of birth weights <1000 g, 1001 to 1500 g, 1501 to 2500 g, and >2501 g were 5.07%, 1.32%, 0.36%, and 0.29%, respectively.

What Are the Associated Morbidities and Mortality?

Neurodevelopmental Impairment (NDI)

Neurodevelopmental impairment or delay is a common long-term complication of ICI, even in the absence of documented fungal meningitis. In ELBW infants, NDI is reported in as many as 57% for candidemia and 53% for *Candida* meningitis. Empiric therapy on the day cultures are sent or prompt antifungal therapy within 2 days of the blood culture may help decrease NDI. One study demonstrated improved outcomes when antifungals were started within 2 days versus approximately 5 days of when the blood culture was obtained, and another study showed a decrease in the combined outcome of NDI or death with empiric antifungal therapy started the day cultures were sent.[47,48]

Survival

Mortality is high in premature infants with candiduria as well as candidemia. In a study of ELBW infants, all-cause mortality was 28% for *Candida* BSI, 26% for *Candida* UTI, 50% for other sterile sites (meningitis and peritonitis), and 57% if two or more culture sites were involved (BSI + UTI or UTI + meningitis).[22] Attributable mortality (the difference between ICI infected and noninfected patients) was 20%.

Survival rates are better in larger infants. In ELBW infants with ICI, all-cause mortality has been reported at 26% compared with 13% in infants without candidiasis. Infants >1000 g with ICI had a much lower mortality rate of 2%, compared with 0.4% in uninfected infants.[49] The *Candida* species causing the infection also affects survival. *C. albicans* is more virulent than non-*albicans* species. In VLBW infants, *Candida*-associated mortality was 44% in infants with *C. albicans* candidemia compared with 19% with *C. parapsilosis* sepsis.[19]

Survival is improved in candidemia cases with prompt removal of a central venous catheter. Survival alone[50,51] or the combined outcome of survival and NDI was improved when empiric antifungal therapy was started the day blood cultures were sent.[47]

Invasive *Candida* Infections (Fig. 7.4)

Congenital Cutaneous Candidiasis

CCC presents most commonly at birth, but can occur within the first week. Dermatologic findings include desquamating maculopapular, papulopustular, and/or erythematous rashes. Findings in a recent study included desquamation alone (scaling, peeling, flaking, or exfoliation) or other rashes (Fig. 7.5).[2] CCC can occur with or without dissemination, such as pneumonia or BSI. Without prompt identification and treatment, dissemination to the blood, urine, or CSF can occur, with rates ranging from 11% in term infants to 33% in infants 1000 to 2500 g and 66% in ELBW infants.[52] Skin biopsies demonstrate a high burden of yeast with invasion into the epidermis and dermis with inflammation and injury, including granulomas, focal necrosis, and hemorrhage.[53] For these reasons, preterm and term infants should be treated promptly at the time of rash presentation with systemic antifungal therapy and for a minimum of 14 days. Delaying systemic treatment, solitary use of topical therapy (nystatin), or treating for <10 days is associated with *Candida* dissemination to the bloodstream.[2]

In evaluating a diffuse CCC rash in the first week of life, aerobic skin cultures for both fungal and bacterial organisms need to be obtained to identify the source of infection. Examination of the umbilical cord for yellow plaques and placenta can aid in the diagnosis as well. Both should be sent for specific fungal staining as well as aerobic culture. Additionally, blood culture, urine culture if older than 48 hours, and CSF if no rash on the back is present should be performed. Most experts would defer the lumbar puncture if there is cutaneous involvement on the back due to invasion into the dermis and risk of introducing *Candida* into the CSF. Empiric antifungal therapy should be started pending culture results. Differential diagnosis includes staphylococcal as well as other bacterial and fungal skin infections. In certain cases when the rash could be due to bacterial and fungal pathogens, empiric staphylococcal and fungal empiric coverage should be initiated pending culture results.

Diagnosis of CCC is made by the presence of a diffuse CCC rash involving major skin areas of the body, extremities, face or scalp, and/or funisitis, presenting in the first week (≤7 days), with identification of *Candida* species or yeast from (1) skin or mucous membrane cultures, (2) placenta staining or cultures, or (3) umbilical cord staining or cultures.

Cutaneous Candidiasis (CC)

Cutaneous (or mucocutaneous) candidiasis presents as a diffuse rash with similar skin manifestations as CCC, but occurs later, at 8 or more days after birth.[2,49,52] In the era before antifungal prophylaxis, the incidence in VLBW infants was reported to be 7.8%.[49] Risk factors include extreme prematurity, vaginal birth, postnatal steroids, and hyperglycemia.[3,49,53] Similar to CCC, CC in premature infants is an invasive infection of the skin and will disseminate if not systemically treated.[49] Aerobic skin cultures for both fungal and bacterial organisms need to be obtained to identify the nature of the infection. Additionally, blood and urine cultures, plus a lumbar puncture if no rash on the back is present, should be performed. Empiric systemic therapy

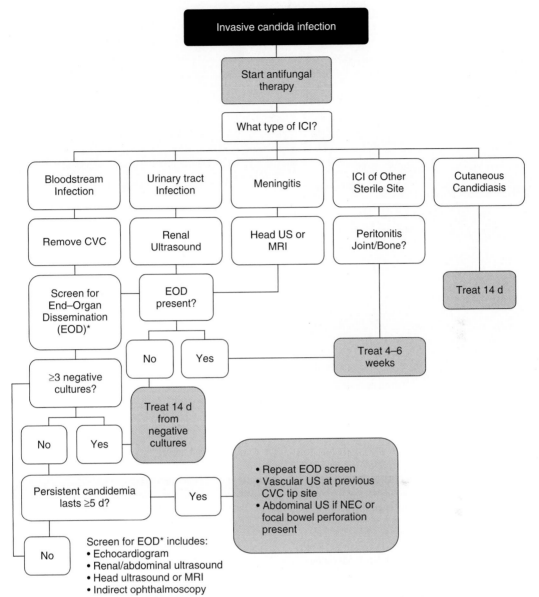

Figure 7.4 Diagnosis and evaluation of invasive *Candida* infections. *CVC,* Central venous catheter; *EOD,* end-organ dissemination; *ICI,* invasive *Candida* infections; *MRI,* magnetic resonance imaging; *NEC,* necrotizing enterocolitis; *US,* ultrasound. If bowel disease, such as NEC or focal bowel perforation, is present or part of the patient's history, a complete abdominal ultrasound for abscess should be performed.

should be started at the time of skin presentation and treatment should be continued for a minimum of 14 days in premature infants.

Candidemia

Compared with bacteremia, candidemia is associated with prolonged positivity of blood cultures with a median of 3 days even in the absence of end-organ dissemination.[28] Signs of *Candida* bloodstream infections are similar to those with bacteremia, with candidemia having some unique patterns related to thrombocytopenia (Table 7.2). VLBW infants with candidemia (as well as those with gram-negative bacteremia) have lower initial platelet counts, lower platelet nadirs, and a greater duration of thrombocytopenia compared with those with gram-positive sepsis.[54] The percentage decrease from baseline at presentation is also greater with candidemia (50%) compared

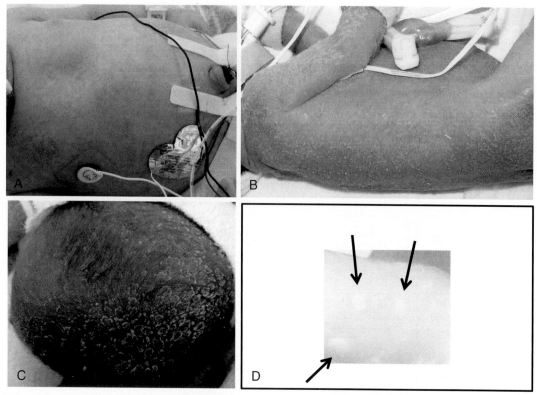

Figure 7.5   Congenital cutaneous candidiasis. (A) Macular papular rash. (B) White-yellow flaking rash on erythematous base. (C) Desquamation with a dry, cracking, scaly rash. (D) White-yellow plaques of the umbilical cord.

Table 7.2   PRESENTING SIGNS OF CANDIDEMIA IN VERY LOW BIRTH WEIGHT INFANTS[80]

Common (>50%)	Frequent (≈33%)
Thrombocytopenia <100,000/μL (84%) Immature-to-total neutrophil ratio ≥0.2 (77%) ↑ C-reactive protein (CRP) (1-3)-Beta-D-glucan >125 pg/dL ↑ Apnea and/or bradycardia ↑ Oxygen requirement ↑ Assisted ventilation	Lethargy and/or hypotonia Gastrointestinal signs (e.g., gastric residuals, distention, bloody stools)
Less Common (10%–15%)	**Can Occur (3%)**
Hypotension Hyperglycemia Elevated white blood cell count >20,000/μL Metabolic acidosis	Absolute neutrophil count <1500/μL

Adpated from Fanaroff AA, Korones SB, Wright LL, et al. Incidence, presenting features, risk factors and significance of late onset septicemia in very low birth weight infants. The National Institute of Child Health and Human Development Neonatal Research Network. *Pediatr Infect Dis J.* 1998;17:593–598.

with gram-positive infection. Between *Candida* species, *C. albicans* and *C. parapsilosis* present with lower platelet counts and more apnea compared with *C. glabrata*.[55] Most importantly, candidemia can be associated with disseminated disease (see Fig. 7.1). Evaluation of cardiac, renal, ophthalmologic, and central nervous systems is warranted even if there is only one blood culture positive for *Candida*. These can be performed at presentation or 5 to 7 days into treatment. Reevaluation for end-organ dissemination should occur with persistent candidemia (>5 to 7 days).

Renal Candidiasis

Candida infection of the kidneys may result from ascending UTI via the urethra or via direct seeding from the bloodstream. Colonization and proliferation are augmented by proteinuria, nitrogenous compounds, acidic pH (preterm infant urine is alkalotic), hydrophobic *Candida* cells, and the presence of Enterobacteriaceae such as *Escherichia coli*. SAPs and phospholipases play a role in the renal system as well attacking structural and immunologic defenses leading to tissue injury and invasion.[56] Risk factors for candiduria include vaginal birth, lower mean birth weight and gestational age, male gender, and prolonged initial courses of empiric antibiotic therapy.[57]

Urinary Tract Infection

Late-onset sepsis evaluations should include a urine culture obtained via sterile catheterization.[58] Infection is most commonly defined as growth of ≥10,000 CFU/mL from a sterile catheterization or ≥1000 CFU/mL in urine obtained by suprapubic bladder aspiration. Some experts and studies have not found colony counts useful in diagnosis and instead, have found that the presence of any *Candida* in the urine is associated with significant infection and outcomes.[22,57,59] *Candida* UTIs may occur alone or in conjunction with *Candida* sepsis. Others have considered lower colony-forming units (CFUs) not infection, but colonization at a high-risk site and preemptive treatment could be considered. Empiric antifungal therapy should be started with subsequent sepsis evaluations if urine colonization is known pending culture results. UTIs and sepsis have similar presentations.[60] Elevated creatinine levels without other causes may be another sign of a UTI. Renal ultrasonography is warranted for all *Candida* UTIs to evaluate for abscess formation. In the absence of antifungal prophylaxis, candiduria can occur in up to 2.4% of VLBW and 6% of ELBW infants.[1,12,22] In ELBWs, high mortality occurs with *Candida* UTI alone (26%) and is similar to candidemia alone (28%).[22] Additionally, neurodevelopmental impairment is increased with candiduria alone to a similar degree to candidemia. These findings emphasize the need for prompt treatment for a minimum duration of 14 days.

Renal Abscess

Renal fungal abscess formation may occur in infants with candiduria via an ascending infection or dissemination to the kidneys with candidemia.[56] Two studies of candiduria from 1982–1993 and 2001–2003 found that renal abscesses developed in 42% (36 screened) and 58% (26 screened) of infants with candiduria (± candidemia), whereas a more recent study during 2004–2007 found the incidence to be 0% (0 of 23 evaluated) with candiduria alone and 22% (2 of 9) with concordant *Candida* infection.[57] One study found normal ultrasound examinations in a third of patients who developed renal abscesses 8 to 39 days later, which may have been related to antifungal dosing used or delay in treatment. Between these two study periods, antifungal prophylaxis, pharmacokinetic and safety studies of appropriate initial antifungal dosing (e.g., amphotericin B deoxycholate at 1 mg/kg compared with 0.25 mg/kg in the previous era), and increased empiric antifungal therapy may have attenuated formation of renal abscesses. These studies have small numbers but suggest that in infants with candiduria, prompt initial antifungal therapy has improved outcomes, so renal imaging should be performed at presentation and repeated in cases with persistent candiduria.

Central Nervous System (CNS) Candidiasis and Sequelae

Meningitis and Encephalitis

Meningitis, encephalitis, or abscess formation may complicate candidemia or occur separately. About 50% of meningitis cases occur without documented candidemia.[28,61] Lumbar puncture at the time of sepsis evaluation before the initiation of antifungal therapy is important, as CSF cell counts and chemistries often are not abnormal with CNS infections in studies with a mixture of lumbar punctures performed before and after antifungal treatments.[62] This may be due to the timing of the lumbar puncture, the neonatal host response, or the location of the CNS infection (spinal fluid versus brain tissue).

Central Nervous System Abscess

In cases of candidemia or CNS fungal disease, neuroimaging (ultrasonography or magnetic resonance imaging [MRI]) is needed to evaluate for abscess formation. Animal studies have demonstrated CNS involvement in cases of fungal sepsis.[63] Ultrasonography can be performed initially and continues to improve in quality, but a small study (performed between 1990 and 1994) found it only to be ≈50% sensitive compared with other neuroimaging or autopsy.[48] Studies have also found an association between ICI and periventricular leukomalacia in premature infants, possibly related to release of cytokines, which may damage the periventricular white matter.

Gastrointestinal Disease

Peritonitis

ICI can complicate NEC or focal bowel perforation. If exploratory laparotomy or drains are placed, cultures should be obtained to determine what organisms are present. Peritonitis may initially present with or without erythema as part of abdominal symptomatology. Identification of pathogens in the peritoneal cavity is critical to appropriate management of bowel perforation or peritonitis and to prevent abscess formation. *Candida* species are the predominant organism causing peritonitis in 44% of focal bowel perforation cases and in 15% of the perforated NEC cases.[64] Although radiographs are the most common study identifying bowel perforation, some cases may be missed, and ultrasound or exploratory laparotomy may be needed if clinically indicated.

Studies in the era before antifungal prophylaxis demonstrated candidemia complicating 16.5% of cases of NEC. Culture of the rectum, stool, or oral flora in infants with diagnosis of NEC should be performed to evaluate for presence of Candida species or yeast. If isolated, systemic antifungal therapy should be initiated in addition to the antibacterial treatment of NEC. This may not be needed in infants who have been on antifungal prophylaxis since birth.

Respiratory Disease

Pneumonia

Pneumonia remains a difficult diagnosis in ventilated infants with chronic lung disease, as radiologic findings of infection, atelectasis, fluid, and scarring are often similar. Respiratory tract colonization usually occurs 1 to 2 weeks after skin and GI colonization and is associated with a high risk for ICI.[6] Preemptive treatment prevents dissemination in intubated ELBW infants when *Candida* is detected in the lungs by culture, PCR, or *Candida* mannan antigen.[65,66]

Endocarditis and Infected Vascular Thrombi

Candida endocarditis and infected vascular thrombi, the most common complications of candidemia (5.5%–15.2%), are associated with higher mortality than candidemia alone.[67,68] Central vascular catheters are a risk factor as local trauma to valvular, endocardial, or endothelial tissue, leading to thrombus formation and infection at the time of insertion and/or at any time while in situ. When antifungal therapy alone is unsuccessful in resolving the endocarditis or thrombus, thrombolytic or anticoagulation therapy has been used in some cases, but the suitability of these measures depends on the infant's gestational age and accompanying conditions.

Endophthalmitis and Retinopathy of Prematurity

Endophthalmitis presents most commonly as an intraocular dissemination from the bloodstream, but also could be a rare complication of retinopathy of prematurity (ROP) surgery or local trauma.[69] Endophthalmitis progresses from a chorioretinal lesion that subsequently elevates and breaks free in the vitreous, appearing as a white fluffy ball. It can present as solitary or multiple yellow-white elevated lesions in the posterior retina and vitreous. The clear cell-free vitreous becomes hazy due to an influx of inflammatory cells. Retinal endophthalmitis rates have decreased significantly, likely due to more rapid diagnosis, treatment, and prevention of ICIs.[70]

Even in the absence of visible retinal abscesses or chorioretinitis, *Candida* sepsis increases the risk for severe ROP, and screening for retinal pathology, if not already indicated by gestational age or birth weight criteria, is recommended in preterm infants with candidemia.[70]

End-Organ Dissemination

By the time an ICI becomes clinically apparent, *Candida* often has disseminated to form abscesses in tissues, organs, or body fluids. The adherence properties of *Candida* predispose to endocarditis, endophthalmitis, dermatitis, peritonitis, osteomyelitis, and septic arthritis. Fungal abscesses may form in the CNS, kidneys, liver, spleen, skin, bowel, and peritoneum (see Figs. 7.1 and 7.4). One meta-analysis (1979–2002) found the incidence of endocarditis to be 5%, endophthalmitis 3%, renal involvement 5%, and CNS abscesses 4%.[4] End-organ dissemination is higher in ELBW infants and in infants with persistent candidemia for >5 to 7 days.[67,68,71]

End-organ dissemination is reduced by prompt removal of central vascular catheters and initiation of antifungal therapy as soon as blood cultures become positive.[68] In addition, antifungal prophylaxis, empiric therapy, better antifungal dosing, and improved culturing techniques and diagnostics have contributed to a decline in the incidence of end-organ dissemination.[12,28,72]

Screening and Diagnosis of End-Organ Dissemination With ICI (Fig. 7.4)

With documented candidemia, initial screening for end-organ dissemination should include an echocardiogram, renal ultrasound, cranial ultrasound, and ophthalmologic examination. If there is significant bowel pathology such as NEC or focal bowel perforation, a complete abdominal ultrasound should be performed to rule out peritoneal, liver, or splenic involvement. If signs of septic arthritis (joint swelling) or osteomyelitis (swelling or immobility) are present, a clinical diagnosis can be made and antifungal treatment provided for 4 to 6 weeks. Joint aspiration may help with diagnosis in the absence of candidemia. Evaluation with bone scan or MRI may help define the extent of involvement, but imaging should not be used to rule out joint or bone involvement in infants. If candidemia persists, end-organ dissemination is even more likely, and the initial screening tests should be repeated along with additional surveillance after 5 to 7 days to include (1) ultrasound at the location of the tip of any prior central catheters for infected thrombus, (2) complete abdominal ultrasound for abscesses (laparotomy is sometimes considered if high clinical suspicion), and (3) cranial ultrasound/MRI to detect brain dissemination. Abscesses that are amenable to drainage or surgery should be removed.

Are Cultures Perfect?

The best method for diagnosing ICIs remains culture of blood, urine, CSF, and peritoneal fluid or other sterile body fluids. Obtaining sufficient blood culture volumes (≥1 mL) and performing urine and CSF fluid cultures at the time of evaluation for sepsis remain critical to making prompt diagnoses. Although neonatal infections may have low colony counts, they are above the detection limit with newer blood culture methods.[73] On average, neonatal blood cultures demonstrate growth by 37 hours, and 97% of blood cultures are positive by 72 hours.[74] Prior antifungal therapy does affect time to positivity. Clinical diagnosis has greatly improved as laboratories have become more skilled at culturing *Candida*, identifying *Candida* species, and performing susceptibility testing. Although some in vitro studies found lack of growth of *Candida* in blood cultures, clinical neonatal studies demonstrate high reliability when appropriate culture volumes and methods are used.[68] The frequent occurrence of multiple positive blood cultures also aids in diagnosis of candidemia. In 110 ICIs in NICU patients (1989–1999), 97% were diagnosed by cultures, with only three patients not diagnosed until autopsy.

How Good Are the Newer Laboratory Diagnostic Adjunctive Tests?

Adjunctive laboratory tests have not replaced cultures, but they can be useful in identifying high-risk patients who would benefit from early empiric antifungal therapy (pending culture results) and in monitoring response to antifungal therapy. Polymerase chain reaction (PCR) and fungal cell wall polysaccharides such as (1-3)-beta-D-glucan (BDG) and mannan can be extremely helpful in detecting non-bloodstream infections and determining the need for extension of treatment. They are currently not better than cultures in identifying true infections; costs per yield are high if included in each infection evaluation, especially because preventative measures have resulted in very few (≈1 in 500) sepsis evaluations in premature infants yielding evidence of fungal infection.

BDG levels are helpful if there is uncertainty in deciding the need for empiric antifungal therapy and in following response to therapy as levels decrease over time with antifungal therapy. Various cutoff points have been recommended for interpreting BDG levels in infants. Serum BDG levels are higher in infants with ICI (364 pg/mL [IQR 131–976] vs. 89 pg/mL [IQR 30–127] in noninfected infants) and decrease significantly with antifungal therapy, to 58 pg/mL [IQR 28–81].[75] The cutoff for BDG should be higher (>125 pg/mL) for infants than adults (>80 pg/mL) due to the effect that colonization and other infections (gram-negative and coagulase-negative *Staphylococcus*) may have on BDG levels. BDG levels in infants infected with coagulase-negative staphylococci were 116 pg/mL (46–128) and 118 pg/mL (52–304) in infants without bacteremia. One challenge is that BDG can be elevated to the same degree with fungal colonization as with ICI, and studies have not critically examined this effect.[76] Infants colonized at certain high-risk sites (e.g., the respiratory tract) may benefit from empiric treatment.[65,66] One study used mannan levels ≥0.5 ng/mL in endotracheal lavage aspirates as a criterion for preemptive treatment and significantly decreased ICI.[66] Further study of preemptive treatment at certain BDG levels may be beneficial.

BDG may also give false-positive results after transfusion of blood products in adults and infants.[77] A study of 133 VLBWs found BDG to be higher in transfused (red blood cells or fresh frozen plasma) infants (170 pg/mL, 65–317) compared with nontransfused infants (57 pg/mL, 34–108; $P < 0.001$).

Another method that may help with the decision to start early empiric therapy is direct fluorescent assay in buffy coat.[78] This test is a fluorescent stain that binds to structures containing cellulose and chitin. This diagnostic test has been successfully used for identifying hyphae and spores, and results are obtained after only 1 to 2 hours.

Molecular techniques, including PCR and DNA microarray technology, may identify fungi and their antifungal susceptibilities more quickly and with higher sensitivity than is possible with blood cultures. Fungal PCR to detect the gene for 18S ribosomal RNA (rRNA) in preterm infants has yielded promising results but requires additional study.[79] PCR is useful when fungal infection suspicion is high despite negative cultures. PCR can detect candidemia as well as non—bloodstream infections, including *Candida* peritonitis or candiduria, but also previous candidal infections and endotracheal colonization. Similar to adjunctive tests, the ability of PCR to distinguish infection from colonization has not been critically studied.

Other markers of fungal disease include anti-*Candida* antibodies, D-arabinitol (a candidal metabolite), and fungal chitin synthase. These markers are similarly challenging to study, as they may be present with bloodstream infections, non—bloodstream infections, or colonization alone.

REFERENCES

1. Kaufman D, Fairchild KD. Clinical microbiology of bacterial and fungal sepsis in very-low-birth-weight infants. *Clin Microbiol Rev*. 2004;17:638–680.
2. Kaufman DA, Coggins SA, Zanelli SA, et al. Congenital cutaneous candidiasis: prompt systemic treatment is associated with improved outcomes in neonates. *Clin Infect Dis*. 2017;published online ahead of print. Avaialble at: https://doi.org/10.1093/cid/cix119.
3. Baley JE, Silverman RA. Systemic candidiasis: cutaneous manifestations in low birth weight infants. *Pediatrics*. 1988;82:211–215.
4. Benjamin DK Jr, Poole C, Steinbach WJ, et al. Neonatal candidemia and end-organ damage: a critical appraisal of the literature using meta-analytic techniques. *Pediatrics*. 2003;112:634–640.
5. Baley JE, Kliegman RM, Boxerbaum B, et al. Fungal colonization in the very low birth weight infant. *Pediatrics*. 1986;78:225–232.
6. Kaufman DA, Gurka MJ, Hazen KC, et al. Patterns of fungal colonization in preterm infants weighing less than 1000 grams at birth. *Pediatr Infect Dis J*. 2006;25:733–737.
7. Manzoni P, Stolfi I, Pugni L, et al. A Multicenter, Randomized trial of prophylactic fluconazole in preterm neonates. *N Engl J Med*. 2007;356:2483–2495.
8. Manzoni P, Farina D, Antonielli d'Oulx E, et al. An association between anatomic site of *Candida* colonization and risk of invasive candidiasis exists also in preterm neonates in neonatal intensive care unit. *Diagn Microbiol Infect Dis*. 2006;56:459–460.
9. Manzoni P, Farina D, Leonessa M, et al. Risk factors for progression to invasive fungal infection in preterm neonates with fungal colonization. *Pediatrics*. 2006;118:2359–2364.
10. Manzoni P, Farina D, Galletto P, et al. Type and number of sites colonized by fungi and risk of progression to invasive fungal infection in preterm neonates in neonatal intensive care unit. *J Perinat Med*. 2007;35:220–226.
11. Rowen JL, Rench MA, Kozinetz CA, et al. Endotracheal colonization with *Candida* enhances risk of systemic candidiasis in very low birth weight neonates. *J Pediatr*. 1994;124:789–794.
12. Kaufman D, Boyle R, Hazen KC, et al. Fluconazole prophylaxis against fungal colonization and infection in preterm infants. *N Engl J Med*. 2001;345:1660–1666.
13. Saiman L, Ludington E, Dawson JD, et al. Risk factors for *Candida* species colonization of neonatal intensive care unit patients. *Pediatr Infect Dis J*. 2001;20:1119–1124.
14. Bliss JM, Basavegowda KP, Watson WJ, et al. Vertical and horizontal transmission of *Candida albicans* in very low birth weight infants using DNA fingerprinting techniques. *Pediatr Infect Dis J*. 2008;27:231–235.
15. Rutter N. Clinical consequences of an immature barrier. *Semin Neonatol*. 2000;5:281–287.
16. Yost CC, Cody MJ, Harris ES, et al. Impaired neutrophil extracellular trap (NET) formation: a novel innate immune deficiency of human neonates. *Blood*. 2009;113:6419–6427.
17. Arboleya S, Binetti A, Salazar N, et al. Establishment and development of intestinal microbiota in preterm neonates. *FEMS Microbiol Ecol*. 2012;79:763–772.
18. Wagner RD, Pierson C, Warner T, et al. Biotherapeutic effects of probiotic bacteria on candidiasis in immunodeficient mice. *Infect Immun*. 1997;65:4165–4172.
19. Manzoni P, Meyer M, Stolfi I, et al. Bovine lactoferrin supplementation for prevention of necrotizing enterocolitis in very-low-birth-weight neonates: a randomized clinical trial. *Early Hum Dev*. 2014; 90(suppl 1):S60–S65.
20. Romeo MG, Romeo DM, Trovato L, et al. Role of probiotics in the prevention of the enteric colonization by *Candida* in preterm newborns: incidence of late-onset sepsis and neurological outcome. *J Perinatol*. 2011;31:63–69.
21. Cotten CM, McDonald S, Stoll B, et al. The association of third-generation cephalosporin use and invasive candidiasis in extremely low birth-weight infants. *Pediatrics*. 2006;118:717–722.
22. Benjamin DK Jr, Stoll BJ, Gantz MG, et al. Neonatal candidiasis: epidemiology, risk factors, and clinical judgment. *Pediatrics*. 2010;126:e865–e873.
23. Saiman L, Ludington E, Pfaller M, et al. Risk factors for candidemia in neonatal intensive care unit patients. The National Epidemiology of Mycosis Survey study group. *Pediatr Infect Dis J*. 2000;19: 319–324.
24. Stoll BJ, Temprosa M, Tyson JE, et al. Dexamethasone therapy increases infection in very low birth weight. *Pediatrics*. 1999;104:e63.
25. Botas CM, Kurlat I, Young SM, et al. Disseminated candidal infections and intravenous hydrocortisone in preterm infants. *Pediatrics*. 1995;95:883–887.
26. Watterberg KL, Gerdes JS, Cole CH, et al. Prophylaxis of early adrenal insufficiency to prevent bronchopulmonary dysplasia: a multicenter trial. *Pediatrics*. 2004;114:1649–1657.
27. Corpeleijn WE, de Waard M, Christmann V, et al. Effect of donor milk on severe infections and mortality in very low-birth-weight infants: the Early Nutrition Study randomized clinical trial. *JAMA Pediatr*. 2016;170:654–661.
28. Benjamin DK Jr, Stoll BJ, Fanaroff AA, et al. Neonatal candidiasis among extremely low birth weight infants: risk factors, mortality rates, and neurodevelopmental outcomes at 18 to 22 months. *Pediatrics*. 2006;117:84–92.
29. Feja KN, Wu F, Roberts K, et al. Risk factors for candidemia in critically ill infants: a matched case-control study. *J Pediatr*. 2005;147:156–161.
30. Barton M, O'Brien K, Robinson JL, et al. Invasive candidiasis in low birth weight preterm infants: risk factors, clinical course and outcome in a prospective multicenter study of cases and their matched controls. *BMC Infect Dis*. 2014;14:327.

7

31. Hawser SP, Douglas LJ. Biofilm formation by *Candida* species on the surface of catheter materials in vitro. *Infect Immun*. 1994;62:915–921.

32. Krysan DJ, Sutterwala FS, Wellington M. Catching fire: *Candida albicans*, macrophages, and pyroptosis. *PLoS Pathog*. 2014;10:e1004139.

33. Bendel CM, Hess DJ, Garni RM, et al. Comparative virulence of *Candida albicans* yeast and filamentous forms in orally and intravenously inoculated mice. *Crit Care Med*. 2003;31:501–507.

34. Cleary IA, Reinhard SM, Lazzell AL, et al. Examination of the pathogenic potential of *Candida albicans* filamentous cells in an animal model of haematogenously disseminated candidiasis. *FEMS Yeast Res*. 2016;16:fow011.

35. Leidich SD, Ibrahim AS, Fu Y, et al. Cloning and disruption of caPLB1, a phospholipase B gene involved in the pathogenicity of *Candida albicans*. *J Biol Chem*. 1998;273:26078–26086.

36. Naglik JR, Challacombe SJ, Hube B. *Candida albicans* secreted aspartyl proteinases in virulence and pathogenesis. *Microbiol Mol Biol Rev*. 2003;67:400–428.

37. Swanson JR, Gurka MJ, Kaufman DA. Risk factors for invasive fungal infection in premature infants: enhancing a targeted prevention approach. *J Pediatric Infect Dis Soc*. 2014;3:49–56.

38. Chitnis AS, Magill SS, Edwards JR, et al. Trends in *Candida* central line-associated bloodstream infections among NICUs, 1999–2009. *Pediatrics*. 2012;130:e46–e52.

39. Fridkin SK, Kaufman D, Edwards JR, et al. Changing incidence of *Candida* bloodstream infections among NICU patients in the United States: 1995–2004. *Pediatrics*. 2006;117:1680–1687.

40. Pammi M, Holland L, Butler G, et al. *Candida parapsilosis* is a significant neonatal pathogen: a systematic review and meta-analysis. *Pediatr Infect Dis J*. 2013;32:e206–e216.

41. Stoll BJ, Hansen N, Fanaroff AA, et al. Late-onset sepsis in very low birth weight neonates: the experience of the NICHD Neonatal Research Network. *Pediatrics*. 2002;110:285–291.

42. Burwell LA, Kaufman D, Blakely J, et al. Antifungal prophylaxis to prevent neonatal candidiasis: a survey of perinatal physician practices. *Pediatrics*. 2006;118:e1019–e1026.

43. Kaufman DA, Morris A, Gurka MJ, et al. Fluconazole prophylaxis in preterm infants: a multicenter case-controlled analysis of efficacy and safety. *Early Hum Dev*. 2014;90(suppl 1):S87–S90.

44. Kaufman DA. Aiming for Zero: Preventing invasive *Candida* infections in extremely preterm infants. *Neoreviews*. 2011;12:e381–e392.

45. Weitkamp JH, Ozdas A, Lafleur B, et al. Fluconazole prophylaxis for prevention of invasive fungal infections in targeted highest risk preterm infants limits drug exposure. *J Perinatol*. 2008;28: 405–411.

46. Kossoff EH, Buescher ES, Karlowicz MG. Candidemia in a neonatal intensive care unit: trends during fifteen years and clinical features of 111 cases. *Pediatr Infect Dis J*. 1998;17:504–508.

47. Greenberg RG, Benjamin DK Jr, Gantz MG, et al. Empiric antifungal therapy and outcomes in extremely low birth weight infants with invasive candidiasis. *J Pediatr*. 2012;161:264–269.

48. Friedman S, Richardson SE, Jacobs SE, et al. Systemic *Candida* infection in extremely low birth weight infants: short term morbidity and long term neurodevelopmental outcome. *Pediatr Infect Dis J*. 2000;19:499–504.

49. Faix RG, Kovarik SM, Shaw TR, et al. Mucocutaneous and invasive candidiasis among very low birth weight (less than 1,500 grams) infants in intensive care nurseries: a prospective study. *Pediatrics*. 1989;83:101–107.

50. Procianoy RS, Eneas MV, Silveira RC. Empiric guidelines for treatment of *Candida* infection in high-risk neonates. *Eur J Pediatr*. 2006;165:422–423.

51. Makhoul IR, Kassis I, Smolkin T, et al. Review of 49 neonates with acquired fungal sepsis: further characterization. *Pediatrics*. 2001;107:61–66.

52. Darmstadt GL, Dinulos JG, Miller Z. Congenital cutaneous candidiasis: clinical presentation, pathogenesis, and management guidelines. *Pediatrics*. 2000;105:438–444.

53. Rowen JL, Atkins JT, Levy ML, et al. Invasive fungal dermatitis in the < or = 1000-gram neonate. *Pediatrics*. 1995;95:682–687.

54. Guida JD, Kunig AM, Leef KH, et al. Platelet count and sepsis in very low birth weight neonates: is there an organism-specific response? *Pediatrics*. 2003;111:1411–1415.

55. Fairchild KD, Tomkoria S, Sharp EC, et al. Neonatal *Candida glabrata* sepsis: clinical and laboratory features compared with other *Candida* species. *Pediatr Infect Dis J*. 2002;21:39–43.

56. Fisher JF, Kavanagh K, Sobel JD, et al. *Candida* urinary tract infection: pathogenesis. *Clin Infect Dis*. 2011;52(suppl 6):S437–S451.

57. Wynn JL, Tan S, Gantz MG, et al. Outcomes following candiduria in extremely low birth weight infants. *Clin Infect Dis*. 2012;54:331–339.

58. Robinson JL, Davies HD, Barton M, et al. Characteristics and outcome of infants with candiduria in neonatal intensive care—a Paediatric Investigators Collaborative Network on Infections in Canada (PICNIC) study. *BMC Infect Dis*. 2009;9:183.

59. Kauffman CA, Fisher JF, Sobel JD, et al. *Candida* urinary tract infections–diagnosis. *Clin Infect Dis*. 2011;52(suppl 6):S452–S456.

60. Bauer S, Eliakim A, Pomeranz A, et al. Urinary tract infection in very low birth weight preterm infants. *Pediatr Infect Dis J*. 2003;22:426–430.

61. Cohen-Wolkowiez M, Smith PB, Mangum B, et al. Neonatal *Candida* meningitis: significance of cerebrospinal fluid parameters and blood cultures. *J Perinatol*. 2007;27:97–100.

62. Garges HP, Moody MA, Cotten CM, et al. Neonatal meningitis: what is the correlation among cerebrospinal fluid cultures, blood cultures, and cerebrospinal fluid parameters? *Pediatrics*. 2006;117: 1094–1100.

63. Hope WW, Mickiene D, Petraitis V, et al. The pharmacokinetics and pharmacodynamics of micafungin in experimental hematogenous *Candida* meningoencephalitis: implications for echinocandin therapy in neonates. *J Infect Dis*. 2008;197:163–171.

64. Coates EW, Karlowicz MG, Croitoru DP, et al. Distinctive distribution of pathogens associated with peritonitis in neonates with focal intestinal perforation compared with necrotizing enterocolitis. *Pediatrics*. 2005;116:e241–e246.

65. Vendettuoli V, Tana M, Tirone C, et al. The role of *Candida* surveillance cultures for identification of a preterm subpopulation at highest risk for invasive fungal infection. *Pediatr Infect Dis J*. 2008;27: 1114–1116.

66. Posteraro B, Sanguinetti M, Boccia S, et al. Early mannan detection in bronchoalveolar lavage fluid with preemptive treatment reduces the incidence of invasive *Candida* infections in preterm infants. *Pediatr Infect Dis J*. 2010;29:844–848.

67. Chapman RL, Faix RG. Persistently positive cultures and outcome in invasive neonatal candidiasis. *Pediatr Infect Dis J*. 2000;19:822–827.

68. Noyola DE, Fernandez M, Moylett EH, et al. Ophthalmologic, visceral, and cardiac involvement in neonates with candidemia. *Clin Infect Dis*. 2001;32:1018–1023.

69. Baley JE, Ellis FJ. Neonatal candidiasis: ophthalmologic infection. *Semin Perinatol*. 2003;27:401–405.

70. Noyola DE, Bohra L, Paysse EA, et al. Association of candidemia and retinopathy of prematurity in very low birthweight infants. *Ophthalmology*. 2002;109:80–84.

71. Barton M, Shen A, O'Brien K, et al. Early-onset invasive candidiasis in extremely low birth weight infants: perinatal acquisition predicts poor outcome. *Clin Infect Dis*. 2017;64:921–927.

72. Kaufman D, Boyle R, Hazen KC, et al. Twice Weekly Fluconazole Prophylaxis for Prevention of Invasive Candida Infection in High-risk Infants of <1000 Grams Birth Weight. *J Pediatr*. 2005;147: 172–179.

73. Pappas PG, Kauffman CA, Andes DR, et al. Executive Summary: Clinical Practice Guideline for the Management of Candidiasis: 2016 Update by the Infectious Diseases Society of America. *Clin Infect Dis*. 2016;62:409–417.

74. Schelonka RL, Moser SA. Time to positive culture results in neonatal Candida septicemia. *J Pediatr*. 2003;142:564–565.

75. Goudjil S, Kongolo G, Dusol L, et al. (1-3)-beta-D-glucan levels in candidiasis infections in the critically ill neonate. *J Matern Fetal Neonatal Med*. 2013;26:44–48.

76. Cornu M, Goudjil S, Kongolo G, et al. Evaluation of the (1,3)-beta-D-glucan assay for the diagnosis of neonatal invasive yeast infections. *Med Mycol*. 2017;published online ahead of print. Avaialble at: https://doi.org/10.1093/mmy/myx021.

77. Goudjil S, Chazal C, Moreau F, et al. Blood product transfusions are associated with an increase in serum (1-3)-beta-d-glucan in infants during the initial hospitalization in neonatal intensive care unit (NICU). *J Matern Fetal Neonatal Med*. 2016;1–5.

78. Higareda-Almaraz MA, Loza-Barajas H, Maldonado-Gonzalez JG, et al. Usefulness of direct fluorescent in buffy coat in the diagnosis of *Candida* sepsis in neonates. *J Perinatol*. 2016;36:874–877.

79. Tirodker UH, Nataro JP, Smith S, et al. Detection of fungemia by polymerase chain reaction in critically ill neonates and children. *J Perinatol*. 2003;23:117–122.

80. Fanaroff AA, Korones SB, Wright LL, et al. Incidence, presenting features, risk factors and significance of late onset septicemia in very low birth weight infants. The National Institute of Child Health and Human Development Neonatal Research Network. *Pediatr Infect Dis J*. 1998;17:593–598.

7

When to Perform Lumbar Puncture in Infants at Risk for Meningitis in the Neonatal Intensive Care Unit

Rachel G. Greenberg, MD, MB, MHS, Tamara I. Herrera, MD

8

- Meningitis occurs most commonly in the neonatal period and is associated with significant morbidity and mortality.
- Fifteen percent to thirty-eight percent of infants with meningitis have negative blood cultures. Selective evaluation of infants with culture-proven bacteremia can result in missed diagnoses of meningitis.
- Routine lumbar puncture in well-appearing infants evaluated because of maternal risk factors is not recommended.
- Lumbar puncture can be deferred or omitted from early-onset sepsis evaluation in premature infants with respiratory distress syndrome.
- Lumbar puncture should be performed as part of the evaluation of infants with suspected late-onset infection.
- Lumbar puncture should be deferred in severely ill infants with cardiorespiratory compromise, though empiric therapy should be considered if meningitis is strongly suspected.
- Repeat lumbar punctures in infants receiving adequate antibiotic therapy and showing clinical improvement are not recommended.

Introduction

The neonatal period is the most common time in life for the presentation of bacterial meningitis, with an estimated incidence of approximately 0.3 per 1000 live births in developed countries.[1,2] However, this figure is likely an underestimate, as 30% to 70% of infants who undergo sepsis evaluation do not have a lumbar puncture (LP) performed.[3,4] In developed countries, mortality from meningitis ranges between 10% and 15% for term infants[5] and reaches 25% in premature infants.[6] Although associated mortality has decreased over time, long-term morbidity remains high.[7,8] Identification of meningitis in infants by clinical examination can be difficult, as early signs are often subtle and nonspecific. Examination of the cerebrospinal fluid (CSF) is essential for diagnosis, identification of pathogens, and appropriate choice of therapy.[9]

The role of LP as part of the diagnostic evaluation of neonatal sepsis, especially in premature infants in the first 72 hours after birth, remains controversial.[10] The incidence of meningitis among asymptomatic infants with antepartum risk factors for infection alone[11–15] and premature infants with respiratory distress but no other signs of sepsis[16–18] is extremely low. However, 20% to 30% of infants with culture-proven early-onset sepsis (EOS) have concomitant bacterial meningitis.[19,20] Furthermore, about 15% to 38% of infants with confirmed meningitis have negative blood cultures,[3,19,21–23] suggesting that negative blood cultures cannot exclude meningitis in a sick infant. Therefore, selective evaluation of infants with culture-proven bacteremia results in missed cases of meningitis. The most common reasons for deferring an LP include the low incidence of neonatal meningitis, especially in the first 72 hours after birth in infants at risk for sepsis,[11–13,16–18] the low yield of the procedure,[14,15,24,25] the risk of complications,[26–31] and the fact that very low birth weight (VLBW) infants often have respiratory and cardiovascular compromise with the procedure.[3] However, there are advantages to obtaining an LP promptly. Diagnosing meningitis has implications in management and prognosis, as the duration of therapy needs to be increased and antimicrobial agents with higher degrees of central nervous system (CNS) penetration should be used.[32,33] Initiation of empiric antimicrobial therapy before LP may result in CSF sterilization, leading to underdiagnosis or in unnecessarily prolonged treatment when the possibility of meningitis cannot be excluded.[34] A delay or failure to diagnose meningitis is associated with inappropriate choice in spectrum and duration of antibiotic therapy, partially treated meningitis, increased mortality, and neurologic sequelae.[35]

Increased Susceptibility to Meningitis in Premature Infants

Bacteria can enter the CNS by (1) "receptor-mediated" transcellular movement through meningeal endothelial cells, (2) disruption of intracellular junctions of the cerebral microvasculature, or (3) transport across the blood–brain barrier within leukocytes.[8,36] Infants, especially premature infants, have a number of host defense impairments that increase their vulnerability to serious bacterial, fungal, and viral infections of the CNS.[37] Studies in fetal and neonatal animals have demonstrated immaturity and increased permeability of the blood–brain barrier,[38] which is reflected in the elevated CSF protein content of the premature infant.[39]

Accumulating evidence links intrauterine and postnatal neonatal infections with adverse neurodevelopmental outcomes in premature infants.[40–44] Exposure of the immature brain, and particularly the white matter, to inflammatory mediators causing cytotoxic injury is associated with increased risk for abnormal cognitive and motor functioning.[45] VLBW infants with meningitis are more likely to have major neurologic disability (45% vs. 11%) and subnormal (<70) Mental Developmental Index results (38% vs. 14%) compared with uninfected infants.[46]

Role of Lumbar Puncture in the Evaluation of Early-Onset Sepsis

The Centers for Disease Control and Prevention (CDC) defines EOS as blood or CSF culture-proven infection within the first week after birth,[47] and in hospitalized premature infants, EOS has also been defined as culture-proven infections occurring within the first 3 days after birth.[48,49] The incidence of EOS in the United States is estimated to be 0.77 to 1 per 1000 live births, with the highest incidence among the most premature infants.[4,50] Despite widespread implementation of intrapartum antibiotic prophylaxis (IAP), group B Streptococcus (GBS) remains the most frequent isolated pathogen associated with EOS in the United States and other developed countries among term infants, and *Escherichia coli* has emerged as the most common cause in VLBW infants.[4,48,51] Among infants with early-onset GBS disease, the most commonly identified syndromes are bacteremia without focus (83%), pneumonia (9%), and meningitis (7%).[52] Collection of CSF via LP is needed to rule out meningitis; however, its role in infants with suspected EOS remains controversial, and clinical practice varies greatly by center.[53]

The yield of CSF cultures in asymptomatic infants who undergo evaluation due to perinatal risk factors for infection is extremely low in the first few days after birth.[11,14,15,25] In a retrospective review of 3423 asymptomatic full-term infants evaluated because of maternal risk factors for infection in the first 7 days after birth, no cases of meningitis were observed.[11] A prospective study of 712 asymptomatic infants who underwent LP during the first week after birth for suspected sepsis found 9 (1.3%)

positive CSF cultures; however, only one infant had concomitant bacteremia and a clinical course consistent with meningitis, and the remaining cases were considered contaminants.[15] Consistent with these findings, a review of 506 infants at risk for infection or with suspected sepsis found no cases of meningitis among 263 infants who underwent LP within the first 72 hours after birth.[25] However, the incidence of positive CSF cultures increases with advancing postnatal age; after 7 days of age, the incidence of meningitis in infants evaluated for sepsis may be as high as 10%.[25] Conversely, a retrospective review of 169,849 infants born in U.S. Army hospitals during a 5-year period identified 43 cases of meningitis in the first 72 hours after birth. Of these 43 cases, 5 occurred in premature infants with respiratory distress syndrome (RDS), 8 were born at term with no specific CNS symptoms and negative blood cultures, and 3 had positive blood cultures, but were asymptomatic.[35] Those findings were worrisome because it suggested that meningitis can occur in infants with negative blood cultures who appeared completely well. However, the retrospective nature of that case series makes that observation questionable. Taking the available evidence into account, it is likely safe to omit routine LPs in well-appearing infants evaluated because of maternal risk factors (Table 8.1).

Similarly, the incidence of meningitis in premature infants with RDS is low.[17,18] In a retrospective review of 238 infants born between 23 and 40 weeks gestation admitted with RDS and evaluated for suspected sepsis within the first 24 hours after birth, no cases of meningitis were found among 203 CSF cultures collected.[17] The authors suggested reserving LPs for infants with RDS with positive blood cultures or infants with other concomitant signs after 24 hours of age, such as hypothermia or hyperthermia, poor feeding, or specific CNS signs. Supporting a selective approach in premature infants with RDS, only 4 cases of proven early-onset meningitis were found among 1495 infants 27 to 36 weeks gestation admitted with respiratory distress and evaluated for sepsis with an LP within the first 24 hours after birth.[18] Another retrospective case review of 1390 premature infants ≤34 weeks gestation evaluated for sepsis identified 32 infants with bacteremia in the first 6 hours after birth, but no missed cases of meningitis (confirmed by autopsy in infants who died).[16] Therefore, deferring or omitting LP from EOS evaluation in premature infants with RDS when the clinician believes that the infant's signs correspond to a noninfectious condition is a reasonable approach (see Table 8.1).

Current recommendations by the Committee on Fetus and Newborn suggest performing an LP as part of the evaluation of EOS in (1) infants with culture-proven sepsis, (2) infants with signs of infection when clinically stable, (3) infants with suspected bacteremia based on laboratory findings, and (4) infants with clinical deterioration despite initial antibiotic treatment.[10]

Role of Lumbar Puncture in the Evaluation of Late-Onset Sepsis

Late-onset sepsis (LOS), sepsis occurring after 3 days of age,[54,55] occurs most commonly among VLBW infants. The incidence of LOS in developed countries is 3 per 1000 live births[51] and varies inversely with gestational age and birth weight.[56] Gram-positive organisms are the most commonly isolated pathogens in LOS (63%–70%), with coagulase-negative staphylococci accounting for the majority of episodes, followed by gram-negative organisms (19%–25%), including *E. coli* (6%–8%) and *Klebsiella* spp. (5%–6%).[3,54] With advances in neonatal care improving the survival of extremely premature infants, invasive candidiasis has become an increasingly important cause of morbidity and mortality, affecting approximately 7% to 9% of VLBW infants during hospitalization with a mortality rate >30%.[57,58] About 5% of candidemic infants develop *Candida* meningitis.[58]

Meningitis is more common in infants evaluated for LOS compared with infants evaluated for EOS.[15,25] A fivefold increase in the yield of LP has been observed after the first week after birth.[15] Among infants with late-onset GBS disease, up to 27% may present with meningitis.[52,59] However, the role of LP as part of the evaluation of LOS, and particularly among VLBW infants, is controversial, and clinical practice

Table 8.1 ROLE OF LUMBAR PUNCTURE IN INFANT SEPSIS EVALUATION

Study	Population	Results	Conclusions
Johnson et al. 1997[11]	Full-term infants with suspected sepsis in the first 7 days after birth, N = 5135	11/1712 (0.6%) symptomatic infants had meningitis 0/3423 asymptomatic infants had meningitis	LP unnecessary in asymptomatic full-term infants
Fielkow et al. 1991[14]	Infants with LP in the first 7 days after birth, N = 1073	13/789 (1.6%) symptomatic infants had meningitis 0/284 asymptomatic infants had meningitis	LP is not indicated in asymptomatic infants evaluated for sepsis because of maternal risk factors, including chorioamnionitis
Schwersenski et al. 1991[15]	Infants with LP in the first 7 days after birth, N = 712 Infants with LP after 7 days after birth, N = 114	1/712 (0.1%) infants with suspected sepsis had meningitis with concomitant culture-proven bacteremia 4/114 (3.5%) infants with suspected sepsis had meningitis 3/114 (2.6%) had concomitant culture-proven bacteremia	Incidence of coexistent meningitis and sepsis in the first 7 days after birth is extremely low Routine LP in asymptomatic infants with risk factors for infection in the first 7 days after birth is not justified Incidence of coexistent meningitis and sepsis after the first week after birth is 2.6% Yield of LP is higher when performed for specific indications after 7 days after birth
Ajayi OA et al. 1997[25]	Infants with suspected sepsis in the first 72 hr, between 72 hr and 7 days, and after 7 days after birth, N = 506	0/263 had meningitis in the first 72 hr 9/115 (8%) had meningitis between 72 hr and 7 days after birth 13/128 (10%) had meningitis after 7 days after birth	Change to selective approach did not result in missed cases of meningitis in the first 72 hr after birth LP should be reserved for infants with bacteremia or CNS signs in the evaluation of EOS CSF yield increases with age
Wiswell et al. 1995[35]	Infants 29 to 42 weeks gestation with culture-proven meningitis in the first 72 hr after birth, N = 43	5/43 (12%) premature infants with RDS 3/43 (7%) asymptomatic term infants with bacteremia 8/43 (19%) term infants with no CNS symptoms and negative BC	Using selective criteria to perform LPs in the first 72 hr results in delayed or missed diagnoses of meningitis in 37% of the cases
Eldadah et al. 1987[17]	Infants 23 and 40 weeks gestation with RDS and suspected sepsis in the first 24 hr after birth, N = 238	17/238 (7%) infants had culture-proven bacteremia 0/203 infants had meningitis	Risks of LP may exceed benefits in infants with RDS and no specific signs of CNS infection
Hendricks-Munoz and Shapiro 1990[16]	Infants ≤34 weeks gestation with suspected sepsis in the first 6 hr after birth, N = 1390	32/1390 (2.3%) infants had culture-proven sepsis 0/1390 had meningitis or partially treated meningitis in the first 24 hr 112/123 infants with initial negative BC developed LOS (38% cases of meningitis)	Omission of LP in early sepsis evaluation in premature infants does not result in missed diagnosis of meningitis in the first 24 hr after birth LP is essential in the evaluation of LOS
Weiss et al. 1991[18]	Infants ≤36 weeks gestation with RDS who underwent LP in the first day after birth, N = 1495	4/1495 (0.3%) infants had meningitis 3/1495 (0.2%) had concomitant culture-proven bacteremia	LP should be performed in selected cases in premature infants with RDS

A

Table 8.1   ROLE OF LUMBAR PUNCTURE IN INFANT SEPSIS EVALUATION—cont'd

Study	Population	Results	Conclusions
Kumar et al. 1995[180]	Infants with LP for suspected sepsis, N = 169	5/148 (3.3%) symptomatic infants had meningitis with no culture-proven bacteremia 0/21 asymptomatic infants had meningitis evaluated for maternal risk factors	LP may be omitted in asymptomatic infants with risk factors, but should be performed in infants with clinical sepsis
Stoll et al. 2004[3]	VLBW infants with suspected sepsis after 72 hr after birth, N = 9641	134/9641 (1.4%) infants had meningitis 89/134 (66%) infants with meningitis had culture-proven bacteremia	Meningitis may be underdiagnosed. LP should be part of LOS evaluation among VLBW infants.

BC, Blood culture; *CNS*, central nervous system; *CSF*, cerebrospinal fluid; *EOS*, early-onset sepsis; *LOS*, late-onset sepsis; *LP*, lumbar puncture; *RDS*, respiratory distress syndrome; *VLBW*, very low birth weight.

varies (see Table 8.1). A survey of 69 Australian neonatologists found that only 51% of practitioners performed routine LPs in premature infants with suspected LOS.[60] Some authors have suggested a selective approach to inclusion of LP in the evaluation of LOS, limiting the procedure to infants with neurologic signs; absence of signs of specific organ infection; bacteremia; and presence of risk factors such as central lines, mechanical ventilation, and VLBW.[61] However, there is considerable evidence that meningitis after 72 hours of age may occur in the absence of a positive blood culture, as approximately one third of infants with bacterial meningitis[3,21–23] and one half of infants with *Candida* meningitis[58,62] have negative blood cultures.

An LP might be considered part of the routine evaluation of suspected LOS for the following reasons: (1) the clinical presentation of meningitis is indistinguishable from that of sepsis; (2) meningitis may occur in the absence of a positive blood culture; (3) the incidence of gram-negative or fungal organisms is higher in LOS with increased risk of poor outcomes; (4) late-onset infection due to GBS is more likely to be associated with meningitis; and (5) meningitis is more common in infants evaluated for LOS compared with EOS. Failure to perform an LP in VLBW infants with suspected LOS may result in missed or partially treated cases of meningitis. In this highly vulnerable population, with increased severity of illness and mortality, the risk of potentially devastating outcomes from not performing an LP may be greater than the potential benefit of avoiding an LP.[3,32,63–66] However, some clinicians recommend a more selective approach to LP in infants with suspected LOS to include any infant with a positive blood culture, infants with clinical signs or laboratory data suggestive of sepsis, and infants who do not respond to conventional antibiotic therapy in the usual fashion.

Role of Lumbar Puncture in Viral Meningitis

Although most cases are benign, some viral CNS infections may result in increased morbidity and mortality if not properly diagnosed and treatment is not initiated promptly.[67] *Enterovirus* infection is the most common cause of viral meningitis in young infants and children, particularly during summer and early fall outbreaks.[68,69] Although most cases are benign and self-limited, recent case series have linked neonatal enteroviral infections with periventricular leukomalacia[70,71]; and infants with enterovirus myocarditis showed an increased risk of mortality.[72–74] The clinical presentation of enteroviral sepsis and meningitis is nonspecific and may resemble bacterial sepsis or meningitis.[75] CSF analysis by reverse transcriptase polymerase chain reaction (RT-PCR) is an efficient method for diagnosing enteroviral meningitis, regardless of CSF profile, particularly in infants ≤3 months of age.[76–79]

Neonatal herpes simplex virus (HSV) infection occurs in 1 out of every 3200 live births in the United States[80] and is associated with significant mortality and long-term sequelae among survivors, including seizures, psychomotor retardation, spasticity, and learning disabilities.[81,82] The disease can present in three different patterns: (1) 25% of cases involve multiple visceral organs, with or without CNS compromise (disseminated disease); (2) 30% have CNS disease, with or without skin, eye, or mouth (SEM) involvement; and (3) 45% are localized to the SEM.[83] HSV infection should always be considered in infants with suspected sepsis, particularly if they fail to improve after 48 hours of antibiotic therapy with persistently negative bacterial cultures.[83,84] The American Academy of Pediatrics (AAP) Committee on Infectious Diseases recommends considering HSV infection in infants with fever, irritability, and abnormal CSF findings, particularly in the presence of seizures. CSF PCR is the method of choice for documenting CNS disease in infants with suspected HSV infection.[85–87] Approximately half of all infants with HSV infection have CNS involvement (CNS-isolated disease or disseminated disease with CNS involvement).[88] Given that only 20% of infants with disseminated HSV infection and 50% of infants with CNS disease develop cutaneous vesicles, an LP should be performed for detection of HSV DNA in the CSF in any infant with a suspected HSV infection.[89]

Asymptomatic infants born to mothers with visible genital lesions characteristic of HSV and no previous history of genital HSV should undergo evaluation with HSV CSF PCR at 24 hours of age. However, HSV CSF PCR in infants born to mothers with previous history of genital HSV is only indicated when surface cultures or the blood or surface PCR result is positive.[90]

Clinicians should consider HSV infection in the differential diagnosis of any acutely ill infant and have a low threshold to perform an LP, as the outcome depends on early diagnosis and prompt antiviral therapy.[88] Because persistent HSV DNA detection in the CSF by PCR after completion of antiviral therapy is associated with increased risk of death or moderate to severe neurologic impairment,[85,91,92] all infants with confirmed HSV CNS disease should undergo a repeat LP at the end of treatment to document CSF clearance, and intravenous antiviral therapy should be continued if CSF PCR remains positive.[88,93] Although a positive PCR is highly predictive of HSV infection, a negative result does not eliminate the possibility of CNS disease, and in cases in which HSV cannot be ruled out, antiviral therapy should be initiated or continued.[91,94]

Risks Associated With Lumbar Punctures in Newborn Infants

Concerns about the dangers of LP, particularly in a population with cardiovascular or respiratory instability, are the most common reasons for deferring or omitting the procedure.[3] Studies in animal models have shown an association between performance of an LP during bacteremia and later development of meningitis, possibly due to bacterial invasion of the subarachnoid space after microtrauma.[95,96] However, observational studies in infants and children found that the incidence of meningitis was not significantly different between patients with bacteremia who underwent an LP and those without a diagnostic LP.[97,98] Therefore, an LP in an infant with suspected bacteremia should not be omitted for theoretical concerns of inducing meningitis, as the risk of missing the diagnosis of meningitis is higher than the possibility of meningeal infection derived from the procedure.[99] Although infectious complications are rare, repeated LPs have been associated with lumbar epidural abscess and vertebral osteomyelitis in premature infants with posthemorrhagic hydrocephalus.[28]

Transentorial or transforaminal herniation resulting from raised intracranial pressure after LP is a potential risk[29,30,100]; however, this event is rare in the neonatal period due to the increased compliance of the neonatal skull in the setting of open fontanelles.[101,102] Rare cases of infants presenting with uncal or cerebellar herniation are related to other concomitant disease processes that increase intracranial pressure, such as galactosemia[103] and large cerebral infarcts.[104]

LPs may be associated with later development of epidermoid spinal tumors through the iatrogenic implantation of epidermal fragments into the spinal canal during the procedure,[31,105] especially when performed with a needle with no stylet.[106,107] To avoid this risk, some authors recommend using the smallest needle available with the stylet in place until the skin is punctured.[107,108]

Intramedullary or epidural hemorrhage is a rare but serious complication of LP in infants and children that can cause severe neurologic sequelae such as paraplegia,[109] but usually occurs in the presence of coagulopathy[110,111] and can result from injury to the conus medullaris in premature infants.[112] Recent imaging techniques have demonstrated that CSF leakage into the epidural space after LP is common in infants and reveals a characteristic sonographic appearance.[113] Among 33 infants who underwent LP during the first 21 days after birth, 21 cases of CSF leakage were identified by spinal sonography. Although obliteration of the subarachnoid space may occur when the fluid collection is extensive, complete resorption was observed in all cases with no evident sequelae.

Hypoxemia and clinical deterioration can occur in infants undergoing an LP, especially in those who are premature and VLBW with respiratory insufficiency.[26,114–116] Although drops in mean transcutaneous PO_2 may occur with each of the three most commonly used positions for an LP (lateral flexed, lateral extended, and upright position), the decrease in oxygenation is more prominent in the flexed position, leading some authors to recommend the upright or modified flexed position with neck extension in infants.[26,116] Preoxygenation before the LP has been recommended by some authors[115]; however, excessive oxygen administration may lead to increased morbidities (e.g., retinopathy of prematurity) and should not be routinely used.[117–119]

In addition to the increased risk of complications in premature infants, performing an LP in this population can be technically challenging due to the small anatomic structures. However, successful access of the subarachnoid space has been reported in small infants in the setting of administration of spinal anesthesia.[120–123] In technically challenging cases, the upright position facilitates the procedure, as it provides the largest interspinous space for the vast majority of infants and seems to be sufficiently safe.[121,124]

Are There Any Contraindications to Performing a Lumbar Puncture in the Newborn Infant?

Although thrombocytopenia is a significant risk factor for spinal hemorrhages,[125] reports in infants are scarce, and evidence supporting the appropriate platelet count threshold before inserting a needle or catheter is lacking.[126] To alleviate the risk of bleeding related to the procedure, thrombocytopenia may be corrected with platelet transfusion before the LP or epidural anesthesia. Studies in thrombocytopenic children with oncologic diseases requiring routine LPs reported no procedure-related hemorrhage with platelet counts $<50 \times 10^9/L$.[127–129] Currently, the National Institute for Health and Care Excellence (NICE) guidelines on the management of blood transfusions recommend considering prophylactic platelet transfusions to raise the platelet count above $50 \times 10^9/L$ in patients who are having invasive procedures.[130] Unless thrombocytopenia is profound ($<50 \times 10^9/L$), performing an LP in thrombocytopenic infants is likely safe, and delaying the procedure is not justified.

Skin infection near the site of puncture can increase the risk of spreading the infection with the needle from adjacent soft tissue into the bone, resulting in osteomyelitis.[131–133] Therefore, performing an LP over an area of infection is not recommended. LP should be deferred in severely ill infants with cardiorespiratory compromise, as it may produce hypoxemia and further clinical deterioration.[9] The 2010 NICE clinical guidelines on recognition, diagnosis, and management of bacterial meningitis in children recommend delaying LP when contraindications are present until they no longer exist. In all cases, the decision to perform an LP should not delay the initiation of antibiotic therapy.[134]

Lumbar Punctures in the Setting of Antibiotic Exposure: Are They Useful?

CSF cultures are the gold standard for the diagnosis of meningitis, but interpretation of LP results can be challenging. A significant number of infants are exposed to intrapartum or empiric antibiotics before LP, which can reduce the yield of CSF cultures and obscure the diagnosis of meningitis.[21,34,135] In a retrospective review including 128 children and infants from 1 day to 16 years of age with suspected or confirmed bacterial meningitis, parenteral exposure to third-generation cephalosporins before the performance of an LP resulted in CSF sterilization of meningococcus within 2 hours and pneumococcus within 4 to 10 hours of initiation of therapy.[34] Similarly, CSF cultures may be "falsely negative" in infants born to mothers who received intrapartum antibiotics for chorioamnionitis or GBS colonization. Many antimicrobial agents (including penicillin and ampicillin) cross the placenta, reaching the fetal circulation. Intrapartum antibiotics may interfere with the growth of bacteria and increase the likelihood of false-negative cultures.[21,35,47] The low yield of CSF cultures in the setting of antibiotic exposure may result in an inability to adjust therapy based on antimicrobial susceptibility or unnecessarily prolonged treatment if the possibility of bacterial meningitis cannot be excluded. However, delaying antimicrobial therapy has been associated with short-term morbidity, including seizures, subdural effusions, hemiparesis, and long-term neurologic impairments.[136] To avoid this situation, clinicians often rely on CSF parameters rather than cultures to determine the likelihood of meningitis. However, reference ranges of CSF parameters and those indicative of neonatal meningitis are the subject of debate and may be affected by several factors such as gestational age, postnatal age, antibiotic exposure, and traumatic taps.[137] The mean white blood cell (WBC) count in healthy, uninfected preterm or term infants in most studies is <10 cells/mm^3,[22,138–141] CSF protein concentrations in uninfected term infants are usually <100 mg/dL, whereas premature infants show higher values that vary inversely with gestational age.[140–143] CSF glucose concentrations in normoglycemic and noninfected infants are usually between 70% and 80% of the serum level,[10] with no significant differences between preterm and term infants[140,144]; values are lower in infants with meningitis.[22] CSF parameters collected from the largest cohort to date of premature infants demonstrated a poor positive predictive value (PPV) of WBC count, protein, and glucose levels for the diagnosis of meningitis (4%–10%).[22] Consistent with these findings, CSF glucose and protein values were highly variable in a study including 9111 near-term and term infants with and without meningitis. In addition, meningitis occurred in the presence of normal CSF parameters. Therefore, no single value was found useful to exclude the diagnosis of meningitis.[23] Based on these data, CSF parameters, either alone or in combination, have poor sensitivity and poor PPV for diagnosis of meningitis in both preterm and term infants in the absence of CSF cultures.

CSF parameters were studied among a cohort of 13,495 infants who underwent at least one LP for the evaluation of EOS and LOS due to GBS.[21] Infants with culture-proven GBS meningitis showed an increase in WBC count (271/mm^3 vs. 6/mm^3) and protein levels (322 mg/dL vs. 114 mg/dL) and a decrease in glucose concentrations (13 mg/dL vs. 49 mg/dL) compared with infants without meningitis. Because GBS meningitis also occurred among infants exposed to intrapartum prophylaxis and in the setting of negative blood cultures (20%), clinicians should not disregard the risk of GBS disease in the setting of IAP or when blood cultures are negative for GBS.[21]

The interpretation of the CSF WBC count in infants exposed to antibiotics is also complicated by the possibility of traumatic LPs, which occurs in up to 50% of cases.[145,146] When the CSF is contaminated with more than 10×10^9/L red cells, CSF WBC counts tend to be lower than predicted by calculations based on the red blood cell (RBC) to WBC ratio, disguising a true leukocytosis and masking the diagnosis of meningitis.[147] Although adjusting WBC counts based on CSF and peripheral RBC counts overestimates the number of WBC originating from the peripheral blood and underestimates CSF WBC, potentially leading to missed cases of meningitis,[145] the observed-to-predicted ratio, obtained by dividing the observed CSF WBC by the predicted CSF WBC, may help identify cases of meningitis despite CSF abnormalities in the setting of a traumatic LP.[148,149]

In summary, prenatal or empiric antibiotic exposure may decrease the sensitivity of CSF cultures, increasing the likelihood of false-negative results that can result in missed cases of meningitis. CSF parameters in the neonatal population are highly variable and may be further compromised by antibiotic exposure as well as traumatic taps. Although some CSF values are suggestive of meningitis, the PPV is poor, and meningitis can occur in the presence of normal WBC, protein, and glucose counts. Therefore, CSF cultures remain the gold standard for diagnosis even in the setting of antibiotic exposure and traumatic taps.

Repeating Lumbar Punctures in Infants With Meningitis: Is It Necessary?

Repeating an LP during the course of therapy in an infant with culture-proven meningitis has been the subject of debate. Some experts have recommended repeating LP in all patients 24 to 48 hours after initiation of antibiotic therapy to document CSF sterilization, as persistence of positive cultures despite treatment may result in a greater risk of complications and poor outcomes.[150,151] The rationale for repeating CSF examination has been well documented. A cohort study including 118 infants with culture-proven meningitis and repeat CSF cultures reported that clearance of infection occurred between 2 and 7 days after antibiotics were begun for different organisms. The presence of a second positive culture was associated with increased mortality.[152] With the emergence of antibiotic-resistant bacterial strains, a repeat LP might also be useful to guide antibiotic therapy in infants with no clinical improvement after 48 hours of appropriate antibiotic therapy.[153] Because rapid progression of meningitis has been observed, some authors suggested that repeating an LP may be justified when the first CSF culture is negative but the clinical picture and other laboratory tests are discordant.[154–157] However, published recommendations do not support repeating the LP routinely.[134,158] The AAP guidelines on Diagnosis and Management of Meningitis recommend repeating CSF examination in infants with no clinical evidence of improvement by 24 to 72 hours after the beginning of therapy.[158] In agreement with this, the NICE in 2010 issued guidelines on the management of meningitis and discouraged repeat LPs in infants who are receiving adequate antibiotic therapy and show clinical improvement. Furthermore, they do not recommend an LP before discontinuing therapy if the infant is clinically well.[134] Clinical practice appears to adhere to these guidelines; a survey among 109 pediatricians and neonatologists indicated that the majority of practitioners (82%) did not repeat LP and preferred a more selective approach based on the clinical findings in the infant.[159]

LPs are sometimes performed after treatment of meningitis to confirm cure by CSF normalization. Different criteria have been proposed for the assessment of CSF findings in the setting of repeated LPs at the end of antibiotic therapy ranging from normal to "acceptable" cell counts, protein, and glucose levels.[160] However, several authors have demonstrated that despite efficient antibiotic therapy, CSF pleocytosis and abnormally elevated protein concentration are commonly observed when treatment is discontinued.[160–162] Among infants with meningitis who cleared the infection and had at least one abnormal value at the time of the last positive culture, only 4% were found to eventually normalize CSF WBC counts, protein, and glucose levels.[152] Because the ranges of glucose and protein levels and cell counts at the end of treatment vary widely, CSF findings may lead to unnecessary intervention in uninfected infants while failing to recognize those still infected.[160,163] A retrospective study that included 165 infants >1 month of age with end-of-treatment LP found that 13 infants with no late complications or relapse were considered treatment failures based on "abnormal" findings in CSF, leading to additional courses of antibiotics, repeated LPs, and more hospital days. In addition, two patients who had signs consistent with complications of their meningitis had reassuring end-of-treatment CSF findings.[160] Consistent with these findings, a review of 47 children between 2 months and 15 years of age with culture-proven meningitis showed that persistence of CSF abnormalities was not associated with complications of the disease but with prolonged antibiotic treatment beyond 13 days.[163] Based on this evidence, the performance of LP at the end of treatment as a "test of cure" or to define length of therapy is not recommended.

Lumbar Punctures in Infants With Intraventricular Drainage Device–Associated Infection

Posthemorrhagic hydrocephalus is a major complication of intracranial hemorrhage in premature infants associated with significant morbidity and mortality, as well as poor neurodevelopmental outcomes among survivors.[164–166] Two temporary devices are commonly used before the permanent insertion of a ventriculoperitoneal (VP) shunt: The ventricular reservoir or ventricular access device is a CSF reservoir connected to a catheter inserted into the ventricles that allows decompression of the ventricular system by serial tapping, and the ventriculosubgaleal shunt consists of a large subgaleal pocket connected to a ventricular catheter that allows continuous CSF diversion.[167]

Infection is a common complication of intraventricular drainage devices (IVDDs) with a reported incidence between 8% and 11%,[168–170] with risk factors including prematurity,[171,172] gestational age at procedure,[168] and previous meningitis.[168,172] Shunt infections are a major source of morbidity and economic burden, with greater need for additional surgical procedures and longer hospital stays.[173,174] They are associated with neurodevelopmental disability[166] and a mortality rate that approaches 10%.[175]

In a cohort of 9704 infants who underwent LP, which included 181 infants with either a VP shunt or CSF reservoir placement, no significant differences were observed in WBC counts, protein, and glucose levels between those with or without drainage devices.[176] As noted earlier, CSF values in infants with devices were not useful in identifying infants with meningitis. Although CSF eosinophilia was previously considered a marker of infection in infants with IVDDs,[177] recent reports have found no clinical significance in the rise of this parameter for the diagnosis of infection.[176,178] In a case-control study of infants <34 weeks gestation with CSF reservoirs who underwent serial taps (5- to 8-day intervals), there was a wide variation in all CSF parameters in infants with negative or positive cultures with abnormal values even in the absence of infection.[170] In addition, the percentages of CSF neutrophils and protein were higher at insertion and declined significantly with subsequent taps, whereas RBC count, glucose, and proportion of lymphocytes and eosinophils showed no significant changes. The authors found that cutoff values of CSF WBC counts of >42/mm^3 and protein >250 mg/dL in later taps after the insertion of IVDDs may result in a sensitivity of almost 90%. However, CSF testing from IVDD in the absence of suspected infection is not recommended due to the limited diagnostic value.[170,176] Moreover, routine culture of shunt components removed at revision in the absence of clinical infection is not recommended, as evidence shows that bacteriologically positive cultures in asymptomatic infants in the majority of cases represents a contaminant and has no therapeutic implications.[179]

Summary

Meningitis is associated with significant morbidity and mortality in the neonatal population. CSF culture obtained via LP is the gold-standard method for the diagnosis of meningitis, and early initiation of antibiotic treatment is of paramount importance to reduce mortality and poor neurodevelopmental outcomes. The most common reason for not performing an LP is that the perceived low incidence of meningitis does not justify the risk of the procedure in an infant with respiratory or cardiovascular compromise. However, despite potential adverse events, LP is not associated with increased mortality. Although clinical practice varies, the current recommendation is to perform an LP routinely in all infants with bacteremia or neurologic signs/symptoms in the neonatal intensive care unit, regardless of gestational age, with

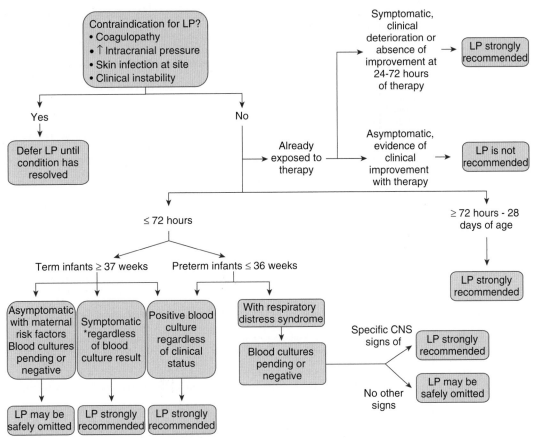

Figure 8.1 Summary of recommendations of performance of lumbar puncture in the evaluation of infants at risk for meningitis. *CNS,* central nervous system; *LP,* lumbar puncture. *Fever or hypothermia, irritability, hypotonia, poor feeding, apnea, hypotension, seizures, and bulging anterior fontanel.

suspected EOS or LOS. Before performing an LP, the infant must be clinically stable (Fig. 8.1). Repeating the LP during the course of treatment is only justified if there is no clinical evidence of improvement 24 to 72 hours after initiation of therapy, and it is not recommended at the end of treatment to confirm cure in bacterial meningitis.

REFERENCES

1. Heath PT, Okike IO. Neonatal bacterial meningitis: an update. *Paediatr Child Health.* 2010;20:526–530.
2. Okike IO, Johnson AP, Henderson KL, et al. Incidence, etiology, and outcome of bacterial meningitis in infants aged <90 days in the United Kingdom and Republic of Ireland: prospective, enhanced, national population-based surveillance. *Clin Infect Dis.* 2014;59:e150–e157.
3. Stoll BJ, Hansen N, Fanaroff AA, et al. To tap or not to tap: high likelihood of meningitis without sepsis among very low birth weight infants. *Pediatrics.* 2004;113:1181–1186.
4. Stoll BJ, Hansen NI, Sánchez PJ, et al. Early onset neonatal sepsis: the burden of group b streptococcal and e. coli disease continues. *Pediatrics.* 2011;127:817–826.
5. Heath PT, Okike IO, Oeser C. Neonatal meningitis: can we do better? *Adv Exp Med Biol.* 2011;719:11–24.
6. Gaschignard J, Levy C, Romain O, et al. Neonatal bacterial meningitis: 444 cases in 7 years. *Pediatr Infect Dis J.* 2011;30:212–217.
7. de Louvois J, Halket S, Harvey D. Neonatal meningitis in England and Wales: sequelae at 5 years of age. *Eur J Pediatr.* 2005;164:730–734.
8. Polin RA, Harris MC. Neonatal bacterial meningitis. *Semin Neonatol.* 2001;6:157–172.
9. Riordan FA, Cant AJ. When to do a lumbar puncture. *Arch Dis Child.* 2002;87:235–237.
10. Polin RA. Committee on Fetus and Newborn: Management of neonates with suspected or proven early-onset neonatal sepsis. *Pediatrics.* 2012;129:1006–1015.
11. Johnson CE, Whitwell JK, Pethe K, et al. Term newborns who are at risk for sepsis: are lumbar punctures necessary? *Pediatrics.* 1997;99:E10.

12. Mecredy RL, Wiswell TE, Hume RF. Outcome of term gestation neonates whose mothers received intrapartum antibiotics for suspected chorioamnionitis. *Am J Perinatol.* 1993;10:365–368.

13. Ray B, Mangalore J, Harikumar C, et al. Is lumbar puncture necessary for evaluation of early neonatal sepsis? *Arch Dis Child.* 2006;91:1033–1035.

14. Fielkow S, Reuter S, Gotoff SP. Cerebrospinal fluid examination in symptom-free infants with risk factors for infection. *J Pediatr.* 1991;119:971–973.

15. Schwersenski J, McIntyre L, Bauer CR. Lumbar puncture frequency and cerebrospinal fluid analysis in the neonate. *Am J Dis Child.* 1991;145:54–58.

16. Hendricks-Munoz KD, Shapiro DL. The role of the lumbar puncture in the admission sepsis evaluation of the premature infant. *J Perinatol.* 1990;10:60–64.

17. Eldadah M, Frenkel LD, Hiatt IM, et al. Evaluation of routine lumbar punctures in newborn infants with respiratory distress syndrome. *Pediatr Infect Dis J.* 1987;6:243–246.

18. Weiss MG, Ionides SP, Anderson CL. Meningitis in premature infants with respiratory distress: role of admission lumbar puncture. *J Pediatr.* 1991;119:973–975.

19. Visser VE, Hall RT. Lumbar puncture in the evaluation of suspected neonatal sepsis. *J Pediatr.* 1980;96:1063–1067.

20. Hoque MM, Ahmed AS, Chowdhury MA, et al. Septicemic neonates without lumbar puncture: what are we missing? *J Trop Pediatr.* 2006;52:63–65.

21. Ansong AK, Smith PB, Benjamin DK, et al. Group B streptococcal meningitis: cerebrospinal fluid parameters in the era of intrapartum antibiotic prophylaxis. *Early Hum Dev.* 2009;85:S5–S7.

22. Smith PB, Garges HP, Cotton CM, et al. Meningitis in preterm neonates: importance of cerebrospinal fluid parameters. *Am J Perinatol.* 2008;25:421–426.

23. Garges HP, Moody MA, Cotten CM, et al. Neonatal meningitis: what is the correlation among cerebrospinal fluid cultures, blood cultures, and cerebrospinal fluid parameters? *Pediatrics.* 2006;117:1094–1100.

24. MacMahon P, Jewes L, de Louvois J. Routine lumbar punctures in the newborn—are they justified? *Eur J Pediatr.* 1990;149:797–799.

25. Ajayi OA, Mokuolu OA. Evaluation of neonates with risk for infection/suspected sepsis: Is routine lumbar puncture necessary in the first 72 hours of life? *Trop Med Int Health.* 1997;2:284–288.

26. Weisman LE, Merenstein GB, Steenbarger JR. The effect of lumbar puncture position in sick neonates. *Am J Dis Child.* 1983;137:1077–1079.

27. Teele DW, Dashefsky B, Rakusan T, et al. Meningitis after lumbar puncture in children with bacteremia. *N Engl J Med.* 1981;305:1079–1081.

28. Bergman I, Wald ER, Meyer JD, et al. Epidural abscess and vertebral osteomyelitis following serial lumbar punctures. *Pediatrics.* 1983;72:476–480.

29. Addy DP. When not to do a lumbar puncture. *Arch Dis Child.* 1987;62:873–875.

30. Slack J. Coning and lumbar puncture. *Lancet.* 1980;2:474–475.

31. Potgieter S, Dimin S, Lagae L, et al. Epidermoid tumours associated with lumbar punctures performed in early neonatal life. *Dev Med Child Neurol.* 1998;40:266–269.

32. McIntyre P, Isaacs D. Lumbar puncture in suspected neonatal sepsis. *J Paediatr Child Health.* 1995;31:1–2.

33. Adams-Chapman I, Bann CM, Das A, et al. Neurodevelopmental outcome of extremely low birth weight infants with Candida infection. *J Pediatr.* 2013;163:961–7e3.

34. Kanegaye JT, Soliemanzadeh P, Bradley JS. Lumbar puncture in pediatric bacterial meningitis: defining the time interval for recovery of cerebrospinal fluid pathogens after parenteral antibiotic pretreatment. *Pediatrics.* 2001;108:1169–1174.

35. Wiswell TE, Baumgart S, Gannon CM, et al. No lumbar puncture in the evaluation for early neonatal sepsis: will meningitis be missed? *Pediatrics.* 1995;95:803–806.

36. Pong A, Bradley JS. Bacterial meningitis and the newborn infant. *Infect Dis Clin N Am.* 1999;13:711–733.

37. Camacho-Gonzalez A, Spearman PW, Stoll BJ. Neonatal infectious diseases: evaluation of neonatal sepsis. *Pediatr Clin N Am.* 2013;60:367–389.

38. Saunders NR, Dreifuss JJ, Dziegielewska KM, et al. The rights and wrongs of blood-brain barrier permeability studies: a walk through 100 years of history. *Front Neurosci.* 2014;8:404.

39. Bauer CH, New MI, Miller JM. Cerebrospinal fluid protein values of premature infants. *J Pediatr.* 1965;66:1017–1022.

40. Dammann O, Leviton A. Brain damage in preterm newborns: might enhancement of developmentally regulated endogenous protection open a door for prevention? *Pediatrics.* 1999;104:541–550.

41. Perlman JM. White matter injury in the preterm infant: an important determination of abnormal neurodevelopment outcome. *Early Hum Dev.* 1998;53:99–120.

42. Jacobsson B. Infectious and inflammatory mechanisms in preterm birth and cerebral palsy. *Eur J Obstet Gynecol Reprod Biol.* 2004;115:159–160.

43. Schlapbach LJ, Aebischer M, Adams M, et al. Impact of sepsis on neurodevelopmental outcome in a Swiss National Cohort of extremely premature infants. *Pediatrics.* 2011;128:e348–e357.

44. Mitha A, Foix-L'Helias L, Arnaud C, et al. Neonatal infection and 5-year neurodevelopmental outcome of very preterm infants. *Pediatrics.* 2013;132:e372–e380.

45. Adams-Chapman I, Stoll BJ. Neonatal infection and long-term neurodevelopmental outcome in the preterm infant. *Cur Opin Infect Dis.* 2006;19:290–297.

46. Doctor BA, Newman N, Minich NM, et al. Clinical outcomes of neonatal meningitis in very-low birth-weight infants. *Clin Pediatr (Phila).* 2001;40:473–480.

47. Verani JR, McGee L, Schrag SJ. Prevention of perinatal group B streptococcal disease–revised guidelines from CDC, 2010. *MMWR Recomm Rep.* 2010;59:1–36.

48. Stoll BJ, Hansen N, Fanaroff AA, et al. Changes in pathogens causing early-onset sepsis in very-low-birth-weight infants. *N Engl J Med*. 2002;347:240–247.
49. Hornik CP, Fort P, Clark RH, et al. Early and late onset sepsis in very-low-birth-weight infants from a large group of neonatal intensive care units. *Early Hum Dev*. 2012;88:S69–S74.
50. Weston EJ, Pondo T, Lewis MM, et al. The burden of invasive early-onset neonatal sepsis in the United sSates, 2005–2008. *Pediatr Infect Dis J*. 2011;30:937–941.
51. Vergnano S, Menson E, Kennea N, et al. Neonatal infections in England: the NeonIN surveillance network. *Arch Dis Child Fetal Neonatal*. 2011;Ed 96:F9–F14.
52. Phares CR, Lynfield R, Farley MM, et al. Epidemiology of invasive group B streptococcal disease in the United States, 1999-2005. *JAMA*. 2008;299:2056–2065.
53. Patrick SW, Schumacher RE, Davis MM. Variation in lumbar punctures for early onset neonatal sepsis: a nationally representative serial cross-sectional analysis, 2003-2009. *BMC Pediatr*. 2012;12:134.
54. Shane AL, Stoll BJ. Neonatal sepsis: progress towards improved outcomes. *J Infect*. 2014;68(suppl 1):S24–S32.
55. Stoll BJ, Hansen N, Fanaroff AA, et al. Late-onset sepsis in very low birth weight neonates: the experience of the NICHD Neonatal Research Network. *Pediatrics*. 2002;110:285–291.
56. Chu A, Hageman JR, Schreiber M, et al. Antimicrobial therapy and late onset sepsis. *NeoReviews*. 2012;13:e94–e102.
57. Benjamin DK Jr, Stoll BJ, Gantz MG, et al. Neonatal candidiasis: epidemiology, risk factors, and clinical judgment. *Pediatrics*. 2010;126:e865–e873.
58. Benjamin DK Jr, Stoll BJ, Fanaroff AA, et al. Neonatal candidiasis among extremely low birth weight infants: risk factors, mortality rates, and neurodevelopmental outcomes at 18 to 22 months. *Pediatrics*. 2006;117:84–92.
59. Jordan HT, Farley MM, Craig A, et al. Revisiting the need for vaccine prevention of late-onset neonatal group B streptococcal disease: a multistate, population-based analysis. *Pediatr Infect Dis J*. 2008;27:1057–1064.
60. Joshi P, Barr P. The use of lumbar puncture and laboratory tests for sepsis by Australian neonatologists. *J Paediatr Child Health*. 1998;34:74–78.
61. Flidel-Rimon O, Leibovitz E, Eventov Friedman S, et al. Is lumbar puncture (LP) required in every workup for suspected late-onset sepsis in neonates? *Acta Paediatr*. 2011;100:303–304.
62. Cohen-Wolkowiez M, Smith PB, Mangum B, et al. Neonatal Candida meningitis: significance of cerebrospinal fluid parameters and blood cultures. *J Perinatol*. 2007;27:97–100.
63. Zea-Vera A, Turin CG, Rueda MS, et al. [Use of lumbar puncture in the evaluation of late-onset sepsis in low birth weight neonates]. *Rev Peru Med Exp Salud Publica*. 2016;33:278–282.
64. Malbon K, Mohan R, Nicholl R. Should a neonate with possible late onset infection always have a lumbar puncture? *Arch Dis Child*. 2006;91:75–76.
65. Millichap J. Lumbar puncture in late onset neonatal infection. *Pediatr Neurol Briefs*. 2006;20:6–7.
66. Kaul V, Harish R, Ganjoo S, et al. Importance of obtaining lumbar puncture in neonates with late onset septicemia a hospital based observational study from north-west India. *J Clin Neonatol*. 2013;2:83–87.
67. Norris CM, Danis PG, Gardner TD. Aseptic meningitis in the newborn and young infant. *Am Fam Physician*. 1999;59:2761–2770.
68. Romero JR, Newland JG. Viral meningitis and encephalitis: traditional and emerging viral agents. *Semin Pediatr Infect Dis*. 2003;14:72–82.
69. March B, Eastwood K, Wright IM, et al. Epidemiology of enteroviral meningoencephalitis in neonates and young infants. *J Paediatr Child Health*. 2014;50:216–220.
70. Verboon-Maciolek MA, Groenendaal F, Cowan F, et al. White matter damage in neonatal enterovirus meningoencephalitis. *Neurology*. 2006;66:1267–1269.
71. Callen J, Paes BA. A case report of a premature infant with coxsackie B1 meningitis. *Adv Neonatal Care*. 2007;7:238–247.
72. Schlapbach LJ, Ersch J, Balmer C, et al. Enteroviral myocarditis in neonates. *J Paediatr Child Health*. 2013;49:E451–E454.
73. Freund MW, Kleinveld G, Krediet TG, et al. Prognosis for neonates with enterovirus myocarditis. *Arch Dis Child Fetal Neonatal*. 2010;Ed 95:F206–F212.
74. Morriss FH, Lindower JB, Bartlett HL, et al. Neonatal Enterovirus infection: case series of clinical sepsis and positive cerebrospinal fluid polymerase chain reaction test with myocarditis and cerebral white matter injury complications. *AJP Reports*. 2016;6:e344–e351.
75. Hawkes MT, Vaudry W. Nonpolio enterovirus infection in the neonate and young infant. *Paediatrics & Child Health*. 2005;10:383–388.
76. Hysinger EB, Mainthia R, Fleming A. Enterovirus meningitis with marked pleocytosis. *Hosp Pediatr*. 2012;2:173–176.
77. Mulford WS, Buller RS, Arens MQ, et al. Correlation of cerebrospinal fluid (CSF) cell counts and elevated CSF protein levels with enterovirus reverse transcription-PCR results in pediatric and adult patients. *J Clin Microbiol*. 2004;42:4199–4203.
78. Graham AK, Murdoch DR. Association between cerebrospinal fluid pleocytosis and enteroviral meningitis. *J Clin Microbiol*. 2005;43:1491.
79. Klein-Kremer A, Nir V, Eias K, et al. ClinicaliInvestigation: The presence of viral meningitis without pleocytosis among pediatric patients. *Open J Pediatr*. 2014;04:276–282.
80. Brown ZA, Wald A, Morrow RA, et al. Effect of serologic status and cesarean delivery on transmission rates of herpes simplex virus from mother to infant. *JAMA*. 2003;289:203–209.
81. Overall JC Jr. Herpes simplex virus infection of the fetus and newborn. *Pediatr Ann*. 1994;23:131–136.

82. Rudnick CM, Hoekzema GS. Neonatal herpes simplex virus infections. *Am Fam Physician*. 2002;65: 1138–1142.

83. Martin RJ, Fanaroff AA, Walsh MC. *Fanaroff and Martin's Neonatal-perinatal medicine: diseases of the fetus and infant*, 2010, 841–845.

84. Amel Jamehdar S, Mammouri G, Sharifi Hoseini MR, et al. Herpes simplex virus infection in neonates and young infants with sepsis. *Iran Red Crescent Med J*. 2014;16:e14310.

85. Malm G, Forsgren M. Neonatal herpes simplex virus infections: HSV DNA in cerebrospinal fluid and serum. *Arch Dis Child Fetal Neonatal*. 1999;Ed 81:F24–F29.

86. Anderson NE, Powell KF, Croxson MC. A polymerase chain reaction assay of cerebrospinal fluid in patients with suspected herpes simplex encephalitis. *J Neurol Neurosurg Psychiatry*. 1993;56:520–525.

87. Rowley AH, Whitley RJ, Lakeman FD, et al. Rapid detection of herpes-simplex-virus DNA in cerebrospinal fluid of patients with herpes simplex encephalitis. *Lancet*. 1990;335:440–441.

88. Kimberlin DW, Lin CY, Jacobs RF, et al. Natural history of neonatal herpes simplex virus infections in the acyclovir era. *Pediatrics*. 2001;108:223–229.

89. Malm G. Neonatal herpes simplex virus infection. *Semin Fetal Neonatal Med*. 2009;14:204–208.

90. Kimberlin DW, Baley J, Brady MT, et al. Guidance on management of asymptomatic neonates born to women with active genital herpes lesions. *Pediatrics*. 2013;131:e635–e646.

91. Kimberlin DW, Lakeman FD, Arvin AM, et al. Application of the polymerase chain reaction to the diagnosis and management of neonatal herpes simplex virus disease. National Institute of Allergy and Infectious Diseases Collaborative Antiviral Study Group. *J Infect Dis*. 1996;174:1162–1167.

92. Mejias A, Bustos R, Ardura MI, et al. Persistence of herpes simplex virus DNA in cerebrospinal fluid of neonates with herpes simplex virus encephalitis. *J Perinatol*. 2009;29:290–296.

93. Kimberlin D. Herpes simplex virus, meningitis and encephalitis in neonates. *Herpes*. 2004;11(suppl 2):65a–76a.

94. Troendle-Atkins J, Demmler GJ, Buffone GJ. Rapid diagnosis of herpes simplex virus encephalitis by using the polymerase chain reaction. *J Pediatr*. 1993;123:376–380.

95. Petersdorf RG, Swarner DR, Garcia M. Studies on the pathogenesis of meningitis. II. Development of meningitis during pneumococcal bacteremia. *J Clin Invest*. 1962;41:320–327.

96. Weed LH, Wegeforth P, Ayer JB, et al. The production of meningitis by release of cerebrospinal fluid: During an experimental septicemia: preliminary note. *JAMA*. 1919;72:190–193.

97. Pray LG. LUmbar puncture as a factor in the pathogenesis of meningitis. *Am J Dis Child*. 1941;62: 295–308.

98. Eng RH, Seligman SJ. Lumbar puncture-induced meningitis. *JAMA*. 1981;245:1456–1459.

99. Williams J, Lye DC, Umapathi T. Diagnostic lumbar puncture: minimizing complications. *Intern Med J*. 2008;38:587–591.

100. Harper JR, Lorber J, Hillas Smith G, et al. Timing of lumbar puncture in severe childhood meningitis. *Br Med J (Clin Res Ed)*. 1985;291:651–652.

101. Davies PA, Rudd PT. Neonatal meningitis. *Clin Devel Med*. 1994;132:83.

102. Polin RA. *Workbook in Practical Neonatology*. 5th ed. 2015:335.

103. Kalay S, Öztekin O, Tezel G, et al. Cerebellar herniation after lumbar puncture in galactosemic newborn. *AJP Reports*. 2011;1:43–46.

104. Thibert RL, Burns JD, Bhadelia R, et al. Reversible uncal herniation in a neonate with a large MCA infarct. *Brain Dev*. 2009;31:763–765.

105. Ziv ET, Gordon McComb J, Krieger MD, et al. Iatrogenic intraspinal epidermoid tumor: two cases and a review of the literature. *Spine (Phila 1976)*. 2004;29:E15–E18.

106. Batnitzky S, Keucher TR, Mealey J Jr, et al. Iatrogenic intraspinal epidermoid tumors. *JAMA*. 1977;237:148–150.

107. Shaywitz BA. Epidermoid spinal cord tumors and previous lumbar punctures. *J Pediatr*. 1972;80: 638–640.

108. Halcrow SJ, Crawford PJ, Craft AW. Epidermoid spinal cord tumour after lumbar puncture. *Arch Dis Child*. 1985;60:978–979.

109. Adler MD, Comi AE, Walker AR. Acute hemorrhagic complication of diagnostic lumbar puncture. *Pediatr Emerg Care*. 2001;17:184–188.

110. Faillace WJ, Warrier I, Canady AI. In an Infant with Previously Undiagnosed Hemophilia A: Treatment and Peri-operative Considerations. *Clin Pediatr*. 1989;28:136–138.

111. Cromwell LD, Kerber C, Ferry PC. Spinal cord compression and hematoma: an unusual complication in a hemophiliac infant. *AJR Am J Roentgenol*. 1977;128:847–849.

112. Tubbs RS, Smyth MD, Wellons JC, et al. Intramedullary hemorrhage in a neonate after lumbar puncture resulting in paraplegia: a case report. *Pediatrics*. 2004;113:1403–1405.

113. Kiechl-Kohlendorfer U, Unsinn KM, Schlenck B, et al. Cerebrospinal fluid leakage after lumbar puncture in neonates: incidence and sonographic appearance. *AJR Am J Roentgenol*. 2003;181:231–234.

114. Sun S, Vangvanichyakorn K, Aranda Z, et al. Harmful effect of lumbar puncture in newborn infants. *Pediatr Res*. 1981;15:684.

115. Fiser DH, Gober GA, Smith CE, et al. Prevention of hypoxemia during lumbar puncture in infancy with preoxygenation. *Pediatr Emerg Care*. 1993;9:81–83.

116. Gleason CA, Martin RJ, Anderson JV, et al. Optimal position for a spinal tap in preterm infants. *Pediatrics*. 1983;71:31–35.

117. Weinberger B, Laskin DL, Heck DE, et al. Oxygen toxicity in premature infants. *Toxicol Appl Pharmacol*. 2002;181:60–67.

118. Shahzad T, Radajewski S, Chao CM, et al. Pathogenesis of bronchopulmonary dysplasia: when inflammation meets organ development. *Mol Cell Pediatr*. 2016;3:23.

119. Hartnett ME. Pathophysiology and mechanisms of severe retinopathy of prematurity. *Ophthalmology*. 2015;122:200–210.
120. Williams RK, Abajian JC. High spinal anaesthesia for repair of patent ductus arteriosus in neonates. *Pediatr Anesth*. 1997;7:205–209.
121. Webster AC, McKishnie JD, Kenyon CF, et al. Spinal anaesthesia for inguinal hernia repair in high-risk neonates. *Can J Anaesth*. 1991;38:281–286.
122. Nickel US, Meyer RR, Brambrink AM. Spinal anesthesia in an extremely low birth weight infant. *Paediatr Anaesth*. 2005;15:58–62.
123. Libby A. Spinal anesthesia in preterm infant undergoing herniorrhaphy. *Aana j*. 2009;77:199–206.
124. Oncel S, Gunlemez A, Anik Y, et al. Positioning of infants in the neonatal intensive care unit for lumbar puncture as determined by bedside ultrasonography. *Arch Dis Child Fetal Neonatal*. 2013;Ed 98:F133–F135.
125. Evans RW. Complications of lumbar puncture. *Neurol Clin*. 1998;16:83–105.
126. Estcourt LJ, Ingram C, Doree C, et al. Use of platelet transfusions prior to lumbar punctures or epidural anaesthesia for the prevention of complications in people with thrombocytopenia. *Cochrane Database Syst Rev*. 2016;(12):Cd011980.
127. Foerster MV, Pedrosa Fde P, da Fonseca TC, et al. Lumbar punctures in thrombocytopenic children with cancer. *Paediatr Anaesth*. 2015;25:206–210.
128. van Veen JJ, Vora AJ, Welch JC. Lumbar puncture in thrombocytopenic children. *Brit J Haematol*. 2004;127:233–234.
129. Howard SC, Gajjar A, Ribeiro RC, et al. Safety of lumbar puncture for children with acute lymphoblastic leukemia and thrombocytopenia. *JAMA*. 2000;284:2222–2224.
130. Pasquali SK, Sanders SP, Li JS. Oral antihypertensive trial design and analysis under the pediatric exclusivity provision. *Am Heart J*. 2002;144:608–614.
131. Wald ER. Risk factors for osteomyelitis. *Am J Med*. 1985;78:206–212.
132. Findlay L, Kemp FH. Osteomyelitis of the spine following lumbar puncture. *Arch Dis Child*. 1943;18: 102–105.
133. Feinbloom RI, Halaby FA. Acute pyogenic spondylitis in infancy: a case report to emphasize the potential risk in lumbar puncture. *Clin Pediatri*. 1966;5:683–684.
134. NICE: Meningitis (bacterial) and meningococcal septicaemia in under 16s: recognition, diagnosis and management. 2010.
135. Feldman WE. Effect of prior antibiotic therapy on concentrations of bacteria in CSF. *Am J Dis Child*. 1978;132:672–674.
136. Lebel MH, McCracken GH Jr. Delayed cerebrospinal fluid sterilization and adverse outcome of bacterial meningitis in infants and children. *Pediatrics*. 1989;83:161–167.
137. Srinivasan L, Harris MC, Shah SS. Lumbar puncture in the neonate: challenges in decision making and interpretation. *Semin Perinatol*. 2012;36:445–453.
138. Byington CL, Kendrick J, Sheng X. Normative cerebrospinal fluid profiles in febrile infants. *J Pediatr*. 2011;158:130–134.
139. Kestenbaum LA, Ebberson J, Zorc JJ, et al. Defining cerebrospinal fluid white blood cell count reference values in neonates and young infants. *Pediatrics*. 2010;125:257–264.
140. Nascimento-Carvalho CM, Moreno-Carvalho OA. Normal cerebrospinal fluid values in full-term gestation and premature neonates. *Arq Neuropsiquiatr*. 1998;56:375–380.
141. Ahmed A, Hickey SM, Ehrett S, et al. Cerebrospinal fluid values in the term neonate. *Pediatr Infect Dis J*. 1996;15:298–303.
142. Shah SS, Ebberson J, Kestenbaum LA, et al. Age-specific reference values for cerebrospinal fluid protein concentration in neonates and young infants. *J Hosp Med*. 2011;6:22–27.
143. Bonadio WA, Stanco L, Bruce R, et al. Reference values of normal cerebrospinal fluid composition in infants ages 0 to 8 weeks. *Pediatr Infect Dis J*. 1992;11:589–591.
144. Srinivasan L, Shah SS, Padula MA, et al. Cerebrospinal fluid reference ranges in term and preterm infants in the neonatal intensive care unit. *J Pediatr*. 2012;161:729–734.
145. Greenberg RG, Smith PB, Cotten CM, et al. Traumatic lumbar punctures in neonates: test performance of the cerebrospinal fluid white blood cell count. *Pediatr Infect Dis J*. 2008;27:1047–1051.
146. Schreiner RL, Kleiman MB. Incidence and effect of traumatic lumbar puncture in the neonate. *Dev Med Child Neurol*. 1979;21:483–487.
147. Osborne JP, Pizer B. Effect on the white cell count of contaminating cerebrospinal fluid with blood. *Arch Dis Child*. 1981;56:400–401.
148. Bonadio WA, Smith DS, Goddard S, et al. Distinguishing cerebrospinal fluid abnormalities in children with bacterial meningitis and traumatic lumbar puncture. *J Infect Dis*. 1990;162:251–254.
149. Mazor SS, McNulty JE, Roosevelt GE. Interpretation of traumatic lumbar punctures: who can go home? *Pediatrics*. 2003;111:525–528.
150. Heath PT, Nik Yusoff NK, Baker CJ. Neonatal meningitis. *Arch Dis Child Fetal Neonatal*. 2003;88: 173–178.
151. Freij BJ, McCracken Jr GH. *Acute Infections. Avery's Neonatology: Pathophysiology and Management of The Newborn*. 5th ed. Philadelphia: Lippincott, Williams and Wilkins; 1999:1207–1211.
152. Greenberg RG, Benjamin DK, Cohen-Wolkowiez M, et al. Repeat lumbar punctures in infants with meningitis in the neonatal intensive care unit. *J Perinatol*. 2011;31:425–429.
153. Tunkel AR, Scheld WM. Issues in the management of bacterial meningitis. *Am Fam Physician*. 1997;56:1355–1362.
154. Kindley AD, Harris F. Repeat lumbar puncture in the diagnosis of meningitis. *Arch Dis Child*. 1978;53:590–592.

8

155. Rapkin RH. Repeat lumbar punctures in the diagnosis of meningitis. *Pediatrics*. 1974;54:34–37.
156. Fischer GW, Brenz RW, Alden ER, et al. Lumbar punctures and meningitis. *Am J Dis Child*. 1975;129:590–592.
157. Heckmatt JZ. Coliform meningitis in the newborn. *Arch Dis Child*. 1976;51:569–575.
158. Klein JO, Feigin RD, McCracken GH Jr. Report of the Task Force on Diagnosis and Management of Meningitis. *Pediatrics*. 1986;78:959–982.
159. Agarwal R, Emmerson AJB. Should repeat lumbar punctures be routinely done in neonates with bacterial meningitis? Results of a survey into clinical practice. *Arch Dis Child*. 2001;84:450.
160. Durack DT, Spanos A. End-of-treatment spinal tap in bacterial meningitis. Is it worthwhile? *JAMA*. 1982;248:75–78.
161. Chartrand SA, Cho CT. Persistent pleocytosis in bacterial meningitis. *J Pediatr*. 1976;88:424–426.
162. Bonadio WA, Smith D. Cerebrospinal fluid changes after 48 hours of effective therapy for Hemophilus influenzae type B meningitis. *Am J Clin Pathol*. 1990;94:426–428.
163. Jacob J, Kaplan RA. Bacterial meningitis. Limitations of repeated lumbar puncture. *Am J Dis Child*. 1977;131:46–48.
164. Murphy BP, Inder TE, Rooks V, et al. Posthaemorrhagic ventricular dilatation in the premature infant: natural history and predictors of outcome. *Arch Dis Child Fetal Neonatal*. 2002;Ed 87:F37–F41.
165. Adams-Chapman I, Hansen NI, Stoll BJ, et al. Neurodevelopmental outcome of extremely low birth weight infants with posthemorrhagic hydrocephalus requiring shunt insertion. *Pediatrics*. 2008;121: e1167–e1177.
166. Resch B, Gedermann A, Maurer U, et al. Neurodevelopmental outcome of hydrocephalus following intra-/periventricular hemorrhage in preterm infants: short- and long-term results. *Childs Nerv Syst*. 1996;12:27–33.
167. Robinson S. Neonatal posthemorrhagic hydrocephalus from prematurity: pathophysiology and current treatment concepts: A review. *J Neurosurg Pediatr*. 2012;9:doi:103171/201112PEDS11136.
168. Spader HS, Hertzler DA, Kestle JR, et al. Risk factors for infection and the effect of an institutional shunt protocol on the incidence of ventricular access device infections in preterm infants. *J Neurosurg Pediatr*. 2015;15:156–160.
169. Drake JM, Kestle JR, Milner R, et al. Randomized trial of cerebrospinal fluid shunt valve design in pediatric hydrocephalus. *Neurosurgery*. 1998;43:294–303, discussion -5.
170. Bajaj M, Lulic-Botica M, Natarajan G. Evaluation of cerebrospinal fluid parameters in preterm infants with intraventricular reservoirs. *J Perinatol*. 2012;32:786–790.
171. Bruinsma N, Stobberingh EE, Herpers MJ, et al. Subcutaneous ventricular catheter reservoir and ventriculoperitoneal drain-related infections in preterm infants and young children. *Clin Microbiol Infect*. 2000;6:202–206.
172. McGirt MJ, Zaas A, Fuchs HE, et al. Risk factors for pediatric ventriculoperitoneal shunt infection and predictors of infectious pathogens. *Clin Infect Dis*. 2003;36:858–862.
173. Kanik A, Sirin S, Kose E, et al. Clinical and economic results of ventriculoperitoneal shunt infections in children. *Turk Neurosurg*. 2015;25:58–62.
174. Morina Q, Kelmendi F, Morina A, et al. Ventriculoperitoneal shunt complications in a developing country: a single institution experience. *Med Arch*. 2013;67:36–38.
175. Vinchon M, Dhellemmes P. Cerebrospinal fluid shunt infection: risk factors and long-term follow-up. *Childs Nerv Syst*. 2006;22:692–697.
176. Lenfestey RW, Smith PB, Moody MA, et al. Predictive value of cerebrospinal fluid parameters in neonates with intraventricular drainage devices. *J Neurosurg*. 2007;107:209–212.
177. Wiersbitzky SK, Ahrens N, Becker T, et al. The diagnostic importance of eosinophil granulocytes in the CSF of children with ventricular-peritoneal shunt systems. *Acta Neurol Scand*. 1998;97:201–203.
178. Lan CC, Wong TT, Chen SJ, et al. Early diagnosis of ventriculoperitoneal shunt infections and malfunctions in children with hydrocephalus. *J Microbiol Immunol Infect*. 2003;36:47–50.
179. Steinbok P, Cochrane DD, Kestle JR. The significance of bacteriologically positive ventriculoperitoneal shunt components in the absence of other signs of shunt infection. *J Neurosurg*. 1996;84:617–623.
180. Kumar P, Sarkar S, Narang A. Role of routine lumbar puncture in neonatal sepsis. *J Paediatr Child Health*. 1995;31:8–10.

CHAPTER 9

Biomarkers in the Diagnosis of Neonatal Sepsis

James Lawrence Wynn, MD, J. Lauren Ruoss, MD

- Biomarkers to detect sepsis are of increasing interest but have not replaced standard microbial cultures for neonatal sepsis.
- Development of biomarkers is limited by a lack of definition for neonatal sepsis.

Introduction

Globally, sepsis results in over 1 million neonatal deaths annually, which has resulted in targeted interventions from the Centers for Disease Control, World Health Organization, and the Bill & Melinda Gates Foundation to reduce this unacceptable burden.[1,2] In developed countries, four of every ten infants that develop sepsis die or develop lifelong major disabilities.[3,4] Neonatal sepsis may occur early after birth (<3 days of life, early-onset sepsis [EOS]) or late (≥3 days after birth, late-onset sepsis [LOS]). Where antenatal intrapartum antibiotic prophylaxis has been implemented, the burden of group B streptococcus (GBS) has been greatly reduced, yet the mortality for culture-positive EOS remains high at 30% in developed countries.[5] Similarly, the implementation of interventions aimed at reducing bloodstream infections has had a positive impact, but a substantial LOS burden remains for our most immature infants.[6] Static risk factors, including gestational age (GA), very low birth weight (VLBW), central venous lines, and prolonged exposure to early antibiotics, are associated with a greater risk of developing LOS.[6–8] The presence of these static risk factors in a high-risk population in the setting of equivocal early clinical signs often prompts evaluation, including ancillary laboratory testing and frequently empiric antimicrobial treatment. As Machiavelli surmised so elegantly in 1532 (*The Prince, N. Machiavelli, 1532*), "hectic fever (sepsis) at its inception is difficult to recognize but easy to treat; left untended [it] becomes easy to recognize but difficult to treat." Despite decades of research aimed at the identification of an ideal, accurate, and early diagnostic test(s) to identify septic infants,[4] little progress has made its way to the bedside clinician's toolkit. Diagnostic biomarkers to detect infection can be *direct* (detect live pathogen or a pathogen's molecular traits) or *indirect* (measure the host's response). A limitation in accuracy and reproducibility of diagnostic biomarkers has led to significant controversy over which markers should be used and the recognition that neonatal sepsis is variably defined.[9] In adult and pediatric populations, consensus definitions for sepsis have been established to better align investigators toward the goal of clinical improvement.[10,11] The critical importance of a consensus definition

Conflict of interest statement: The authors have declared that no conflicts of interest exist.

Disclosure of funding: National Institutes of Health (NIH)/National institutes of General Medical Science (GM106143).

Acknowledgments: None

for neonatal sepsis, particularly for researchers, has been reviewed in detail elsewhere.[12,13] In this chapter, we will review the advantages and limitations of several types of biomarkers used to diagnose neonatal sepsis, but the use of a variable definition for the primary outcome (sepsis) is a significant limitation of all studies discussed.

Pathogen Biomarkers

Pathogen detection is classically accomplished by isolation and growth of the organism from a normally sterile site. A positive blood culture remains the "gold standard" for neonatal sepsis despite having many disadvantages, which have been recently reviewed.[12–15] Limitations of culture-based methods have prompted exploration using highly sensitive molecular modalities that target detection of pathogen-specific nucleic acids. Real-time polymerase chain reaction (PCR) (organism specific versus multiplex assays), PCR followed by post-PCR processing (including array-based hybridization or mass spectroscopy), and beacon-based fluorescence in situ hybridization (FISH) are used to detect bacterial-specific ribosome subunit DNA (16sRNA DNA).[16] These technologies are promising because of the potential for rapid results and a requirement for only a small amount of blood to accurately detect pathogen nucleic acids.[17] FISH-based detection of 16sRNA DNA can identify bacteria within 45 minutes with high sensitivity (94%) and specificity (100%).[18] Use of PCR to detect 16sRNA DNA has a large range of sensitivities and specificities compared with blood cultures in diagnosis of neonatal sepsis, with sensitivities as low as 41%.[16,17,19–22] Chan et al. showed that although PCR detected 16sRNA DNA in blood from 5 infants with blood culture–negative sepsis it was negative in 9/42 culture-positive infections (4 were coagulase-negative *Staphylococcus*).[19] Jordan et al. showed PCR could detect bacteria using only 200 microliters of blood with a high sensitivity (96%) and specificity (99%) compared with blood cultures.[23] A meta-analysis of 23 studies found that molecular assays that targeted 16sRNA DNA, including real-time PCR and broad-range conventional PCR, had pooled mean sensitivity of only 90% with a specificity of 96%, with real-time PCR being the most sensitive.[16] Due to the heterogeneity of these studies, including varying GA, different methodologies of DNA extraction used, inclusion of different disease states (LOS vs. EOS), and arbitrary definition of sepsis, interpretation of the results is challenging. The authors concluded that the molecular assays reviewed could not replace standard microbial cultures because the sensitivity was <98%.[16] Post-PCR mass spectroscopy may also be used to rapidly identify pathogens; however, similar to FISH and PCR alone, sensitivity was <90%.[24] Collectively, the broad range of reported sensitivities, cost, and technical difficulty of the assays have limited the widespread use of molecular assays for pathogen detection.[19,20] In the VIRIoN study, respiratory viruses detected by PCR were positive in 6% of neonatal sepsis evaluations, highlighting the utility of molecular methods to detect pathogens other than bacteria.[25] Viral infection may play a significant role in neonatal events that prompt antibiotic treatment and may in part explain why as many as 91% of neonatal sepsis evaluations are culture negative.[26] The limitations of pathogen biomarker detection prompt clinicians to rely heavily on clinical presentation or biomarkers produced by the host to diagnose neonatal sepsis.

Host Response

The host immune response to sepsis begins with the development of a local inflammatory response that underlies and precedes the manifestation of clinical signs and leads to detectable immune system responses (biomarkers). Pathogen-associated molecular patterns, including cell surface components and nucleic acids, as well as components of damaged host cells (damage-associated molecular patterns) are sensed by sentinel immune cells via several classes of pathogen recognition receptors (e.g., Toll-like receptors).[27] Activation of these receptors leads to intracellular signaling via second messenger systems and ultimately to gene expression of acute-phase proteins that promulgate the inflammatory response, including cytokines and chemokines. These acute-phase proteins subsequently lead to activation of the local endothelial environment by promoting production of cytokines, chemokines, and vasodilators such as nitric oxide. These mediators recruit and activate circulating white blood cells (WBCs), including an increase in expression of cell surface molecules that facilitate their exit from the bloodstream into the infected area. When the infection is severe or no longer locally confined, exaggerated activation of endothelium and the resultant systemic inflammation result in significant clinical signs and more dramatic changes in ancillary laboratory test results. These host immune response mediators produced during infection and their actions are the primary targets of host-based biomarker testing for sepsis.

Acute-Phase Response Proteins

Acute-phase proteins produced early after the onset of infection and circulating in the blood include interleukin (IL) proteins, chemokines, and proinflammatory cytokines. Three commonly studied biomarkers include IL-6, IL-8, and tumor necrosis factor (TNF)-α. The benefits of measuring these biomarkers include rapid rate of rise, short half-life, limited changes in the setting of noninfectious conditions such as respiratory distress syndrome,[28] and elevation across gestational ages.[29] IL-6 increases in the early stages of the infection, but the sensitivity decreases over time due to its short half-life of 12 to 24 hours.[4,28,30] Small studies have shown that IL-8 can be used to diagnose EOS and as a marker of antibiotic effectiveness.[31,32] In 105 infants (25–37 weeks) with suspected sepsis (LOS and EOS), Laborada et al. showed that IL-6, IL-8, C-reactive protein (CRP), and immature to total (I/T) were significantly higher at the onset of infection in the septic group (n = 48) compared with the nonseptic group (n = 57).[33] This study also showed that IL-6, IL-8, and TNF-α in isolation had low sensitivities (66%–76%) and specificities (60%–73%); however, when IL-6 and CRP were combined, the sensitivity and specificity increased (89% and 73%, respectively). IL-6, IL-8, and TNF-α were poor markers of infection at 24 hours, with low sensitivity (49%–63%) and specificity (72%–79%), most likely secondary to their short half-lives. In a meta-analysis of 13 studies, IL-6 had a pooled sensitivity (79%) and specificity (84%) with an area under the curve (AUC) of 0.89 for neonatal sepsis.[34] A meta-analysis of TNF-α found that the pooled sensitivity and specificity for EOS (66% and 76%) was lower than for LOS (68% and 88%).[35] This study also compared TNF-α, procalcitonin (PCT), and CRP for diagnosing LOS and found that PCT had the highest sensitivity but lowest specificity, whereas CRP had the lowest sensitivity and comparable specificity to TNF-α. The authors concluded that the ability to predict LOS using TNF-α is similar to CRP and PCT, which are more readily available biomarkers. A limitation of pooling these studies together for comparison is that the accuracy of these biomarkers is significantly affected by the timing of sepsis (EOS versus LOS), timing of laboratory test draws, use of single versus serial measurements, and age of the infant. Several studies have evaluated the diagnostic utility of chemokine/cytokine profiles, alone or in conjunction with other inflammatory response proteins, in infants with EOS, LOS,[36] and in extremely low birth weight infants with bacterial and fungal sepsis.[37] Proteins involved in cell adhesion and inflammation (i.e., P-selectin, E-selectin, IL-2 soluble receptor α, IL-18, IL-10, transforming growth factor-β, and CRP) were elevated in infants with EOS and LOS compared with healthy controls.[36,37] Of those proteins, IL-18 showed the greatest degree of change from uninfected infants; significant elevation of IL-18 has been shown in other cohorts of human infants with sepsis.[37,38] IL-18 is a proinflammatory member of the IL-1 cytokine family that is released in response to infection. It plays a role in both innate and adaptive immunity[39] and is elevated in in vivo murine models of GBS[40] and polymicrobial sepsis.[38] Larger studies are needed to better understand the utility of these biomarkers in the diagnosis of neonatal sepsis.

PCT is a hormokine made by monocytes and hepatocytes in response to stimulation by TNF-α, IL-1β, IL-2, or IL-6.[41] PCT has a delayed rise in concentration of 2 to 4 hours after onset of infection and increases at 6 to 8 hours, with a peak at 12 to 24 hours.[42,43] PCT is not affected by maternal antibiotic administration[44] and can be used to monitor the effect of antibiotic coverage because it plateaus and then decreases after antibiotic treatment.[45] PCT interpretation is challenging for EOS because of an unexplained physiologic increase after birth, peaking at 10 ng/mL on day of life 1, with decline by day of life 2 to 4.[44–47] In an observational study of 762 VLBW and normal birth weight infants evaluated for LOS, PCT was higher in infants with blood culture–positive sepsis compared with culture-negative sepsis.[42] This study also showed that the predictive utility of PCT varied with birth weight with a PCT <2.4 ng/mL indicating absence of infection in infants weighing >1500 g at birth (sensitivity 58%, specificity 79%) and >2.4 ng/mL indicating infection in VLWBs with low positive predictive value (PPV, 50%), sensitivity (62%), and specificity (84%).[42] Results of studies that compared PCT with CRP in the setting of EOS have also been controversial, where varying sensitivities and specificities occurred most likely secondary to the timing of evaluation and the definition of sepsis used.[45,48] A meta-analysis of 29 studies found that the overall pooled sensitivity (81%) and specificity (79%) for PCT to diagnose EOS or LOS was low, with an AUC of 0.87.[44] When evaluating EOS and LOS studies separately, the authors found a higher sensitivity and specificity in the LOS group (90% sensitivity, 88% specificity, AUC 0.95) in comparison to the EOS group (76% sensitivity, 76% specificity, AUC 0.78). This finding is most likely attributed to the natural physiologic increase in PCT after birth, as well as the delay of rise of PCT after onset of infection. The results of the Neonatal Procalcitonin Intervention Study (NeoPInS) study, a multicenter randomized superiority and noninferiority trial, will shed light on whether PCT can be used to guide treatment in EOS.[49]

CRP is commonly used in the evaluation of neonatal sepsis. Pathogen-induced IL-6 production by macrophages acts on the hepatocyte to produce CRP. It takes approximately 4 to 6 hours for CRP production to begin after stimulation by IL-6, and production peaks 24 to 48 hours after a single stimulus.[50] However, the long half-life of CRP (18 hours) and 1000-fold dynamic range (0.3 mg/L–300 mg/L) make this biomarker useful to demonstrate the presence of systemic inflammation when measured serially. CRP has multiple advantages, including the small amount of blood needed, rapid results, and absence of an effect of maternal antibiotic administration on neonatal blood levels.[45,46,51] However, CRP is a nonspecific and late marker of inflammation with a low sensitivity at the onset of the infection, which limits its prospective diagnostic utility.[9,52] CRP is affected by multiple causes of inflammation other than neonatal infection, including maternal infection, prolonged rupture of membranes, delivery room resuscitation, and noninfectious causes of neonatal inflammation.[9] Although >10 mg/L is commonly used as a cutoff for CRP,[9,53] suggested normative values for CRP change based on timing of afterbirth with 5 mg/L at birth, 14 mg/L at 24 hours, and 9.7 mg/L at 48 hours.[54] Studies that have evaluated the accuracy of CRP to diagnose neonatal sepsis have produced a large range of sensitivities (35%–94%) and specificities (60%–96%), which most likely reflect that the accuracy of this diagnostic test is affected by the timing of when it was drawn, whether serial measurements were used, and whether it was used in EOS versus LOS.[55] In addition, early CRP levels may not be useful to indicate appropriate antibiotic coverage because the level may continue to rise until 48 hours.[45,46,52] Kocabas et al. compared the diagnostic abilities of single measurements of PCT, CRP, IL-6, IL-8, and TNF-α at the time of evaluation to diagnose neonatal sepsis. All markers demonstrated a high AUC (ranging from 0.9–1.00) with the exception of CRP, which had an AUC of 0.68. TNF-α and PCT had high sensitivities and specificities (>96%) compared with CRP's low sensitivity, leading to the conclusion that CRP was not as useful as PCT or TNF-α at diagnosing neonatal sepsis.[56] Benitz et al. showed that, although CRP had dismal PPV, serially normal CRPs obtained 24 hours apart at least 8 hours after onset of infection had a remarkably high negative predictive value (NPV 99.7%).[50] Serial CRPs can be used to identify the presence and severity of inflammation, but the slow-response kinetics of CRP production do not readily support its use to screen for infection.

WBC and WBC Indices

Despite large epidemiologic reports that show limited sensitivity for this long-used diagnostic testing method, the complete blood count (CBC) and differential is, in practice, the most commonly used biomarker for identification of sepsis.[4,57] Its advantages include the wide availability, small amount of blood needed, and rapid results. However, the components of the CBC are affected by age, maternal history (specifically pregnancy-induced hypertension), venous versus arterial blood draw, delivery mode, altitude, and gender, in addition to causes of inflammation other than infection.[9,57–59] These limitations may, in part, account for its low sensitivity for EOS[58] and low PPV.[60] Newman et al. studied 67,623 infants ≥34 weeks estimated gestational age who had an EOS evaluation and found that the CBC was more predictive of infection if drawn >4 hours after birth.[58] Although obtaining a CBC >4 hours after birth improved its reliability, the authors cautioned that "even when the CBC is optimally interpreted, decisions about antibiotic treatment should remain highly dependent on maternal risk factors and newborn symptoms of infection." Hornik et al. evaluated the accuracy of the CBC in 203,918 infants with EOS or LOS and found that although some CBC parameters were associated with infection, no parameter possessed adequate sensitivity to accurately rule out EOS or LOS.[61,62] The odds of sepsis were increased if the WBC count was low (compared with infants for whom it was high),[58,61,63] but the WBC was "normal" in 60% of infants with a positive blood culture.[61] Newman et al. found that the absolute neutrophil count (ANC) was more predictive if drawn >4 hours after birth,[58] however Hornik et al. showed 59% of blood culture positive infants with EOS had an ANC between 1–10,000/mm^3.[62] Murphy et al. studied 3213 infants with sepsis evaluations and found that serial I/T of >0.2 was a more reliable marker of infection than WBC or absolute neutrophil count alone.[64] Other studies reported a better sensitivity and NPV with I/T compared with other components of the CBC, but noted that I/T alone was not accurate enough to rule in or out an infection.[57,58,61] Van der Meer et al. asked 756 laboratory technicians from 157 unique hospital laboratories to review a slide presentation of 100 individual Giemsa-stained cells taken from a peripheral blood smear of a septic patient and assigned each cell a leukocyte type (manual differential). Striking intralaboratory and interlaboratory variation in interpretations for neutrophils (15%–72%, SD 11%) and for band forms (4%–64%, SD 11%) were reported, which suggests the interpretation of the band count and thus the I/T ratio may limit use of the I/T ratio as a definition criterion.[65] Although components of the CBC are the most commonly used laboratory marker to evaluate for infection, in isolation they do not have the sensitivity and specificity to rule out neonatal sepsis, and the I/T ratio should be used with extreme caution given the high rate of interreader variability.[60]

WBC Surface Markers

Infection leads to activation of WBCs through upregulation of cell surface receptors and cell surface markers, including neutrophil CD64 (nCD64), CD11b, CD14, and human leukocyte antigens. Of the cell surface markers, CD64 (FcγRI), a receptor that binds the Fc portion of gamma immunoglobulin, is the most well studied and has shown significant promise. CD64 expression rises rapidly at the onset of an infection and stays elevated for a minimum of 24 hours and can be measured rapidly in a small amount of blood.[29,66] However, fluorescence-activated cell sorting (flow cytometry) is required to identify cell surface markers, including CD64, which requires specialized, often costly laboratory equipment as well as highly trained laboratory staff that may not be available in all centers.[67] CD64 is not affected by other clinical conditions, including respiratory distress syndrome, transient tachypnea of the newborn, or prolonged rupture of membranes, but CD64 expression may be higher in preterm infants compared with term infants.[68,69] Streimish et al. found that among 749 infants, CD64 showed high sensitivity and modest specificity for EOS (100% and 68%) with lower sensitivity but better specificity for LOS (75% and 77%).[67] CD64 had better predictive value when compared with CRP at time of diagnosis, likely secondary to its rapid rise at the onset of an infection.[70] A meta-analysis evaluated the utility of CD64 to diagnose neonatal sepsis and included 17 studies with 3478 infants.[71] The pooled sensitivity (77%) and specificity (74%) were lower than the results of the meta-analysis for PCT as a diagnostic biomarker, suggesting PCT may be superior.[44] The sensitivity and specificity were also higher in the culture-positive sepsis group compared with the clinical sepsis group (blood culture negative plus clinical signs) and in term infants (80%, 85%) compared with preterm infants (74%, 69%). A higher sensitivity was shown for EOS in comparison to LOS, but with a lower specificity. The conclusion of this analysis was that CD64 could not reliably be used to diagnose neonatal sepsis.[71] The results suggest this marker may be better in term infants with EOS as an adjunct to other laboratory tests.

CD11b is a neutrophil cell surface protein that facilitates adhesion, migration, phagocytosis, chemotaxis, cellular activation, and cytotoxicity.[72,73] Use of this integrin as a biomarker is supported by the rapid increase in surface expression with a peak at 2 hours after the onset of infection.[74] In umbilical cord blood inoculated with GBS, CD11b expression had a higher sensitivity (95%) and specificity (100%) compared with CD64 expression (specificity of 48%) for detecting the most common GBS strains.[74] Adib et al. found that in septic infants (27–38 weeks), CD11b demonstrated low sensitivity (75%) but high specificity (100%), and when combined with CRP the sensitivity increased to 100%.[75] CD14 is present on macrophages, monocytes, and neutrophils; leads to a cascade of events releasing cytokines (TNF-α, IL-6, IL-8); and may be increased in the setting of physiologic stressors other than infection.[76] Presepsin is a fragment of soluble CD14 (sCD14) that reflects active bacterial phagocytosis.[77] Presepsin levels drawn in healthy term and preterm infants did not differ by GA but were higher than what was observed in adults.[78] Another study compared presepsin levels in premature infants with and without LOS and found that at time of evaluation presepsin was higher in the LOS group (100% sensitivity and 67% specificity).[79] Presepsin, CD11b, and CD64 may be useful as adjunct laboratory tests in conjunction with other biomarkers.

Metabolomic, Proteomic, and Transcriptomic Biomarker Approaches

Metobolomics is defined as "the quantitative measurement of the metabolic response of living systems to pathophysiologic stimuli or genetic modification,"[80] and the study of metabolomics is facilitated by mass spectrometry to rapidly detect metabolites.[81] Strikingly, the plasma metabolome and proteome were not different between survivors in any group of the sepsis continuum (sepsis, severe sepsis, septic shock) among adults.[82] In contrast, significant defects in mitochondrial function (defect in fatty acid beta oxidation) and mobilization of energetic substrates (including citrate, malate, pyruvate, dihydroxyacetone, lactate, phosphate, and gluconeogenic amino acids) were increased in adult sepsis nonsurvivors. The authors suggested that sepsis survivors mobilized various energetic substrates to use in aerobic catabolism, resulting in decreased plasma concentrations, whereas sepsis nonsurvivors failed to use these fully. Based on the results of the study the authors created an algorithm using clinical markers and metabolites to predict mortality. Mickiewicz et al. used nuclear magnetic resonance spectroscopy–based metabolomics to show that serum metabolites could be used to diagnose and predict morbidity and mortality in pediatric patients with septic shock[80] and were useful to differentiate children with sepsis requiring care in a pediatric intensive care unit (PICU) from children with or without sepsis who can be safely cared for outside a PICU.[83] Stewart et al. evaluated the serum proteome and metabolome of infants with necrotizing enterocolitis (NEC) and LOS compared with controls and found that no unique protein or metabolite could be identified from infants with NEC or LOS.[81] However, Fanos et al. found that there were alterations in urine metabolites in infants with sepsis compared with uninfected controls, including increased glucose, lactate, and acetate, and decreased 2,3,4-trihydroxybutyric acid, ribitol, ribonic acid, and citrate.[84] Ng et al. used an unbiased mass spectroscopy-based proteomic approach on neonatal plasma samples to discover biomarkers for sepsis and/or NEC using a case-control discovery phase followed by prospective study of an independent cohort to generate a composite biomarker that delivered an AUC of 0.93 (95% CI 0.87–0.98, $P < 0.001$).[85]

Transcriptomic profiling can identify diagnostic and prognostic gene signatures and novel therapeutic targets, uncover mechanisms behind differential sepsis outcomes, and reveal rapid and dynamic shifts in transcription patterns associated with various phases of sepsis.[86-90] Using transcriptomic profiling on whole blood, Wynn et al. showed term (completed at least 36 weeks' gestation) infants with septic shock manifested a unique host response compared with other pediatric patient groups (toddlers and school-age children)[86] and that timing of sepsis after birth was a critical determinant of the host response to sepsis in premature infants.[91] Using genome-wide transcriptomic profiling on neonatal whole blood, Cernada et al. and Hilgendorf et al. identified profiles that discriminated septic from nonseptic infants, and Smith et al. identified a 52-gene classifier that predicted sepsis.[92-94] Although more investigation is clearly needed to identify unique metabolites to support a predictive algorithm in neonatal sepsis, metabolomics, proteomic, and transcriptomic approaches hold significant promise to reveal previously unknown or unsuspected differences between states of health and disease and molecular endotypes among diseased patients. Importantly, the sensitivity of these techniques can amplify heterogeneity among even similar study subjects, which underscores the critical need to establish a consensus definition of sepsis to reduce variability in research studies to maximize the diagnostic and prognostic utility of these approaches.[12]

Despite advances in the management of infants, mortality and morbidity due to sepsis remain unacceptably high.[3,95] Diagnostic and management decisions regarding neonatal sepsis remain controversial, but before this controversy can be settled there needs to be a consensus on the definition of neonatal sepsis.[12] Despite the heterogeneity of this diagnosis and the population it affects, a consensus statement would allow for improved trials to better evaluate available tools.[13] In the era of precision medicine, the ability to accurately predict who is at risk for sepsis and define why they are at increased risk based on molecular phenotyping would revolutionize how we approach the septic infant.

Summary

Biomarkers that target pathogen products using molecular assays are an expanding field but have not surpassed the use of standard microbial cultures in infants evaluated for sepsis. Biomarkers of host response to infection, including acute-phase reactants, cytokine/chemokines, leukocyte count, and cell surface marker expression, as well as "-omic" approaches, may help with diagnosis and prognosis of septic infants. The greatest barrier to achieving accurate diagnostic and prognostic biomarkers for neonatal sepsis remains the absence of a consensus definition of sepsis.

REFERENCES

1. Lawn JE, Cousens S, Zupan J, et al. 4 million neonatal deaths: when? Where? Why? *Lancet*. 2005;365:891–900.
2. Liu L, Johnson HL, Cousens S, et al. Global, regional, and national causes of child mortality: an updated systematic analysis for 2010 with time trends since 2000. *Lancet*. 2012;379:2151–2161.
3. The INIS Collaborative Group, Brocklehurst P, Farrell B, et al. Treatment of neonatal sepsis with intravenous immune globulin. *N Engl J Med*. 2011;365:1201–1211.
4. Celik HT, Portakal O, Yigit S, et al. Efficacy of new leukocyte parameters versus serum C-reactive protein, procalcitonin, and interleukin-6 in the diagnosis of neonatal sepsis. *Pediatr Int*. 2016;58:119–125.
5. Cortese F, Scicchitano P, Gesualdo M, et al. Early and late infections in newborns: where do we stand? A review. *Pediatr Neonatol*. 2016;57:265–273.
6. Stoll BJ, Hansen N, Fanaroff AA, et al. Late-onset sepsis in very low birth weight neonates: the experience of the NICHD Neonatal Research Network. *Pediatrics*. 2002;110:285–291.
7. Stoll BJ, Hansen NI, Bell EF, et al. Neonatal outcomes of extremely preterm infants from the NICHD Neonatal Research Network. *Pediatrics*. 2010;126:443–456.
8. Fanaroff AA, Korones SB, Wright LL, et al. Incidence, presenting features, risk factors and significance of late onset septicemia in very low birth weight infants. The National Institute of Child Health and Human Development Neonatal Research Network. *Pediatr Infect Dis J*. 1998;17:593–598.
9. Chiesa C, Panero A, Osborn JF, et al. Diagnosis of neonatal sepsis: a clinical and laboratory challenge. *Clin Chem*. 2004;50:279–287.
10. Seymour CW, Liu VX, Iwashyna TJ, et al. Assessment of Clinical Criteria for Sepsis: For the Third International Consensus Definitions for Sepsis and Septic Shock (Sepsis-3). *JAMA*. 2016;315:762–774.
11. Goldstein B, Giroir B, Randolph A, et al. International pediatric sepsis consensus conference: definitions for sepsis and organ dysfunction in pediatrics. *Pediatr Crit Care Med*. 2005;6:2–8.
12. Wynn JL, Wong HR, Shanley TP, et al. Time for a neonatal-specific consensus definition for sepsis. *Pediatr Crit Care Med*. 2014;15:523–528.

13. Wynn JL. Defining neonatal sepsis. *Curr Opin Pediatr*. 2016;28:135–140.
14. Abiramalatha T, Santhanam S, Mammen JJ, et al. Utility of neutrophil volume conductivity scatter (VCS) parameter changes as sepsis screen in neonates. *J Perinatol*. 2016;36:733–738.
15. Bizzarro MJ, Raskind C, Baltimore RS, et al. Seventy-five years of neonatal sepsis at Yale: 1928-2003. *Pediatrics*. 2005;116:595–602.
16. Pammi M, Flores A, Leeflang M, et al. Molecular assays in the diagnosis of neonatal sepsis: a systematic review and meta-analysis. *Pediatrics*. 2011;128:e973–e985.
17. Frayha HH, Kalloghlian A. Gram-specific quantitative polymerase chain reaction for diagnosis of neonatal sepsis: implications for clinical practice. *Crit Care Med*. 2009;37:2487–2488.
18. Sakarikou C, Parisato M, Lo Cascio G, et al. Beacon-based (bbFISH(R)) technology for rapid pathogens identification in blood cultures. *BMC Microbiol*. 2014;14:99.
19. Chan KY, Lam HS, Cheung HM, et al. Rapid identification and differentiation of Gram-negative and Gram-positive bacterial bloodstream infections by quantitative polymerase chain reaction in preterm infants. *Crit Care Med*. 2009;37:2441–2447.
20. Jordan JA, Durso MB, Butchko AR, et al. Evaluating the near-term infant for early onset sepsis: progress and challenges to consider with 16S rDNA polymerase chain reaction testing. *J Mol Diagn*. 2006;8:357–363.
21. Wu YD, Chen LH, Wu XJ, et al. Gram stain-specific-probe-based real-time PCR for diagnosis and discrimination of bacterial neonatal sepsis. *J Clin Microbiol*. 2008;46:2613–2619.
22. Shang S, Chen G, Wu Y, et al. Rapid diagnosis of bacterial sepsis with PCR amplification and microarray hybridization in 16S rRNA gene. *Pediatr Res*. 2005;58:143–148.
23. Jordan JA, Durso MB. Comparison of 16S rRNA gene PCR and BACTEC 9240 for detection of neonatal bacteremia. *J Clin Microbiol*. 2000;38:2574–2578.
24. Srinivasan L, Harris MC. New technologies for the rapid diagnosis of neonatal sepsis. *Curr Opin Pediatr*. 2012;24:165–171.
25. Ronchi A, Michelow IC, Chapin KC, et al. Viral respiratory tract infections in the neonatal intensive care unit: the VIRIoN-I study. *J Pediatr*. 2014;165:690–696.
26. Hornik CP, Fort P, Clark RH, et al. Early and late onset sepsis in very-low-birth-weight infants from a large group of neonatal intensive care units. *Early Hum Dev*. 2012;88(suppl 2):S69–S74.
27. Wynn JL, Wong HR. Pathophysiology and Treatment of Septic Shock in Neonates. *Clin Perinatol*. 2010;37:439–479.
28. Chiesa C, Pellegrini G, Panero A, et al. C-reactive protein, interleukin-6, and procalcitonin in the immediate postnatal period: influence of illness severity, risk status, antenatal and perinatal complications, and infection. *Clin Chem*. 2003;49:60–68.
29. Ng PC, Lee CH, Lam CW, et al. Transient adrenocortical insufficiency of prematurity and systemic hypotension in very low birthweight infants. *Arch Dis Child Fetal Neonatal Ed*. 2004;89:F119–F126.
30. Volante E, Moretti S, Pisani F, et al. Early diagnosis of bacterial infection in the neonate. *J Matern Fetal Neonatal Med*. 2004;16(suppl 2):13–16.
31. Franz AR, Steinbach G, Kron M, et al. Reduction of unnecessary antibiotic therapy in newborn infants using interleukin-8 and C-reactive protein as markers of bacterial infections. *Pediatrics*. 1999;104:447–453.
32. Nupponen I, Andersson S, Jarvenpaa AL, et al. Neutrophil CD11b expression and circulating interleukin-8 as diagnostic markers for early-onset neonatal sepsis. *Pediatrics*. 2001;108:E12.
33. Laborada G, Rego M, Jain A, et al. Diagnostic value of cytokines and C-reactive protein in the first 24 hours of neonatal sepsis. *Am J Perinatol*. 2003;20:491–501.
34. Shahkar L, Keshtkar A, Mirfazeli A, et al. The role of IL-6 for predicting neonatal sepsis: a systematic review and meta-analysis. *Iran J Pediatr*. 2011;21:411–417.
35. Lv B, Huang J, Yuan H, et al. Tumor necrosis factor-alpha as a diagnostic marker for neonatal sepsis: a meta-analysis. *ScientificWorldJournal*. 2014;2014:471463.
36. Kingsmore SF, Kennedy N, Halliday HL, et al. Identification of diagnostic biomarkers for infection in premature neonates. *Mol Cell Proteomics*. 2008;7:1863–1875.
37. Sood BG, Shankaran S, Schelonka RL, et al. Cytokine profiles of preterm neonates with fungal and bacterial sepsis. *Pediatr Res*. 2012;72:212–220.
38. Wynn JL, Wilson CS, Hawiger J, et al. Targeting IL-17A attenuates neonatal sepsis mortality induced by IL-18. *Proc Natl Acad Sci USA*. 2016;113:E2627–E2635.
39. Mickiewicz B, Tam P, Jenne CN, et al. Integration of metabolic and inflammatory mediator profiles as a potential prognostic approach for septic shock in the intensive care unit. *Crit Care*. 2015;19:11.
40. Cusumano V, Midiri A, Cusumano VV, et al. Interleukin-18 is an essential element in host resistance to experimental group B streptococcal disease in neonates. *Infect Immun*. 2004;72:295–300.
41. Oberhoffer M, Stonans I, Russwurm S, et al. Procalcitonin expression in human peripheral blood mononuclear cells and its modulation by lipopolysaccharides and sepsis-related cytokines in vitro. *J Lab Clin Med*. 1999;134:49–55.
42. Auriti C, Fiscarelli E, Ronchetti MP, et al. Procalcitonin in detecting neonatal nosocomial sepsis. *Arch Dis Child Fetal Neonatal Ed*. 2012;97:F368–F370.
43. Dandona P, Nix D, Wilson MF, et al. Procalcitonin increase after endotoxin injection in normal subjects. *J Clin Endocrinol Metab*. 1994;79:1605–1608.
44. Vouloumanou EK, Plessa E, Karageorgopoulos DE, et al. Serum procalcitonin as a diagnostic marker for neonatal sepsis: a systematic review and meta-analysis. *Intensive Care Med*. 2011;37:747–762.
45. Kordek A, Torbe A, Tousty J, et al. The Determination of Procalcitonin Concentration in Early-Onset Neonatal Infection: A Valuable Test Regardless of Prenatal Antibiotic Therapy. *Clin Pediatr (Phila)*. 2016.

46. Chiesa C, Natale F, Pascone R, et al. C reactive protein and procalcitonin: reference intervals for preterm and term newborns during the early neonatal period. *Clin Chim Acta*. 2011;412:1053–1059.

47. Stocker M, Fontana M, El Helou S, et al. Use of procalcitonin-guided decision-making to shorten antibiotic therapy in suspected neonatal early-onset sepsis: prospective randomized intervention trial. *Neonatology*. 2010;97:165–174.

48. van Rossum AM, Wulkan RW. Oudesluys-Murphy AM: Procalcitonin as an early marker of infection in neonates and children. *Lancet Infect Dis*. 2004;4:620–630.

49. Stocker M, Hop WC, van Rossum AM. Neonatal Procalcitonin Intervention Study (NeoPInS): Effect of Procalcitonin-guided decision making on duration of antibiotic therapy in suspected neonatal early-onset sepsis: A multi-centre randomized superiority and non-inferiority Intervention Study. *BMC Pediatr*. 2010;10:89.

50. Benitz WE, Han MY, Madan A, et al. Serial serum C-reactive protein levels in the diagnosis of neonatal infection. *Pediatrics*. 1998;102:E41.

51. Patil S, Dutta S, Attri SV, et al. Serial C reactive protein values predict sensitivity of organisms to empirical antibiotics in neonates: a nested case-control study. *Arch Dis Child Fetal Neonatal Ed*. 2016.

52. Hofer N, Zacharias E, Muller W, et al. An update on the use of C-reactive protein in early-onset neonatal sepsis: current insights and new tasks. *Neonatology*. 2012;102:25–36.

53. Haque KN. Definitions of bloodstream infection in the newborn. *Pediatr Crit Care Med*. 2005;6:S45–S49.

54. Chiesa C, Signore F, Assumma M, et al. Serial measurements of C-reactive protein and interleukin-6 in the immediate postnatal period: reference intervals and analysis of maternal and perinatal confounders. *Clin Chem*. 2001;47:1016–1022.

55. Ng PC, Lam HS. Diagnostic markers for neonatal sepsis. *Curr Opin Pediatr*. 2006;18:125–131.

56. Kocabas E, Sarikcioglu A, Aksaray N, et al. Role of procalcitonin, C-reactive protein, interleukin-6, interleukin-8 and tumor necrosis factor-alpha in the diagnosis of neonatal sepsis. *Turk J Pediatr*. 2007;49:7–20.

57. Polin RA, Committee on F, Newborn. Management of neonates with suspected or proven early-onset bacterial sepsis. *Pediatrics*. 2012;129:1006–1015.

58. Newman TB, Puopolo KM, Wi S, et al. Interpreting complete blood counts soon after birth in newborns at risk for sepsis. *Pediatrics*. 2010;126:903–909.

59. Christensen RD, Lambert DK, Schmutz N, et al. Fatal bowel necrosis in two polycytemic term neonates. *Fetal Pediatr Pathol*. 2008;27:41–44.

60. Benitz WE. Adjunct laboratory tests in the diagnosis of early-onset neonatal sepsis. *Clin Perinatol*. 2010;37:421–438.

61. Hornik CP, Benjamin DK, Becker KC, et al. Use of the complete blood cell count in late-onset neonatal sepsis. *Pediatr Infect Dis J*. 2012;31:803–807.

62. Hornik CP, Benjamin DK, Becker KC, et al. Use of the complete blood cell count in early-onset neonatal sepsis. *Pediatr Infect Dis J*. 2012;31:799–802.

63. Philip AG, Hewitt JR. Early diagnosis of neonatal sepsis. *Pediatrics*. 1980;65:1036–1041.

64. Murphy K, Weiner J. Use of leukocyte counts in evaluation of early-onset neonatal sepsis. *Pediatr Infect Dis J*. 2012;31:16–19.

65. van der Meer W, van Gelder W, de Keijzer R, et al. Does the band cell survive the 21st century? *Eur J Haematol*. 2006;76:251–254.

66. Dilli D, Oguz SS, Dilmen U, et al. Predictive values of neutrophil CD64 expression compared with interleukin-6 and C-reactive protein in early diagnosis of neonatal sepsis. *J Clin Lab Anal*. 2010;24:363–370.

67. Streimish I, Bizzarro M, Northrup V, et al. Neutrophil CD64 as a diagnostic marker in neonatal sepsis. *Pediatr Infect Dis J*. 2012;31:777–781.

68. Fjaertoft G, Hakansson L, Foucard T, et al. CD64 (Fcgamma receptor I) cell surface expression on maturing neutrophils from preterm and term newborn infants. *Acta Paediatr*. 2005;94:295–302.

69. Miyake F, Ishii M, Hoshina T, et al. Analysis of the Physiological Variation in Neutrophil CD64 Expression during the Early Neonatal Period. *Am J Perinatol*. 2016.

70. Choo YK, Cho HS, Seo IB, et al. Comparison of the accuracy of neutrophil CD64 and C-reactive protein as a single test for the early detection of neonatal sepsis. *Korean J Pediatr*. 2012;55:11–17.

71. Shi J, Tang J, Chen D. Meta-analysis of diagnostic accuracy of neutrophil CD64 for neonatal sepsis. *Ital J Pediatr*. 2016;42:57.

72. Srinivasan G, Aitken JD, Zhang B, et al. Lipocalin 2 deficiency dysregulates iron homeostasis and exacerbates endotoxin-induced sepsis. *J Immunol*. 2012;189:1911–1919.

73. Zhou H, Liao J, Aloor J, et al. CD11b/CD18 (Mac-1) is a novel surface receptor for extracellular double-stranded RNA to mediate cellular inflammatory responses. *J Immunol*. 2013;190:115–125.

74. Nakstad B, Sonerud T, Solevag AL. Early detection of neonatal group B streptococcus sepsis and the possible diagnostic utility of IL-6, IL-8, and CD11b in a human umbilical cord blood in vitro model. *Infect Drug Resist*. 2016;9:171–179.

75. Adib M, Ostadi V, Navaei F, et al. Evaluation of CD11b expression on peripheral blood neutrophils for early detection of neonatal sepsis. *Iran J Allergy Asthma Immunol*. 2007;6:93–96.

76. Zhou M, Cheng S, Yu J, et al. Interleukin-8 for diagnosis of neonatal sepsis: a meta-analysis. *PLoS ONE*. 2015;10:e0127170.

77. Arai Y, Mizugishi K, Nonomura K, et al. Phagocytosis by human monocytes is required for the secretion of presepsin. *J Infect Chemother*. 2015;21:564–569.

78. Pugni L, Pietrasanta C, Milani S, et al. Presepsin (Soluble CD14 Subtype): Reference Ranges of a New Sepsis Marker in Term and Preterm Neonates. *PLoS ONE*. 2015;10:e0146020.

79. Topcuoglu S, Arslanbuga C, Gursoy T, et al. Role of presepsin in the diagnosis of late-onset neonatal sepsis in preterm infants. *J Matern Fetal Neonatal Med.* 2016;29:1834–1839.

80. Mickiewicz B, Vogel HJ, Wong HR, et al. Metabolomics as a novel approach for early diagnosis of pediatric septic shock and its mortality. *Am J Respir Crit Care Med.* 2013;187:967–976.

81. Stewart CJ, Nelson A, Treumann A, et al. Metabolomic and proteomic analysis of serum from preterm infants with necrotising entercolitis and late-onset sepsis. *Pediatr Res.* 2016;79:425–431.

82. Langley RJ, Tsalik EL, van Velkinburgh JC, et al. An integrated clinico-metabolomic model improves prediction of death in sepsis. *Sci Transl Med.* 2013;5:195ra95.

83. Mickiewicz B, Thompson GC, Blackwood J, et al. Development of metabolic and inflammatory mediator biomarker phenotyping for early diagnosis and triage of pediatric sepsis. *Crit Care.* 2015;19:320.

84. Fanos V, Caboni P, Corsello G, et al. Urinary (1)H-NMR and GC-MS metabolomics predicts early and late onset neonatal sepsis. *Early Hum Dev.* 2014;90(suppl 1):S78–S83.

85. Ng PC, Ang IL, Chiu RW, et al. Host-response biomarkers for diagnosis of late-onset septicemia and necrotizing enterocolitis in preterm infants. *J Clin Invest.* 2010;120:2989–3000.

86. Wynn JL, Cvijanovich NZ, Allen GL, et al. The Influence of Developmental Age on the Early Transcriptomic Response of Children with Septic Shock. *Molecular Medicine.* 2011;17:1146–1156.

87. Wong HR, Cvijanovich NZ, Allen GL, et al. Validation of a gene expression-based subclassification strategy for pediatric septic shock. *Crit Care Med.* 2011;39:2511–2517.

88. Wong HR, Freishtat RJ, Monaco M, et al. Leukocyte subset-derived genomewide expression profiles in pediatric septic shock. *Pediatr Crit Care Med.* 2010;11:349–355.

89. Wong HR, Odoms K, Sakthivel B. Divergence of canonical danger signals: the genome-level expression patterns of human mononuclear cells subjected to heat shock or lipopolysaccharide. *BMC Immunol.* 2008;9:24.

90. Wong HR, Shanley TP, Sakthivel B, et al. Genome-level expression profiles in pediatric septic shock indicate a role for altered zinc homeostasis in poor outcome. *Physiol Genomics.* 2007;30:146–155.

91. Wynn JL, Guthrie SO, Wong HR, et al. Postnatal Age Is a Critical Determinant of the Neonatal Host Response to Sepsis. *Mol Med.* 2015;21:496–504.

92. Smith CL, Dickinson P, Forster T, et al. Identification of a human neonatal immune-metabolic network associated with bacterial infection. *Nat Commun.* 2014;5:4649.

93. Cernada M, Serna E, Bauerl C, et al. Genome-wide expression profiles in very low birth weight infants with neonatal sepsis. *Pediatrics.* 2014;133:e1203–e1211.

94. Hilgendorff A, Windhorst A, Klein M, et al. Gene expression profiling at birth characterizing the preterm infant with early onset infection. *J Mol Med (Berl).* 2017;95(2):169–180.

95. Bryce J, Boschi-Pinto C, Shibuya K, et al. WHO estimates of the causes of death in children. *Lancet.* 2005;365:1147–1152.

CHAPTER 10

Congenital Zika Syndrome

Maria Elisabeth Moreira, MD, Rosana Richtmann, MD

- A major outbreak of Zika virus infection occurred in Brazil in late 2014.
- Vertical transmission from mother to fetus often resulted in fetal losses or central nervous system infection, causing severe microcephaly and disrupted brain development.
- Diagnosis relies on detection of viral RNA via real-time reverse transcription polymerase chain reaction or identification of an IgM serologic response.
- Prevention strategies include avoidance of mosquito bites and use of condoms.

The Zika Virus

Zika virus (ZIKV) is an arbovirus member of the virus family Flaviriridae (RNA viruses) that is usually transmitted by the female *Aedes aegypti* mosquito. *A. aegypti* is also the main vector for dengue (DENV), West Nile virus (WNV), yellow fever, and chikungunya.[1] ZIKV was first identified in 1947 in a sentinel Rhesus monkey in the Zika forest of Uganda. Although ZIKV has circulated among small groups of people in Africa and Southeast Asia since it was identified in humans in 1952, the first major outbreak of ZIKV was reported in 2007 on Yap Island, where an estimated 73% of the population was infected with ZIKV over the course of several months.[1] Subsequent to the Yap Island outbreak, an outbreak in French Polynesia infected around 60% of the population between October 2013 and April 2014.[2] Since the first reports of autochthonous transmission in Brazil, other countries and territories on four continents have reported vectorborne ZIKV transmission.[3]

ZIKV has two major strains: an Asian and an African strain. The Asian strain, which has been implicated in the outbreaks in French Polynesia and the Americas, has specific mutations that have increased the virus's ability to replicate in human tissues and its pathogenicity,[4] which may explain differences in the speed and scope of the epidemic and in the severity of the outcomes between the African and Asian lineages of ZIKV.[5,6]

Mode of Transmission

The ZIKV can be contracted through the bite of an infected mosquito, through sexual contact, through prenatal transmission from mother to fetus, or through blood transfusion. The risk of transmission by breastfeeding is not clear and needs to be better investigated.[3]

Mechanisms of Vertical Transmission

To reach the human fetus, ZIKV must overcome the placental barrier. Previous studies have indicated that nonplacental macrophages play a key role in the replication

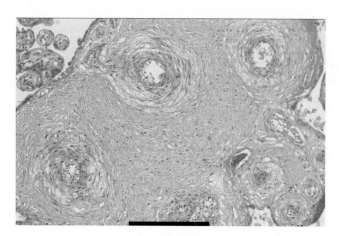

Figure 10.1   Placenta: Thickened vessel walls (hematoxylin-eosin staining).

of DENV, a closely related flavivirus. Because the placenta provides the conduit for vertical transmission of certain viruses and placental Hofbauer cells (HBCs) are fetal-placental macrophages located adjacent to fetal capillaries, several recent studies have examined infection of HBCs by ZIKV. The entire mechanism of the ability of ZIKV to infect and damage a developing fetus is not completely understood, but fetal infection implies that the virus can cross and/or bypass the placental barrier. Vertical transmission of pathogens from mother to fetus can occur by several routes, including infection of endothelial cells in the maternal microvasculature and spread to invasive extravillous trophoblasts (the cells that anchor the villous trees to the uterine wall), trafficking of infected maternal immune cells across the placental barrier, paracellular or transcellular transports from maternal blood across the villous trees and into fetal capillaries, damage to the villous tree and breaks in the syncytiotrophoblast layer, and/or transvaginal ascending infection. Microscopic examination of the placental disc from affected pregnancies, using routine hematoxylin-eosin staining, is revealing secondary and tertiary chorionic villi that were enlarged early in gestation, with focally marked stromal edema. Histologic findings in some placentas included thickened vessel walls in some villi and villous axes due to concentric fibrosis with consequent reduction of their lumens (Fig. 10.1). Occasional focal calcification, fibrosis, fibrin deposition, and mild lymphocytic infiltration were seen in the villous stroma. Some of the enlarged and edematous villi have irregular outlines. Most chorionic villi at all levels demonstrated prominent hyper-cellularity of the villous stroma. These stromal cells have variable appearance, from rounded to spindle shaped, and had the morphologic features of villous stromal macrophages (HBC). The roles of HBC in ZIKV fetus infection have been described in animal models.[7–9]

Hyperplasia of HBC is abnormal and has been reported to occur as a result of a wide variety of pathologic conditions of pregnancy. These include ascending infections, villitis of unknown etiology, and maternal bloodborne infections that cause villitis, including Chagas disease and TORCH infections such as syphilis and cytomegalovirus (CMV). The mechanism(s) by which HBC hyperplasia occurs in response to such stimuli is, at least in part, the result of proliferation of these cells within the chorionic villous stroma. Animal studies had implicated HBC in fetal infection, but this is not completely established in humans.[8,9]

Maternal Infection During Pregnancy

Maternal clinical manifestations of ZIKV infection include fever, headache, arthralgia, myalgia, red eyes (conjunctivitis), and maculopapular rash (usually pruritic), but only one of every four to five people who are infected manifest symptoms (Fig. 10.2). The Pan American Health Organization (PAHO) criteria require, in addition to exanthema, the presence of two other symptoms. This decreases sensitivity and can lead to underreporting of cases. Exanthema may be the only manifestation of

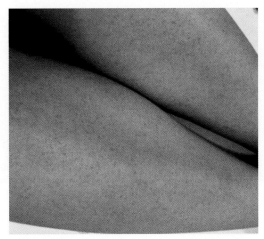

Figure 10.2   Maculopapular rash caused by ZIKV.

ZIKV infection. This differentiates Zika from other arboviral infections, not only by the high frequency (90%–100%) of rash, but also by its timing, appearing in the first 72 hours of infection.[9–11]

Fetal Infection

The Asian strain of ZIKV has been shown to replicate in the placenta and fetal brain,[9] with devastating effects on fetal brain development.[10] The causal relation between ZIKV and miscarriage (pregnancy loss at <20 weeks gestation), fetal loss (pregnancy loss at ≥20 weeks gestation), and a spectrum of fetal anomalies that includes primary microcephaly, now known as congenital Zika syndrome (CZS),[11] has been demonstrated through case-control and cohort studies.[11–13]

Fetal infection by ZIKV presents myriad challenges from an epidemiologic and outbreak control perspective. Acute viremia occurs during the 7 days before onset of symptoms.[14] Between 75% and 80% of those infected have no symptoms. Immunologists are trying to determine the mechanism for ZIKV-associated brain defects: brain defects may be caused directly when maternal blood flow into the placenta begins around 10 week' gestation or indirectly by the placental immune response to ZIKV infection.[15,16]

Neuroimaging investigation contributes to the prenatal detection of microcephaly and other brain abnormalities in cases of intrauterine ZIKV infection. Antenatal neuroimaging is based on two-dimensional and three-dimensional ultrasound (Fig. 10.3) and fetal magnetic resonance imaging (MRI). Although neuropathology associated with intrauterine ZIKV infection is characterized by nonspecific findings of brain disorder, reduced cortical gyration and white-matter hypomyelination or dysmyelination, and cerebellar hypoplasia have been consistently observed in the majority of fetuses and newborns. Fetal images have also shown ventriculomegaly, lissencephaly, and pachygyria (i.e., smooth brains with reduced gyral ridges). Fetal akinesia deformation sequence, or arthrogryposis, has also been frequently found. Other frequent findings were hypoplasia of the cerebellum and cerebellar vermis, with consequent enlargement of the posterior fossa, calcifications in various brain regions, and hypoplasia of the corpus callosum.[13,17,18]

Intrauterine growth restriction and low birth weight have been reported in infants with presumed and confirmed CZS infection. However, its relation to the congenital ZIKV syndrome phenotype and pathogenic mechanism has been not determined.[19]

The Congenital ZIKA Syndrome

Although microcephaly (Fig. 10.4) has been the most frequent clinical manifestation associated with vertical exposure to ZIKV, originating the term *congenital ZIKV*

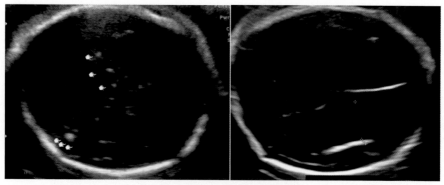

Figure 10.3   Cerebral ultrasound in fetus showing calcifications and Blake cyst.

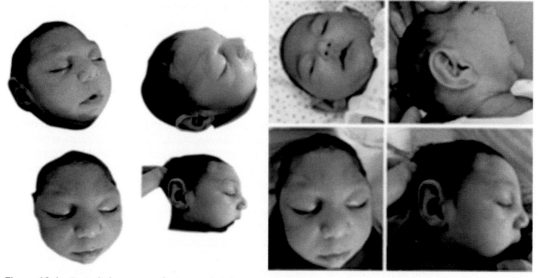

Figure 10.4   Typical phenotype of microcephaly in congenital Zika virus: Biparietal depression, prominent occiput, and redundant nuchal skin.

syndrome, a broad spectrum of neurologic injuries with different clinical manifestations has been observed.[11,12,18] Little is known about the level of neurologic damage in the early years after congenital infection by ZIKV. The association with microcephaly is the most frequently described manifestation, but may only be part of the neuronal dysfunction syndrome, which is characterized by varying levels of global involvement of the cerebral white and gray matter.[19-21] However, the phenotyping of microcephaly is typical. Severe microcephaly (occipital frontal circumference more than 3 standard deviations (SD) below the mean) observed with intrauterine ZIKV infection can be accompanied by findings consistent with fetal brain disruption sequence, characterized by severe microcephaly, overlapping cranial sutures, prominent occipital bone, and redundant scalp skin (Fig. 10.5). Therefore, craniofacial disproportion with biparietal depression, prominent occiput, and excess nuchal skin are components of microcephaly. However, typical microcephaly of the small for gestational age infant has been found mainly in cases where infection is acquired in the first trimester of pregnancy.[13,20,21]

Other severe neurologic sequelae, including motor and cognitive disabilities, seizures, and swallowing difficulties leading to failure to thrive,[11,12] have been reported. Neurologic examination of affected infants has shown hypertonia and spasticity, irritability manifested by excessive crying, dysphagia, and, less frequently, hypotonia. Abnormal activity on electroencephalogram was seen in several infants with presumed

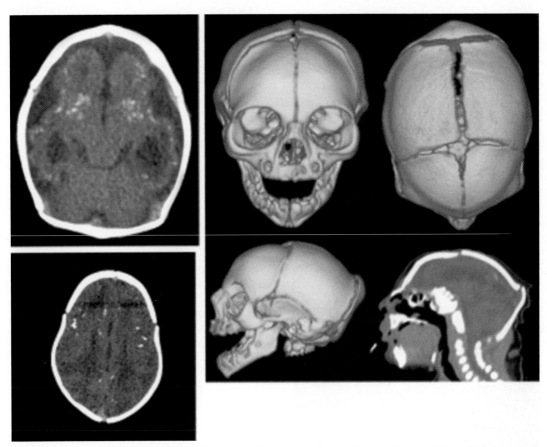

Figure 10.5 Brain computed tomography with calcifications and other abnormalities: Parietal collapse, occipital protrusion, and lissencephaly.

congenital ZIKV infection, and other infants had either focal or multifocal discharges. In addition, tremors and posturing consistent with extrapyramidal dysfunction have been reported.[22]

Ocular Anomalies

Structural eye anomalies (in particular, microphthalmia and coloboma), cataracts, intraocular calcifications, and posterior ocular findings have been reported in infants with presumed and laboratory-confirmed prenatal ZIKV infection. Posterior chamber findings have been the most prevalent. Case series report chorioretinal atrophy, focal pigmentary mottling of the retina, and optic nerve atrophy/anomalies (Figs 10.6 and 10.7). Case reports with more than 20 infants with presumed ZIKV-associated microcephaly report ocular findings in 24% to 55%.[23,24]

Active chorioretinitis, a possible precursor of chorioretinal atrophy, has not been reported in infants with congenital ZIKV infection, and the pattern of ocular findings differs from those in other congenital infections, such as toxoplasmosis and cytomegalovirus. In particular, retinal lesions, including well-defined chorioretinal atrophy and gross pigmentation, generally affecting the macular region, are unique to ZIKV infection.[23,24]

Hearing

Profound sensorineural hearing loss was reported in an infant with characteristic brain imaging findings and cerebrospinal fluid positive for ZIKV IgM, and sensorineural hearing loss was documented in 4 of 69 infants (6%) with microcephaly and laboratory evidence of congenital ZIKV infection.[11,12]

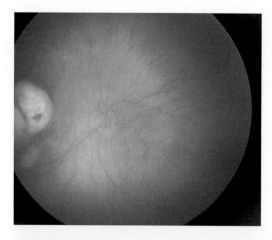

Figure 10.6 Peripapillary atrophy; macular colobomatous chorioretinal atrophy; nasal focal pigment mottling.

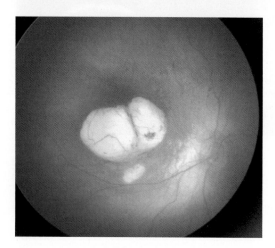

Figure 10.7 Macular colobomatous chorioretinal atrophy; macular focal pigment mottling; peripapillary atrophy.

Neuroimaging

Transfontanel ultrasonography, computed tomography (CT) of the head with and without contrast, and MRI have been used in the evaluation of brain injury. Reported brain abnormalities on CT include intracranial calcifications, corpus callosum abnormalities, abnormal cortical formation, cerebral atrophy, ventriculomegaly, hydrocephaly, and cerebellar abnormalities. On the other hand, a number of infants with normal clinical assessments in early infancy, with normal head circumference at birth, had abnormal nonspecific MRI findings at 3 months of life; a common description was excessive hyperintensity of T_2 signal in the white matter, diffusely in the peritrigonal posterior areas and less evident in the frontal parietal white matter, with hypointense signal in the diffusion sequence. These findings are abnormal and may reflect cortical tract dysfunction.[11,13]

Diagnosis

The diagnosis of ZIKV infection currently relies on the detection of viral RNA via real-time reverse transcription polymerase chain reaction (rRT-PCR) or identification of an IgM serologic response. Given testing limitations, diagnosis and patient counseling are inexact with poor predictive sensitivity (rRT-PCR) and antibody cross-reactivity (IgM).[1,14–16] The incubation period for ZIKV is 3 to 14 days, and in nonpregnant subjects' serum, viremia lasts for 2 to 10 days. Longer periods of viremia and viruria have been observed during pregnancy, presumably because of fetal-placental infection. Virus persists on average 2 weeks longer in urine, and testing for viruria has been shown to improve detection.[17–20]

Because the majority of patients with ZIKV infection (60%–80%) are asymptomatic, identifying patients during the viremic or viruric stage is challenging. Current Centers for Disease Control (CDC) guidelines recommend testing serum or urine by rRT-PCR when a patient presents within 14 days of their last potential exposure to ZIKV or within 14 days of symptoms. Their last potential exposure can be either the date of sexual contact with someone at risk for ZIKV or the last date of travel to a ZIKV endemic region. Strictly adhering to this testing algorithm would, by definition, miss prolonged viremia, which may be a surrogate of fetal-placenta infection.[1,20]

Serologic Testing

Serologic testing is recommended 4 or more days after the onset of clinical illness or ≥14 days from the last potential exposure in asymptomatic patients. An IgM capture enzyme-linked immunosorbent assay is the only Food and Drug Administration–approved serologic test and can be performed on serum and cerebrospinal fluid. Evidence from the serologic response to other flaviviruses, particularly DENV and WNV, suggests that IgM may be present up to 3 months after the exposure; in some patients with West Nile encephalitis, IgM antibodies were detectable more than 1 year after the infection, with one study showing IgM antibodies persisting up to 8 years after the infection.[11,20,25,26]

At present, serologic testing for ZIKV with IgM is currently recommended up to 12 weeks after the exposure. IgG antibodies to ZIKV develop shortly after IgM antibodies and are thought to confer lifelong immunity with higher avidity.[25] In addition to waning titers of IgM isotypes, there is often serologic cross-reactivity with other flaviviruses in patients who have had a recent or prior flavivirus infection, particularly DENV. This complicates the diagnosis, particularly because ZIKV is emerging in areas in which DENV is endemic. Currently, serologic differentiation and confirmation rely on a more cumbersome and less available testing method: the plaque reduction neutralization test (PRNT). The PRNT identifies virus-specific neutralizing antibody titers to various related flaviviruses.[25]

Amniocentesis

A growing body of literature suggests infants with confirmed fetal infection are at an increased risk of intracranial abnormalities. In the setting of a positive ZIKV IgM with positive PRNT, with positive rRT-PCR in maternal serum or urine, or with ultrasound abnormalities, amniocentesis to detect ZIKV RNA via rRT-PCR should be considered to evaluate for vertical transmission. However, the sensitivity, specificity, and a positive and negative predictive value of rRT-PCR on amniotic fluid is unknown, and these potential benefits and limitations should be discussed openly.[26]

Differential Diagnosis

CMV, toxoplasmosis, and rubella need to be investigated in cases of microcephaly and cerebral calcifications.[9]

Supportive Care to Children and Families: Early Intervention in Development

The implementation of programs for early intervention in development in the first years of children born with or at risk of neurodevelopmental disability has shown improved outcomes in their cognitive development and consequently in their quality of life. The effects of initial damage to the development, organization, and function of the nervous system and ultimately to behavior have been extensively documented in various processes of perinatal injury,[27–29] and injuries related to intrauterine exposure to ZIKV can probably be minimized by this type of intervention.

Prevention and Treatment

There is no specific antiviral treatment for ZIKV. Prevention is recommended by the CDC and includes avoidance of mosquito bites (use of repellents, wearing long-sleeved shirts and long pants, taking steps to control mosquitos inside and outside the home) and use of condoms.[30]

REFERENCES

1. Duffy MR, Chen TH, Hancock WT, et al. Zika virus outbreak on Yap Island, Federated States of Micronesia. *N Engl J Med*. 2009;360:2536–2543.
2. Jaenisch T, Rosenberger KD, Brito C, et al. Risk of microcephaly after Zika virus infection in Brazil, 2015 to 2016. *Bull World Health Organ*. 2017;95:191–198.
3. Zika situation report; 2017. Available from: http://www.who.int/emergencies/zika-virus/situation -report/2-february-2017/en/. Accessed February 20, 2017.
4. Wang L, Valderramos SG, Wu A, et al. From mosquitos to humans: genetic evolution of Zika virus. *Cell Host Microbe*. 2016;19:561–565.
5. Musso D. Zika virus transmission from French Polynesia to Brazil. *Emerg Infect Dis*. 2015;21:1887.
6. Fauci AS, Morens DM. Zika virus in the Americas—yet another arbovirus threat. *N Engl J Med*. 2016;374:601–604.
7. Simoni MK, Jurado KA, Abrahams VM, et al. Zika virus infection of Hofbauer cells. *Am J Reprod Immunol*. 2017;77.
8. Rosenberg AZ, Yu W, Hill DA, et al. Placental pathology of Zika virus: viral infection of the placenta induces villous stromal macrophage (Hofbauer cell) proliferation and hyperplasia. *Arch Pathol Lab Med*. 2017;141:43–48.
9. Coyne CB, Lazear HM. Zika virus—reigniting the TORCH. *Nat Rev Microbiol*. 2016;14:707–715.
10. Melo AS, Aguiar RS, Amorim MM, et al. Congenital Zika virus infection: beyond neonatal microcephaly. *JAMA Neurol*. 2016;73:1407–1416.
11. Brasil P, Pereira JP Jr, Moreira ME, et al. Zika virus infection in pregnant women in Rio de Janeiro. *N Engl J Med*. 2016;375:2321–2334.
12. de Araujo TVB, Rodrigues LC, de Alencar Ximenes RA, et al. Association between Zika virus infection and microcephaly in Brazil, January to May, 2016: preliminary report of a case-control study. *Lancet Infect Dis*. 2016;16:1356–1363.
13. Araujo Junior E, Carvalho FH, Tonni G, et al. Prenatal imaging findings in fetal Zika virus infection. *Curr Opin Obstet Gynecol*. 2017;29:95–105.
14. Galliez RM, Spitz M, Rafful PP, et al. Zika virus causing encephalomyelitis associated with immunoactivation. *Open Forum Infect Dis*. 2016;3:ofw203.
15. Morrison TE, Diamond MS. Animal models of Zika virus infection, pathogenesis, and immunity. *J Virol*. 2017;91.
16. Lanciotti RS, Kosoy OL, Laven JJ, et al. Genetic and serologic properties of Zika virus associated with an epidemic, Yap State, Micronesia, 2007. *Emerg Infect Dis*. 2008;14:1232–1239.
17. Beckham JD, Pastula DM, Massey A, et al. Zika virus as an emerging global pathogen: neurological complications of Zika virus. *JAMA Neurol*. 2016;73:875–879.
18. Panchaud A, Stojanov M, Ammerdorffer A, et al. Emerging role of Zika virus in adverse fetal and neonatal outcomes. *Clin Microbiol Rev*. 2016;29:659–694.
19. Meaney-Delman D, Oduyebo T, Polen KN, et al. Prolonged detection of Zika virus RNA in pregnant women. *Obstet Gynecol*. 2016;128:724–730.
20. Driggers RW, Ho CY, Korhonen EM, et al. Zika virus infection with prolonged maternal viremia and fetal brain abnormalities. *N Engl J Med*. 2016;374:2142–2151.
21. Moore CA, Staples JE, Dobyns WB, et al. Characterizing the pattern of anomalies in congenital Zika syndrome for pediatric clinicians. *JAMA Pediatr*. 2017;171:288–295.
22. Carvalho MD, Miranda-Filho DB, van der Linden V, et al. Sleep EEG patterns in infants with congenital Zika virus syndrome. *Clin Neurophysiol*. 2017;128:204–214.
23. de Andrade GC, Ventura CV, Mello Filho PA, et al. Arboviruses and the eye. *Int J Retina Vitreous*. 2017;3:4.
24. de Oliveira Dias JR, Ventura CV, Borba PD, et al. Infants with congenital Zika syndrome and ocular findings from Sao Paulo, Brazil: spread of infection. *Retin Cases Brief Rep*. 2017.
25. Eppes C, Rac M, Dunn J, et al. Testing for Zika virus infection in pregnancy: key concepts to deal with an emerging epidemic. *Am J Obstet Gynecol*. 2017;216:209–225.
26. Cabral-Castro MJ, Cavalcanti MG, Peralta RHS, et al. Molecular and serological techniques to detect co-circulation of DENV, ZIKV and CHIKV in suspected dengue-like syndrome patients. *J Clin Virol*. 2016;82:108–111.
27. Bann CM, Wallander JL, Do B, et al. Home-based early intervention and the influence of family resources on cognitive development. *Pediatrics*. 2016;137.
28. Wallander JL, Biasini FJ, Thorsten V, et al. Dose of early intervention treatment during children's first 36 months of life is associated with developmental outcomes: an observational cohort study in three low/low-middle income countries. *BMC Pediatr*. 2014;14:281.
29. Carlo WA, Goudar SS, Pasha O, et al. Randomized trial of early developmental intervention on outcomes in children after birth asphyxia in developing countries. *J Pediatr*. 2013;162:705–712 e3.
30. Vouga M, Musso D, Van Mieghem T, et al. CDC guidelines for pregnant women during the Zika virus outbreak. *Lancet*. 2016;387:843–844.

Pharmacology

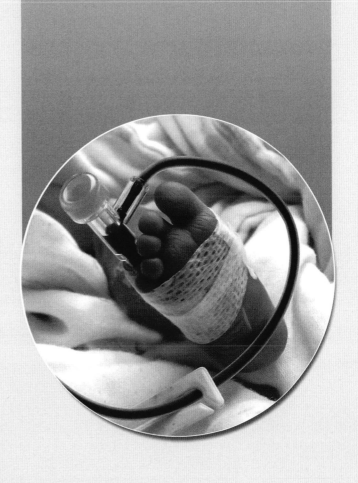

CHAPTER 11

Pharmacokinetic Considerations in Neonates

Adam Frymoyer, MD

- Understanding of the pharmacokinetics of a drug is essential for developing safe and effective dosing strategies in neonates.
- Drug dosing in neonates can be challenging due to large pharmacokinetic variation between patients.
- Consideration of size, maturation & development, and organ pathophysiology can help explain pharmacokinetic variation between neonates and provides a framework for developing evidence-based dosing strategies.
- Therapeutic drug monitoring, when available, is valuable and supports dose individualization in a neonate.

Introduction

Pharmacokinetics explains what the body does with a drug after it is administered and helps provide a description of the time course of the drug in the body. Major processes involved in the pharmacokinetics of a drug include absorption, distribution, metabolism, and excretion. Understanding the movement of a drug in the body helps guide the development of dosing strategies in patients by answering questions of how much, how often, and for how long.

Knowledge about the pharmacokinetics of a drug is essential for its safe and effective use. For example, if the therapeutic window (i.e., range of exposure that results in the desired therapeutic response while minimizing adverse effects) is known, an ideal dosing regimen can be designed to maintain exposure within that therapeutic window throughout the treatment period. If excessive doses are given, the drug may have the desired therapeutic effect, but due to concentrations above the therapeutic window, the risk of adverse effects and toxicity is increased. On the other hand, a dose that is too low, although safe, offers no therapeutic benefit.

The tragedy that can occur because of a lack of knowledge about the pharmacokinetics of a drug in a population of intended use is exemplified by the chloramphenicol experience in neonates. During the 1950s chloramphenicol—a new broad-spectrum antibiotic with good blood–brain barrier penetration—was used in preterm and term neonates at high risk for sepsis. The chloramphenicol dose used in these neonates was extrapolated from that used for adults by adjusting for weight on a linear mg per kg basis. The result was the accumulation of chloramphenicol and its metabolites to toxic levels in some neonates with resulting cardiovascular collapse and even death (aka "gray baby syndrome").[1] Subsequent pharmacokinetic studies performed revealed a markedly longer half-life of chloramphenicol in neonates compared with children and adults (Fig. 11.1).[2] The age dependence of the pharmacokinetics of chloramphenicol is now known to be caused by the reduced capacity for glucuronide conjugation in neonates, the major metabolic pathway for chloramphenicol. To achieve similar exposures to children and adults, neonates require lower and less frequent doses of chloramphenicol. This important lesson

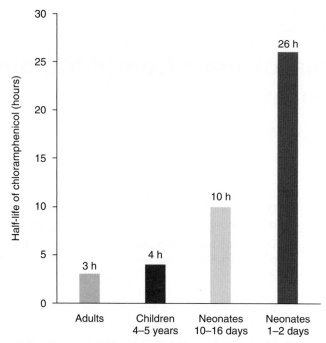

Figure 11.1 Differences in half-life of chloramphenicol by age. Longer half-lives seen in neonates are due to maturational delay in glucuronide conjugation, which is the major metabolic pathway for chloramphenicol. (Data from Weiss CF, Glazko AJ, Weston JK: Chloramphenicol in the newborn infant. A physiologic explanation of its toxicity when given in excessive doses. *N Engl J Med* 1960;262:787–794; Chloramphenicol. In: *WHO model prescribing information: drugs used in bacterial infections.* Geneva, 2001, World Health Organization, p 117–121.)

from the chloramphenicol experience highlights the value of understanding key pharmacokinetic principles behind the safe and effective use of drugs in the neonatal population.

Clinical Pharmacokinetic Principles

Pharmacokinetic Exposure Measures

Fig. 11.2 illustrates several clinically relevant exposure measures during drug dosing. For a drug given intravenously, the maximum concentration (C_{max} or peak) is achieved immediately at the end of the infusion. For antibiotics that have concentration-dependent killing, such as aminoglycosides (gentamicin, tobramycin), achieving a target C_{max} is important for bacteria eradication and treatment success. The minimum concentration (C_{min} or trough) during a dosing strategy occurs at the end of a dosing interval, immediately before the next dose. The C_{min} is relevant for beta-lactam antibiotics (penicillins, cephalosporins, carbapenems, monobactams) that have time-dependent killing in which the goal is to maintain a concentration that exceeds the minimum inhibitory concentration (MIC). The area under the plasma concentration time curve (AUC) is a measure of overall exposure to the drug. AUC is dependent on both the concentration achieved and the duration of exposure. The vancomycin 24 hour AUC over the MIC (AUC_{24}/MIC) has been shown to be a predictor of clinical outcomes when treating methicillin-resistant *Staphylococcus aureus* infections.

The most basic framework that can be used to describe the plasma concentration time course of a drug is a one-compartment model (Fig. 11.3). Although many drugs are more precisely described by a two- or even three-compartment model, a one-compartment model is helpful to illustrate basic pharmacokinetic relationships and potential clinical implications. In a one-compartment model, the two fundamental

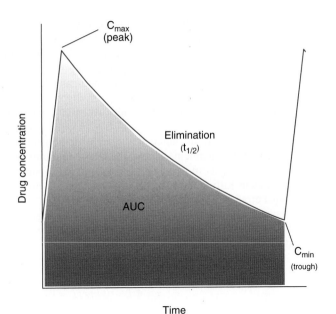

Figure 11.2 Clinically relevant exposure measures during drug dosing. C_{max}, maximum concentration; C_{min}, minimum concentration; AUC, area under the plasma concentration time curve.

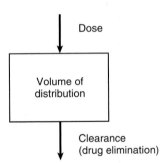

Figure 11.3 Example of a one-compartment model to describe the pharmacokinetics of a drug. Volume of distribution and elimination clearance are the two fundamental parameters of a drug and allow the concentration in the body at any given time after a dose to be calculated. The elimination half-life ($t_{1/2}$) of a drug can be calculated from the volume of distribution and clearance.

parameters of a drug that describe its pharmacokinetics are the volume of distribution (V_d) and elimination clearance (CL).

Volume of Distribution

The volume of distribution (V_d) is a measure of the extent of tissue distribution with units in volume (i.e., liters or milliliters) and relates the amount of drug in the body to the concentration of drug by,

$$\text{Dose} = V_d \times \text{Concentration} \qquad \text{Eq. 11.1}$$

Accordingly,

$$V_d = \frac{\text{Dose}}{\text{Concentration}} \qquad \text{Eq. 11.2}$$

Physiochemical properties of the drug such as plasma protein binding, tissue protein binding, lipid solubility, and pK_a (and ionization state at physiologic pH) all affect the V_d. In addition, patient-specific factors influence the V_d (acid–base status, organ perfusion, disease state). The larger the V_d, the more the drug distributes to all the tissues of the body. The smaller the V_d, the more the drug remains within the vascular system. It is worth highlighting that the V_d is not a "real" physical or physiologic space. For example, digoxin has a large V_d due to its high tissue binding affinity. The average apparent V_d of digoxin in a 2.9-kg neonate is 9.7 L/kg.[3] This is larger than the total body water in a neonate ($\approx$0.8 L/kg), and even total body size.[4]

The clinical relevance of V_d can be demonstrated using an example to calculate the dose for gentamicin—one of the most commonly used antibiotics to treat early- and late-onset sepsis in neonates.[5,6] Gentamicin, an aminoglycoside, has concentration-dependent killing, and the clinical response is predicted by the ratio of maximum concentration over the minimum inhibitory concentration (C_{max}/MIC).[7,8] For a 3-kg neonate who has a typical V_d of 1.4 L (0.46 L/kg),[9] the gentamicin loading dose can be calculated in which a target C_{max} (or peak) plasma concentration of 10 mg/L is desired using Eq. 11.1,

$$\text{Dose} = V_d \times \text{Concentration}$$
$$= 1.4\ L \times 10\ mg/L = 14\ mg\ (4.7\ mg/kg)$$

A loading dose of 4.7 mg/kg will achieve a C_{max} concentration of 10 mg/L. For simplicity in this example, we assumed the dose was given as an instantaneous intravenous bolus and the C_{max} concentration was drawn immediately after the bolus dose. In clinical practice, gentamicin is routinely given as a 30-minute infusion and C_{max} (or peak) is collected 30 minutes after the end of infusion. Nonetheless, the basic principle guiding the recommended gentamicin dose of 4 to 5 mg/kg for a full-term neonate is analogous.

Clearance

The clearance (CL) of a drug relates the rate of elimination to the concentration of the drug in the body by,

$$\text{Rate of Elimination} = CL \times \text{Concentration} \qquad \textbf{Eq. 11.3}$$

Accordingly,

$$CL = \frac{\text{Rate of Elimination}}{\text{Concentration}} \qquad \textbf{Eq. 11.4}$$

The units of CL are volume per time (i.e., L/h or mL/min) and represent the volume of fluid that can be completely cleared of drug per unit time. Conceptually, this is similar to the way that kidney function is measured with glomerular filtration rate (GFR), which is also in units of volume per time (mL/min). The two main organ systems involved in drug clearance are the liver (CL_{liver}) and kidney (CL_{kidney}), but other sites of clearance (CL_{other}) may be present. The total clearance (CL_{total}) by the body is the sum of each clearance pathway.

$$CL_{total} = CL_{liver} + CL_{kidney} + CL_{other} \qquad \textbf{Eq. 11.5}$$

At steady-state, the rate of drug input equals the rate of drug elimination, and Eq.11.3 can then be used to calculate the infusion rate needed to achieve a desired drug concentration at steady-state (C_{ss}) during a continuous infusion:

$$\text{Infusion Rate} = CL \times C_{ss} \qquad \textbf{Eq. 11.6}$$

As an example, the rate for a continuous vancomycin infusion needed to achieve a C_{ss} of 18 mg/L in a 2-kg neonate with clearance of 0.14 L/hr (0.07 L/hr/kg) would be:

$$\text{Infusion Rate} = 0.14\ L/hr \times 18\ mg/L = 2.5\ mg/hr\ (1.25\ mg/kg/hr)$$

If instead the drug is given as an *intermittent* dose (i.e., every 6 hours, every 8 hours, every 12 hours, etc.), the infusion rate in Eq. 11.6 is replaced with

$$\text{Infusion Rate} = \frac{\text{Dose}}{\text{tau}} = CL \times C_{avg,ss} \qquad \text{Eq. 11.7}$$

where Dose is the dose amount, tau is the dosing interval, and $C_{avg,ss}$ is the average concentration in the body during the dosing interval.

It is often more clinically relevant to know the AUC during the dosing interval:

$$AUC_{time} = \frac{\text{Dose}}{\text{Clearance}} \qquad \text{Eq. 11.8}$$

The subscript *time* notes that the AUC is for a defined period. The period is most often the dosing interval (tau) at which the dose is given. AUC_{12hr} would represent the AUC for a dosing interval of every 12 hours. However, the AUC can be calculated for any clinically relevant time period. For example, the AUC over 24 hours (AUC_{24hr}) for a 2-kg neonate receiving vancomycin 15 mg/kg every 12 hours (= 60 mg/24 hr) is

$$AUC_{24hr} = \frac{\text{Dose}_{24hr}}{CL} = \frac{60\ mg}{0.14\ L/hr} = 429\ mg \bullet h/L \qquad \text{Eq. 11.9}$$

The AUC for a given period is not affected by how the dose is divided during the time period (i.e., every 6 hours, every 12 hours, or even as a continuous infusion). Only the total dose given during the time period matters. For example, the AUC_{24hr} in the earlier example is the same whether vancomycin is given as a 1.25 mg/kg/hr continuous infusion, 15 mg/kg q12 hours intermittent dose, or 7.5 mg/kg q6 hours intermittent dose (Table 11.1). In all cases, the patient receives 60 mg/day and the AUC_{24hr} is 429 mg•h/L. However, the peak and trough concentrations achieved are dependent on the dosing interval (Fig. 11.4 and Table 11.1). The longer the dosing interval, the larger the fluctuations in concentrations (i.e., larger difference between peak and trough concentrations). The relationship between the dosing interval and half-life of a drug determines the concentrations achieved.

Elimination Rate Constant, Half-Life, and Steady-State

The elimination rate constant (k_{el}) is the fraction of drug eliminated per unit time. It is not an independent pharmacokinetic parameter because it depends both on clearance and V_d:

$$k_{el} = \frac{\text{Clearance}}{V_d} \qquad \text{Eq. 11.10}$$

Table 11.1 EFFECT OF DOSE INTERVAL ON EXPOSURES AT STEADY-STATE FOR VANCOMYCIN*

Dosing Strategy	Daily Dose	AUC_{24hr} (mg*hr/L)	$C_{avg,ss}$ (mg/L)	Peak (mg/L)	Trough (mg/L)
15 mg/kg q12 hours	30 mg/kg/day	429	17.9	33.0	8.3
7.5 mg/kg q6 hours	30 mg/kg/day	429	17.9	24.8	12.4
Continuous infusion - 1.25 mg/kg/hr	30 mg/kg/day	429	17.9	n/a	n/a

*Exposures represent a typical neonate weighing 2 kg and postmenstrual age of 33 weeks (clearance 0.14 L/h, volume 1.21 L).
AUC_{24hr}, area under the plasma concentration time curve over 24 hours; $C_{avg,ss}$, average concentration during dosing interval at steady-state; Peak, maximum concentration during dosing interval; Trough, minimum concentration during dosing interval.

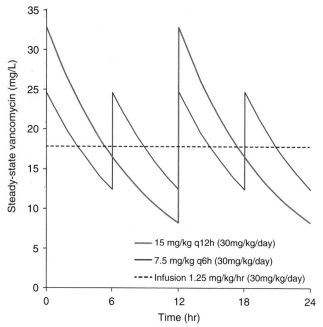

Figure 11.4 Impact of dosing interval on the concentration–time profile of vancomycin at steady-state in a neonate receiving the same daily dose of 30 mg/kg/day. Vancomycin was given as (1) a continuous infusion of 1.25 mg/kg/hr, (2) 15 mg/kg q12 hours, or (3) 7.5 mg/kg q6 hours. The AUC and average concentration over 24 hours are the same for all dose schedules. The peak and trough concentrations are dependent on the dosing interval.

k_{el} can also be calculated directly from concentration data. As seen in Fig. 11.5, the concentration–time curve is linear on the log scale and the k_{el} is the slope of the line given by

$$k_{el} = \frac{\ln C_1 - \ln C_2}{t_2 - t_1}$$ Eq. 11.11

where C_1 and C_2 are the concentrations measured at time one (t_1) and time two (t_2), respectively. When the elimination rate constant is known, the concentration after a single intravenous dose can be calculated at any time (t) by,

$$C(t) = \frac{\text{Dose}}{V_d} \times e^{-k_{el} \cdot t}$$ Eq. 11.12

Although useful for calculations, k_{el} is more difficult to relate from a clinical perspective. The half-life ($t_{1/2}$) is easier to conceptualize and is calculated from k_{el}:

$$t_{1/2} = \frac{0.693}{k_{el}} = 0.693 \times \frac{V_d}{\text{Clearance}}$$ Eq. 11.13

The $t_{1/2}$ represents the time needed to eliminate 50% of the drug in the body. After 3.3 half-lives, 90% of the drug will be eliminated from the body (Table 11.2). The relationship between $t_{1/2}$ (= $0.693/k_{el}$) and dosing interval (tau) will determine the amount of drug accumulated at steady-state with multiple doses by the accumulation index:

$$\text{Accumulation Index} = \frac{1}{1 - e^{-k_{el} \cdot tau}}$$ Eq. 11.14

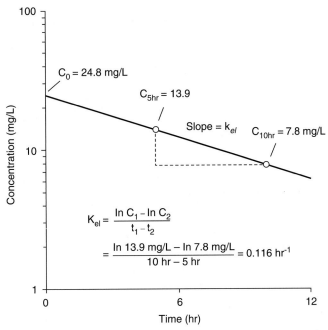

Figure 11.5 The concentration–time curve plotted on the log scale is linear for a drug that follows a one-compartment model. The elimination rate constant (k_{el}) is the slope of the straight line on the log scale.

Table 11.2 RELATIONSHIP BETWEEN HALF-LIFE ($T_{1/2}$) AND AMOUNT OF DRUG ELIMINATED AFTER A DOSE OR ACHIEVEMENT OF STEADY-STATE WITH MULTIPLE DOSES

Half-Lives	% Drug Eliminated or % Steady-State Achieved
1	50%
2	75%
3	87.5%
3.3	90%
4	94%
5	97%
6	98%
7	99%

The shorter the dosing interval relative to the $t_{1/2}$, the more drug accumulation occurs.

By factoring in the accumulation index, the concentration at steady-state after multiple IV doses is calculated by combining Eqs. 11.12 and 11.14:

$$C(t)_{ss} = \frac{Dose}{V_d} \times \frac{e^{-k_{el} \cdot t}}{1 - e^{-k_{el} \cdot tau}}$$

Eq. 11.15

In addition to the amount of accumulation, the $t_{1/2}$ of the drug determines the time it will take to reach steady-state conditions. With multiple or continuous dosing regimens, the amount of drug in the body continues to accumulate until the rate of drug entering the body equals the rate of elimination from the body. Once this equilibrium is achieved, the system is said to be at a steady-state, and the average concentration in the body does not change. It takes 3.3 half-lives to reach

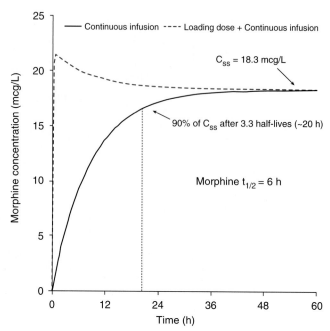

Figure 11.6 Concentration–time curve of morphine during a continuous infusion with and without a loading dose. When no loading dose is given, morphine concentrations increase until steady-state is achieved (C_{ss}). The half-life ($t_{1/2}$) of morphine is 6 hours; therefore, it would take almost 20 hours after starting the infusion to reach 90% of steady-state. When a loading dose is given before the infusion, therapeutic concentrations are achieved more quickly. Pharmacokinetic parameters represent a typical neonate weighing 2.2 kg and postmenstrual age of 33 weeks (clearance 0.6 L/h, volume 5.2 L). Loading dose was 50 µg/kg, and continuous infusion rate was 5 µg/kg/hr.

Table 11.3   EFFECT OF CHANGES IN CLEARANCE AND V_D ON KEY PHARMACOKINETIC PARAMETERS

	AUC	$C_{avg,ss}$	C_{max}	C_{min}	$t_{1/2}$
↑ Clearance	↓	↓	↓	↓	↓
↓ Clearance	↑	↑	↑	↑	↑
↑ V_d	No Δ	No Δ	↓	↑	↑
↓ V_d	No Δ	No Δ	↑	↓	↓

90% of steady-state and 5 half-lives to reach 97% of steady-state (see Table 11.2). A continuous infusion of morphine demonstrates this principle (Fig. 11.6), with increasing drug concentrations over time until a steady-state concentration (C_{ss}) is achieved. The $t_{1/2}$ of morphine is 6 hours in this neonate; therefore, it will take ≈20 hours to reach concentrations that are 90% of steady-state. Inadequate analgesia may result in the neonate before steady-state is achieved. To achieve therapeutic concentrations more rapidly, a loading dose, calculated using Eq. 11.1, can be used. This is demonstrated for the morphine example in Fig. 11.6. For drugs with very long elimination half-lives such as phenobarbital ($t_{1/2}$ = 60–120 hours) and theophylline ($t_{1/2}$ = 20–30 hours), a loading dose is critical when starting therapy, because otherwise the target concentrations required for drug response will not be achieved for several days.[10,11]

Table 11.3 provides a summary of how clearance and V_d affect the pharmacokinetic exposure measures described earlier.

Linear versus Nonlinear Pharmacokinetics

For most drugs used in neonates, CL is constant for the doses used in clinical care. Therefore, from Eq. 11.3 the rate of elimination increases in direct proportion to

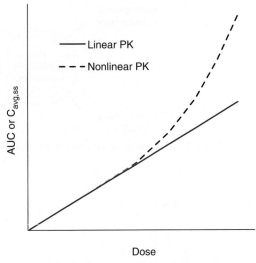

Figure 11.7   Linear versus nonlinear pharmacokinetics. Most drugs have linear pharmacokinetics, which results in drug exposure increasing directly proportional to dose. In contrast, drugs with nonlinear pharmacokinetics have an increase in exposure out of proportion to the increase in dose.

drug concentration. This first-order elimination process results in linear pharmacokinetics, whereby drug exposure in the body is directly proportional to dose (Fig. 11.7). The property of linear pharmacokinetics is applied clinically when adjusting the dose of a drug in a neonate with a known exposure for a given dose. For example, if the AUC_{24hr} at steady-state for vancomycin is measured to be 320 mg•g/L in a neonate after receiving a dose of 15 mg/kg every 12 hours, then to achieve a 25% higher exposure (AUC_{24hr} 400 mg•g/L), a 25% higher dose (18.75 mg/kg every 12 hours) is needed. This proportionality is seen for other exposure measures, such as C_{min} or C_{max} at steady-state, and the same principles for dose adjustment apply.

In contrast, drugs that have nonlinear pharmacokinetics have a less predictable relationship between the dose given and exposure achieved. Nonlinear pharmacokinetics most often result from saturation of a major elimination pathway, and a small change in dose will produce a large increase in exposure after saturation occurs. Fortunately, few drugs used in neonates have nonlinear pharmacokinetics. The most relevant example is phenytoin. Understanding dose–exposure relationships for these drugs is critical, and the use of therapeutic drug monitoring often plays an important role.

Pharmacokinetic Variation in Neonates

From a pharmacokinetic perspective, neonates are not "small adults," nor even "small children," for that matter. As highlighted by the chloramphenicol experience, simple weight-based dose scaling from adults is not appropriate for most drugs. Safe dosing strategies in neonates require an understanding of how they are a unique population. There are many sources of variation in this complex group (Fig. 11.8). Outlining the major factors at play—maturation and development, size, and organ pathophysiology—will provide a fundamental framework for optimization of drug dosing.

Volume of Distribution Considerations

V_d has a linear relationship to weight (*L/kg*). Therefore loading doses scaled by weight (i.e., *mg/kg*) will, in general, be expected to achieve similar peak concentrations across neonates of different sizes. However, unique considerations in the neonate have been shown to affect their V_d. Neonates have a higher total body water content due to increased extracellular water compared with older children and adults (Fig. 11.9). Drugs that are hydrophilic and distribute mainly to the extracellular space

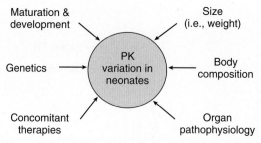

Figure 11.8 Sources of variation in the pharmacokinetics of drugs in neonates.

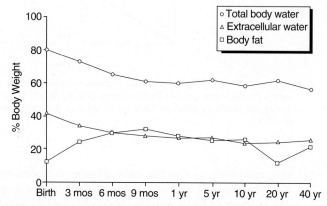

Figure 11.9 Change in water and fat content in body across age. (Figure reproduced from Rakhmanina NY, van den Anker JN: Pharmacological research in pediatrics: from neonates to adolescents. *Adv Drug Deliv Rev* 2006;58:4–14.)

have a higher V_d in neonates. For example, gentamicin has a typical V_d of 0.46 L/h in neonates, 0.24 L/kg in older children, and 0.25 L/kg in adults.[9,12,13] For such drugs, higher loading doses are needed in neonates to achieve the same peak concentration early in the course of therapy. However, as a result of reduced clearance of gentamicin in neonates, attributable to immature kidney function (see Clearance Considerations later), more prolonged dosing intervals are needed to prevent excess accumulation. Conversely, highly lipophilic drugs may have a smaller V_d in neonates. The V_d of propofol increases over the first year of life from 3.7 L/kg in neonates <28 days old to 8.2 L/kg in children 1 to 3 years old.[14,15]

Alterations in V_d are also anticipated in neonates with hypoxic ischemic encephalopathy (HIE) receiving hypothermia. Hypothermia affects tissue perfusion and shunts blood away from muscle, skin, and fat, and a reduction in the V_d of some drugs may result.[16] The V_d of morphine is reported to be 33% less in neonates with HIE receiving hypothermia compared with normothermic neonates without HIE.[17,18] Nevertheless, neonates with HIE receiving hypothermia are complex, and additional alterations in physiology such as tissue pH, tissue binding, lipid solubility, blood–brain barrier, and so forth, may affect drug distribution and even increase V_d.[16] Pharmacokinetic studies of drugs used in this complex population are paramount to understanding their unique dosing needs.

Clearance Considerations

Size

Size is a fundamental predictor of CL, and scaling the clearance of a drug for size is needed to account for these changes. The impact of size is especially relevant in the neonatal population in whom weight can vary >10-fold depending on gestational age and due to the rapid growth that occurs within an individual neonate.

Traditionally, simple linear scaling for weight (i.e., L/h/kg) has been used to account for changes in CL across patients of different sizes. Linear scaling is convenient, as it is easy to calculate and to communicate. Most dosing strategies in neonates and children are expressed on a per kg basis (i.e., mg/kg). However, it is now appreciated that most metabolic processes such as CL do not scale linearly with weight. Metabolic processes that influence CL, such as cardiac output, metabolic rate, enzymatic reactions, and GFR, are more accurately related to weight using allometric scaling and a ¾ power model.[19] In allometric scaling CL and weight are related by

$$CL_{individual} = CL_{popuation} \times \left(\frac{Weight_{individual}}{Weight_{population}} \right)^{0.75}$$ Eq. 11.16

where $CL_{individual}$ is the CL in a patient of $Weight_{individual}$ and $CL_{populaton}$ is the typical CL in the reference population with $Weight_{population}$. The ¾ (0.75) exponent results in a slightly curvilinear change in CL with weight (Fig. 11.10). Scaling of drug clearance using this principle of allometry has been shown to better predict CL and drug dose needs than linear scaling across a range of weights.[20,21] Compared with allometric scaling, linear scaling of weight underestimates CL at lower weights, which may lead to underdosing in older infants and young children (Fig. 11.11). In the example in Fig. 11.11, the CL predicted using linear scaling is lower by >10% for a 40-kg child and >25% for a 20-kg child. The oversimplified use of linear scaling is one reason why children are often reported to have higher CL than adults when expressed on a per kg basis (i.e., *L/h/kg*). However, when weight is scaled via allometry, CL is often the same in children and adults expressed relative to a 70-kg adult (i.e., *L/h/kg*$^{0.75}$ or *L/h/70 kg*).

In neonates, the clinical impact of a lower prediction of CL with linear scaling is hidden by the concomitant effect of incomplete maturation and development, which also lowers clearance in neonates. Therefore the signals of each separate process (size versus maturation and development) are tangled, and misscaling for size could potentially cloud the pharmacokinetic picture. Accurate scaling of weight on CL is helpful to elucidate the signal of other concomitant processes affecting CL (such as maturation and development) and to improve dosing strategies optimized for neonates.

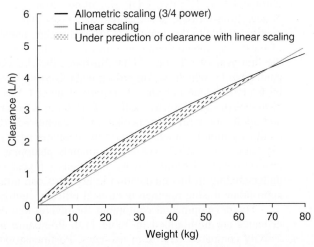

Figure 11.10 Comparison of clearance scaled by weight using an allometric model with a ¾ power exponent (*L/h/kg*$^{3/4}$) versus linear scaling (*L/h/kg*). Linear scaling underpredicts clearance at lower weights compared with the allometric model as highlighted by the shaded area. The difference in clearance is >25% at a weight of 20 kg, and the difference increases as weight decreases. The current example represents vancomycin clearance scaled from a reference 70-kg adult with normal renal function (clearance 4.3 *L/h*).

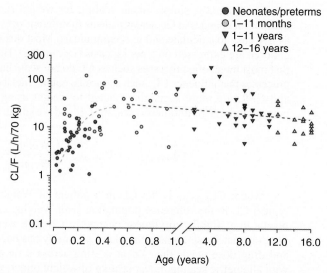

Figure 11.11 Maturation of the clearance of pantoprazole across age. Pantoprazole is metabolized mainly by CYP2C19 and to a lesser extent by CYP3A4. Clearance here represents oral clearance (CL/F) because pantoprazole was given orally. Clearance is weight-adjusted to a 70-kg adult using allometric scaling (*L/h/70 kg*). (Figure reproduced from Jones BL, Van den Anker JN, Kearns GL: Pediatric clinical pharmacology and therapeutics. In: *Principles of clinical pharmacology*, ed 3, San Diego, CA, Academic Press, p 417–436.)

Maturation and Development

Maturation is an ongoing process beginning in utero, continuing through the newborn period, and extending well into childhood. Maturation of the liver and kidney is central to drug CL, as these organs play a key role in the metabolism and elimination of most drugs. Research into the maturation of specific metabolic and elimination processes as they relate to drug pharmacokinetics is rapidly evolving, and typical patterns of liver and kidney maturation are now recognized. With this more in-depth understanding of organ maturation, drug clearance and dosing in neonates can be improved.

The major enzymes involved in hepatic drug metabolism include the cytochrome P450s (CYPs), UDP-glucuronosyltransferases (UGTs), sulfotransferases, N-acetyltransferases, and methyltransferases. The CYPs and UGTs are the most significant due to the quantity of drugs that they metabolize. In general, the activity of most drug-metabolizing enzymes is very low in the neonate and increases over the first year of life. Fig. 11.11 illustrates the changes in clearance across age for pantoprazole, which is primarily metabolized by CYP2C19 and to a lesser extent by CYP3A4. Due to reduced activity of these CYPs in neonates, weight-adjusted clearance (using allometric scaling; *L/h/70 kg*) is lower compared with older children and adults. In a full-term neonate, CL reaches ≈50% of that of an older child or adult by 2 months of age.[22] Therefore, neonates need lower doses to achieve similar exposures (i.e., AUC). Although ultimately pantoprazole is not effective in treating gastroesophageal reflux disease in infants <1 year of age,[23] the pharmacokinetic understanding of this medication in neonates and infants was essential to define an appropriate dosing regimen in clinical efficacy studies.

The developmental continuum for several key drug-metabolizing enzymes in neonates are highlighted in Table 11.4. Premature infants have lower enzymatic activity compared with term neonates. Postmenstrual age (PMA) can be a useful marker of the development status of a neonate and has been applied to help predict maturation of drug clearance for several drugs (Fig. 11.12). Similarly, gestational age and postnatal age can also be used to account for maturational status.

Analogous to hepatic metabolism, renal function and elimination of drugs via the kidney are reduced in neonates. Nephrogenesis is ongoing until 34 weeks gestation,

Table 11.4 DEVELOPMENTAL PATTERNS FOR DRUG-METABOLIZING ENZYMES IN NEONATES

Enzyme	Developmental Pattern	Example Substrate
CYP3A4	Extremely low activity at birth reaching approximately 30%–40% of adult activity by 1 month and full adult activity by 6 months.	Midazolam
CYP2C19	Apparently absent in fetal liver. Low activity in first 2–4 weeks of life, with adult activity reached by approximately 6 months.	Proton pump inhibitors
CYP1A2	Not present in appreciable levels in human fetal liver. Adult levels reached by approximately 4 months and exceeded in children at 1–2 years of age.	Caffeine, theophylline
CYP2C9	Detected at very low levels (1% of adult levels) in early gestation (earliest at 8 weeks). At term, activity increases to approximately 10% of that observed in adults; by 5–6 months of age, activity is approximately 25% of adult.	Phenytoin, indomethacin
UGT (glucuronidation)	Activity appears to be highly variable with limited activity at birth. Adult activity is achieved between 2 months and 3 years of age.	Morphine, chloramphenicol

CYP, Cytochrome P450; *UGT,* UDP-glucuronosyltransferase.
Adapted from Jones BL, Van den Anker JN, Kearns GL: Pediatric clinical pharmacology and therapeutics. In: *Principles of clinical pharmacology,* ed 3, San Diego, CA, 2012, Academic Press, p 417–436.

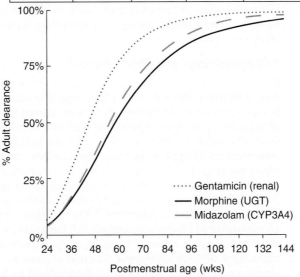

		% Adult clearance		
	Clearance Pathway	PMA 30 weeks	PMA 40 weeks	PMA 50% Adult
Gentamicin	Renal	19%	38%	45 wks
Morphine	UGT	9%	21%	58 wks
Midazolam	CYP3A4	8%	21%	55 wks

····· Gentamicin (renal)
— Morphine (UGT)
— Midazolam (CYP3A4)

Postmenstrual age (wks)

Figure 11.12 Clearance maturation patterns of common drugs used in neonates. *PMA* is postmenstrual age expressed in weeks; a full-term neonate would have a PMA 40 weeks at birth. *CYP,* Cytochrome P450; *UGT,* UDP-glucuronosyltransferase. (Data simulated from Germovsek E, Barker CIS, Sharland M, Standing JF: Scaling clearance in paediatric pharmacokinetics: all models are wrong, which are useful? *Br J Clin Pharmacol* 2017;83:777–790; Holford NHG, Ma SC, Anderson BJ: Prediction of morphine dose in humans. *Paediatr Anaesth* 2012;22:209–222.)

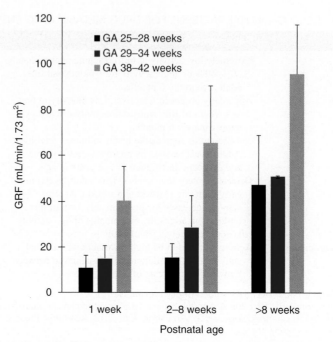

Figure 11.13 Glomerular filtration rate (*GFR*) in neonates by gestational age (*GA*) and postnatal age. (Data from Schwartz GJ, Brion LP, Spitzer A: The use of plasma creatinine concentration for estimating glomerular filtration rate in infants, children, and adolescents. *Pediatr Clin North Am* 1987;34:571–590.)

and premature neonates have a lower GFR than term neonates (Fig. 11.13). After birth, increased renal perfusion leads to rapid changes in GFR in the first week of life. GFR continues to change during the first year of life, with 50% of adult GFR attained by 2 months of age for a full-term neonate (PMA 48 weeks).[24] By 1 year of age, >90% of adult GFR is achieved. Maturation of CL of gentamicin—a renally eliminated drug—follows a pattern similar to GFR maturation (see Fig. 11.12). Dosing strategies in neonates for renally eliminated drugs should account for these maturational changes of kidney function.

Pathophysiology and Organ Function

Critically ill neonates often have altered physiology and organ dysfunction due to their underlying disease state. Identifying neonates with injury to the liver and/or kidney is necessary to identify those with altered drug clearance. Serum creatinine offers a direct measure of renal function and is helpful in considering the need for dose adjustment for drugs eliminated by the kidneys. For example, vancomycin is eliminated unchanged in the urine, and clearance in neonates is predicted by serum creatinine (Fig. 11.14).[25] Lower doses and/or more prolonged dosing intervals are needed in neonates with elevated serum creatinine and reduced renal function. The AAP Redbook dosing recommendations for vancomycin in neonates are now guided by the patient's serum creatinine.[26] For a serum creatinine ≤0.6 *mg/dL*, a dose of 15 *mg/kg* every 12 hours is recommended. For infants with an elevated serum creatinine of 1.0 to 1.2 *mg/dL*, a dose of 15 *mg/kg* every 24 hours is recommended. Unfortunately, biomarkers of liver injury and function are not as sensitive nor as predictive of alterations in the clearance of drugs metabolized by the liver. Nonetheless, neonates with marked hepatic failure as measured by elevated liver enzymes and reduced synthetic function (i.e., albumin, ammonia, and coagulation factors) may warrant dose reductions.

Certain neonatal populations are known to frequently have alterations in drug pharmacokinetics. In addition to injury to the brain, neonates with HIE commonly

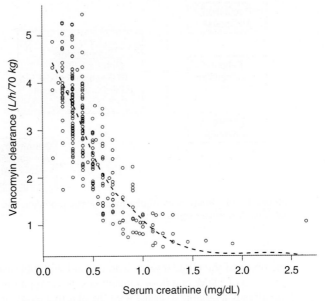

Figure 11.14 Vancomycin clearance in neonates by serum creatinine. Clearance is weight-adjusted to a 70-kg adult using allometric scaling (*L/h/70 kg*). (Data from Frymoyer A, Hersh AL, El-Komy MH, Gaskari S, Su F, Drover DR, Van Meurs K: Association between vancomycin trough concentration and AUC in neonates. *Antimicrob Agents Chemother* 2014;58:6454–6461.)

have hypoxic injury to the liver and kidney. Reduced clearance of both renally eliminated (gentamicin) and hepatically metabolized drugs (morphine, midazolam, phenobarbital) have been demonstrated.[17,27–30] Dose reductions and/or more prolonged dosing intervals are required in this population. Other populations where clearance can be markedly altered include those receiving coronary-pulmonary bypass, extracorporeal membrane oxygenation, or continuous renal replacement therapy. Consultation with a clinical pharmacist and utilization of therapeutic drug monitoring where available are necessary to appropriately guide the drug dosing needs in these populations.

Dosing Strategies and Therapeutic Drug Monitoring

Clinical pharmacokinetic studies in neonates have advanced the evidence-based dosing strategies of many commonly used drugs. Further, the application of population pharmacokinetic modeling and simulation has provided a quantitative framework to enhance the understanding of sources of variation between neonates in clearance and V_d (both known and unknown). The predictive construct offered by the pharmacokinetic models supports the development of customized dosing strategies that are most likely to achieve exposure targets of interest across subgroups of neonates (Fig. 11.15). Incorporation of weight and developmental status into the dose decision making is a critical element of designing a clinically pragmatic dosing strategy. Further adjustments based on underlying injury to organs important in drug metabolism and elimination are also often necessary.

Due to the large pharmacokinetic variation between neonates, even an optimally designed dosing strategy may result in widely different exposures across patients. For narrow therapeutic index drugs, this presents a problem. Therapeutic drug monitoring (TDM) is therefore essential for evaluation of concentration-related toxicity or therapeutic efficacy. Drugs for which TDM is readily available include gentamicin, tobramycin, vancomycin, phenobarbital, theophylline, phenytoin, and digoxin. Pharmacokinetic principles as outlined in this chapter allow further refinement of the dosing strategy for an individual neonate. Of course, such calculations can be time consuming and a burden to clinical workflow. Clinical pharmacists are invaluable

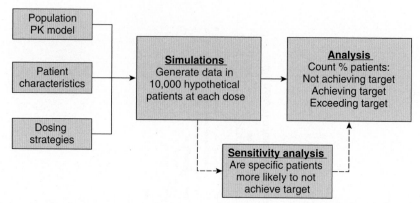

Figure 11.15   Framework of pharmacokinetic modeling and simulation approach to develop optimal dosing strategies.

members of the clinical team who can aid with pharmacokinetic calculations, interpretation of TDM, and dose adjustments. Several pharmacokinetic software programs are already available to assist with the pharmacokinetic calculations and dose adjustment.[31] In addition, with advances in computing power, availability of electronic medical records, and flourishing clinical informatics support, more advanced clinical dosing support tools are being developed to improve user experience, assist in clinical workflow, and provide a seamless integration with the electronic medical record.[32]

REFERENCES

1. Burns LE, Hodgman JE, Cass AB. Fatal circulatory collapse in premature infants receiving chloramphenicol. *N Engl J Med.* 1959;261:1318–1321.
2. Weiss CF, Glazko AJ, Weston JK. Chloramphenicol in the newborn infant. A physiologic explanation of its toxicity when given in excessive doses. *N Engl J Med.* 1960;262:787–794.
3. Wettrell G. Distribution and elimination of digoxin in infants. *Eur J Clin Pharmacol.* 1977;11:329–335.
4. Friis-Hansen B. Body water compartments in children: changes during growth and related changes in body composition. *Pediatrics.* 1961;28:169–181.
5. Jenh AM, Tamma PD, Milstone AM. Extended-interval aminoglycoside dosing in pediatrics. *Pediatr Infect Dis J.* 2011;30:338–339.
6. Nestaas E, Bangstad HJ, Sandvik L, et al. Aminoglycoside extended interval dosing in neonates is safe and effective: a meta-analysis. *Arch Dis Child Fetal Neonatal Ed.* 2005;90:F294–F300.
7. Moore RD, Lietman PS, Smith CR. Clinical response to aminoglycoside therapy: importance of the ratio of peak concentration to minimal inhibitory concentration. *J Infect Dis.* 1987;155:93–99.
8. Moore RD, Smith CR, Lietman PS. Association of aminoglycoside plasma levels with therapeutic outcome in gram-negative pneumonia. *Am J Med.* 1984;77:657–662.
9. DiCenzo R, Forrest A, Slish JC, et al. A gentamicin pharmacokinetic population model and once-daily dosing algorithm for neonates. *Pharmacotherapy.* 2003;23:585–591.
10. *Aminophylline Injection USP [package insert].* Lake Forest, IL: Hospira, Inc; 2009.
11. Pitlick W, Painter M, Pippenger C. Phenobarbital pharmacokinetics in neonates. *Clin Pharmacol Ther.* 1978;23:346–350.
12. McDade EJ, Wagner JL, Moffett BS, et al. Once-daily gentamicin dosing in pediatric patients without cystic fibrosis. *Pharmacotherapy.* 2010;30:248–253.
13. Kirkpatrick CM, Duffull SB, Begg EJ. Pharmacokinetics of gentamicin in 957 patients with varying renal function dosed once daily. *Br J Clin Pharmacol.* 1999;47:637–643.
14. Allegaert K, de Hoon J, Verbesselt R, et al. Maturational pharmacokinetics of single intravenous bolus of propofol. *Paediatr Anaesth.* 2007;17:1028–1034.
15. Murat I, Billard V, Vernois J, et al. Pharmacokinetics of propofol after a single dose in children aged 1–3 years with minor burns. Comparison of three data analysis approaches. *Anesthesiology.* 1996;84:526–532.
16. van den Broek MP, Groenendaal F, Egberts AC, et al. Effects of hypothermia on pharmacokinetics and pharmacodynamics: a systematic review of preclinical and clinical studies. *Clin Pharmacokinet.* 2010;49:277–294.
17. Frymoyer A, Bonifacio SL, Drover DR, et al. Decreased morphine clearance in neonates with hypoxic ischemic encephalopathy receiving hypothermia. *J Clin Pharmacol.* 2017;57:64–76.
18. Knibbe CA, Krekels EH, van den Anker JN, et al. Morphine glucuronidation in preterm neonates, infants and children younger than 3 years. *Clin Pharmacokinet.* 2009;48:371–385.
19. West GB, Brown JH, Enquist BJ. A general model for the origin of allometric scaling laws in biology. *Science.* 1997;276:122–126.

20. Anderson BJ, Holford NH. Mechanism-based concepts of size and maturity in pharmacokinetics. *Annu Rev Pharmacol Toxicol*. 2008;48:303–332.
21. Holford N, Heo YA, Anderson B. A pharmacokinetic standard for babies and adults. *J Pharm Sci*. 2013;102:2941–2952.
22. Knebel W, Tammara B, Udata C, et al. Population pharmacokinetic modeling of pantoprazole in pediatric patients from birth to 16 years. *J Clin Pharmacol*. 2011;51:333–345.
23. van der Pol RJ, Smits MJ, van Wijk MP, et al. Efficacy of proton-pump inhibitors in children with gastroesophageal reflux disease: a systematic review. *Pediatrics*. 2011;127:925–935.
24. Rhodin MM, Anderson BJ, Peters AM, et al. Human renal function maturation: a quantitative description using weight and postmenstrual age. *Pediatr Nephrol*. 2009;24:67–76.
25. Frymoyer A, Hersh AL, El-Komy MH, et al. Association between vancomycin trough concentration and area under the concentration-time curve in neonates. *Antimicrob Agents Chemother*. 2014;58:6454–6461.
26. Kimberlin D, Brady M, Jackson M, et al, eds. *AAP Red Book*. 30th ed. Elk Grove Village, IL.: American Academy of Pediatrics; 2015:1151.
27. Gal P, Toback J, Erkan NV, et al. The influence of asphyxia on phenobarbital dosing requirements in neonates. *Dev Pharmacol Ther*. 1984;7:145–152.
28. Frymoyer A, Meng L, Bonifacio SL, et al. Gentamicin pharmacokinetics and dosing in neonates with hypoxic ischemic encephalopathy receiving hypothermia. *Pharmacotherapy*. 2013;33:718–726.
29. van den Broek MP, van Straaten HL, Huitema AD, et al. Anticonvulsant effectiveness and hemodynamic safety of midazolam in full-term infants treated with hypothermia. *Neonatology*. 2015;107:150–156.
30. Filippi L, la Marca G, Cavallaro G, et al. Phenobarbital for neonatal seizures in hypoxic ischemic encephalopathy: a pharmacokinetic study during whole body hypothermia. *Epilepsia*. 2011;52:794–801.
31. Roberts JA, Abdul-Aziz MH, Lipman J, et al. Individualised antibiotic dosing for patients who are critically ill: challenges and potential solutions. *Lancet Infect Dis*. 2014;14:498–509.
32. Mould DR, D'Haens G, Upton RN. Clinical decision support tools: the evolution of a revolution. *Clin Pharmacol Ther*. 2016;99:405–418.

11

CHAPTER 12

Neonatal Pharmacogenetics

Tamorah Lewis, MD, PhD

- Pharmacogenetics is a tool that can improve predictability of wanted drug effects and unwanted drug toxicities.
- Genetic influences on drug transport, metabolism, and response are not apparent until the relevant protein is sufficiently developmentally expressed.
- There are many examples of pharmacogenetic findings in adults and older pediatric populations that, if studied in infants, could change our current clinical practice.
- Pharmacogenetics can be used to predict which individuals are likely to fall at the extreme ends of drug disposition and drug response.

Introduction to Pharmacogenetics

Drug therapy is an integral part of neonatal medical care, and clinicians strive to optimize treatment. Medical interventions in the neonatal intensive care unit (NICU) are intended to reduce the consequences of preterm birth and severe neonatal illness, with the goal of minimizing long-term sequelae. In addition to the potential benefit of a medication to ameliorate a disease process, most medications carry a risk of toxicity. Many medications used in infants have not been rigorously studied for efficacy or safety, and the pharmacology of these medications is assumed based on studies in populations of older subjects. It is important to study pharmacologic variability in critically ill infants because they are exposed to many drugs, and this exposure increases with decreasing gestational age. On average, NICU infants are exposed to 4 medications, and the extremely low birth weight infant is exposed to 17.[1] In addition, there are unique drug risks in the neonatal population because of critical periods of organ development. The consequences of toxicity in the neonatal period can have lifelong consequences, such as dexamethasone exposure leading to central nervous system injury, nephrotoxicity leading to decreased nephron number, and ototoxicity leading to chronic hearing loss.

Optimizing the use of medications for individual critically ill infants requires knowledge of factors that contribute to variability in drug disposition and response and their integration into dosing strategies. Drug response in infants is highly variable for multiple reasons, including immediate postnatal adaptations in physiology, rapidly developing organ systems, and environmental influences such as diet and microbiome development. Maternal medication and cigarette, alcohol, or illicit drug use during gestation can alter metabolic pathways and drug targets important for postnatal therapy. The degree of prematurity is a major source of variability in drug response, as certain metabolic pathways are immature and drug targets may not have sufficiently developed. Critically ill infants in the NICU are especially vulnerable because medical illness can magnify these sources of pharmacologic variability. For these reasons, it can be difficult to pinpoint the effects of genetic variation on an already very heterogeneous population of patients.

Traditional pharmacology studies in infants have focused on pharmacokinetics and pharmacodynamics, but have largely failed to address genetic variability, one important source of interindividual differences in drug disposition and response. **Pharmacogenetics** describes the role of genetic variability in drug clinical response and toxicity. Pharmacogenetics in infants has to account for unique challenges, including prenatal factors and critical illness. Ontogeny, or organ development, is also a confounding factor because genetic variation cannot be evident if the drug metabolizing enzyme or drug target is not yet developmentally expressed. Yet these challenges should not prevent the field of neonatal pharmacogenetics from moving forward. An improved understanding of genetic predictors of drug response can move the field of neonatology toward personalized medicine and improve the care for individual infants.

When an infant is treated with a medication, we can predict the likely response from prior population studies, but there is value in having a more precise understanding of how *individual* patients will respond based on their stage of development and genotype. Each infant carries genetic polymorphisms, or variations, and this results in individual genes having slightly different nucleotide sequences. When one gene can have many different sequence options, each different sequence is defined an allele (i.e., *CYP2D6*1* and *CYP2D6*2*). The *1 designation indicates the fully functional reference sequence against which all other sequences are assessed. Sequence deviations from this reference sequence are considered variant forms of the gene. Single nucleotide polymorphisms (SNPs) are the most common type of genetic variation, with each human carrying approximately 10 million SNPs in their genome. SNPs can be associated with total loss of activity, partial loss of activity, or in some cases, gain of function. A more extreme version of genetic variation is copy number variations (CNVs). In CNVs, multiple copies of fully functional genes can give rise to greater-than-anticipated activity, as will be described later for *CYP2D6* and codeine. For genes important for drug response, an infant can be either homozygous for the reference allele, heterozygous with one variant allele, or homozygous for the variant allele, and each of these states has the potential to manifest clinically as a different drug response phenotype. Genetic variability is not only pertinent to drug response. Many endogenous compounds are subject to transport in the intestine and liver and metabolism in the liver and kidneys. Important discoveries in the genetics of hyperbilirubinemia have found that polymorphisms in transporters SLCO1B1 and SLCO1B3 and metabolizing enzyme UGT1A1 are predictors of significant jaundice.[2,3] Table 12.1 contains a list of definitions for commonly used pharmacogenetic terms.

Genetic variation differs with ethnic background and geographic origin. Certain SNPs and variant alleles are more common in populations of different races, so in order for pharmacogenetics to benefit all patients, it is important for studies to include a wide range of racial diversity. The adult pharmacogenetic studies of warfarin anticoagulation are an example of this phenomenon. African Americans were underrepresented in the studies looking for candidate genes of warfarin response, and the types and frequency of phenotypically important variants are different between Caucasians and African Americans. CYP2C9 is important for warfarin clearance, and the SNPs discovered in the largely Caucasian populations were not as helpful in explaining the variability in warfarin dose in African Americans. *VKORC1* is an important gene for warfarin response, and the important alleles for this gene occur at different frequencies in Caucasians and African Americans. Thus the early dose-prediction models for warfarin did not perform well in African American populations.[4] Novel gene sequencing studies targeting the minority population revealed novel variants, which when taken into account improved the genetic prediction of warfarin dose needed in this minority population.[5]

Table 12.1 GLOSSARY OF COMMONLY ENCOUNTERED TERMS IN THE GENETIC LITERATURE (ALPHABETICAL ORDER)

Allele	Varying (or variant) forms of a gene at a specific location in the genome.
Exon	Region of a gene encoding for a particular portion of the complete protein.
Gene	The functional and physical unit of heredity passed from parent to offspring. Genes contain information for making a specific protein.
Genetic testing	Generic term for an array of techniques that analyze DNA, RNA, or proteins for general health or medical identification purposes.
Genome	The entirety of an individual's genetic code: approximately 6 billion nucleotides comprising approximately 20,500 genes.
Genomics	Scientific study of a genome, including any or all combinations of genes, their functions, and their interactions with each other and the surrounding environment.
Genotype	An individual's two alleles at specific loci.
Haplotype	Combinations of SNP alleles located close to one another on a chromosome. If close together, haplotypes can be inherited as units or blocks.
Heterozygous	Having two different forms of a particular gene (AB).
Homozygous	Having two identical forms of a particular gene (AA).
Intron	Noncoding sequences of DNA that are removed from the RNA transcript before exportation from the nucleus.
Mutation	Permanent and structural alteration in DNA. Most cause little, if any, harm. If in a critical location, such as the DNA repair genes in *BRCA1* and *BRCA2,* can cause severe disease such as early-onset cancer.
Phenotype	A patient's observable clinical and physiologic characteristics as a result of inherited genotype interacting with their environment.
Polymorphism	The existence of multiple genotypes in a population at one locus. Variants are not caused by mutations in DNA because they occur at a frequency greater than can occur by evolutionary (slow) means. Polymorphisms may take several forms, including SNPs, CNVs, and insertion/deletion (indels).
Promoter	Short stretch of regulatory DNA sequence that signals where transcription should start in a gene (for the RNA polymerase).
SNPs	Single nucleotide polymorphism(s). The difference of a single-base pair at a specific position in the genome between two different individuals in a population. Most are inconsequential, but if in a coding region may cause changes in gene efficiency and/or function.
Variant	Another word for polymorphism.

Table modified from Table 2 Kurnat-Thomas EL: Genetics and genomics: the scientific drivers of personalized medicine. *Annu Rev Nurs Res* 2011;29:27–44.

12

Intersection of Ontogeny and Pharmacogenetics

In order for genetic variation to have a clinical impact, the protein of interest (be it a transporter or metabolizing enzyme) must be sufficiently expressed in the patient. Depending on gestational age and postnatal age, there is a wide range of developmental trajectories in proteins important in drug absorption and metabolism.[6] One classic example of ontogenic change in protein expression and abundance is the transition from fetal hepatic CYP3A7 to postnatal CYP3A4. Fetal CYP3A7 plays a role in steroid metabolism and homeostasis, and expression is the highest in the first trimester and declines with gestation. Hepatic CYP3A4 is low during gestation and shows a 29-fold surge in mRNA shortly after birth, and the mRNA levels exceed adult levels between 2 and 7 months of age.[7] Using enzyme-specific metabolite formation in liver samples, Stevens et al. confirmed a decrease in CYP3A7 during gestation and an increase in CYP3A4 in the perinatal and postnatal period.[8] In addition, they showed that CYP3A4 contributes anywhere between <1% and 36% of the total hepatic CYP3A content between the ages of 0 and 6 months. This developmental trajectory of CYP3A4 is important for drugs used in the NICU.

Clearance of midazolam, a CYP3A4 substrate, matures rapidly over the first months of life.[9] A very thorough pharmacokinetic (PK) modeling study using multiple newborn data sets shows that midazolam clearance in preterm infants between 0.5 and 4 kg is only 2.6% to 28% of adult values.[10] This same study shows a 10-fold

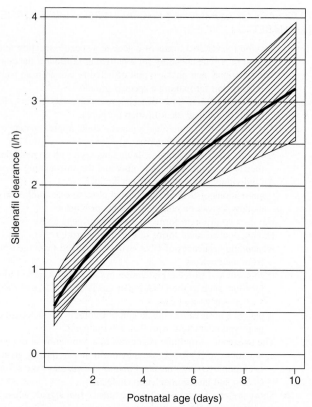

Figure 12.1 Model-predicted relationship between sildenafil clearance and postnatal age for the typical infant. The bold line is the mean and the shaded region is the 90% confidence interval. (Figure modified from Figure 7 in Mukherjee et al.: Population pharmacokinetics of sildenafil in term infants: evidence of rapid maturation of metabolic clearance in the early postnatal period. *Clin Pharmacol Ther* 2009;85[1]:56–63.)

difference in midazolam clearance between infants weighing 1 kg (0.001 L/min) and 10 kg (0.01 L/min); thus, the model predicts that clearance can increase up to 10-fold over the first year of life. The low clearance in newborns likely reflects the lack of CYP3A7 capacity for midazolam metabolism, and the increase over the first months of life likely reflects the increased developmental expression of CYP3A4. Although it is well known that midazolam clearance increases with age, there are no current dosing guidelines that increase the weight-based dose with age, in part because the development of the drug target and the target drug exposure in the central nervous system (CNS) are not well understood. CYP3A4 is also responsible for the majority of sildenafil metabolism. Sildenafil clearance triples over the first week of life[11] (Fig. 12.1), reflecting maturation of the CYP-mediated metabolism. This signifies that achievement of the same plasma concentrations requires a threefold dose escalation over the first week of life. Current dosing guidelines in newborns do not contain this information, likely leading to underdosing as metabolic capacity matures.

Thus genetic variation in drug metabolism will not be apparent until the drug metabolizing enzyme (DME) is sufficiently expressed. Pantoprazole is used to treat symptomatic gastroesophageal reflux disease in the NICU. Ward and colleagues undertook a population pharmacokinetic study in which infants were randomized to two pantoprazole doses and the drug exposure was quantified.[12] In addition, *CYP2C19* and *CYP3A4* genotypes were determined. As can be seen in Fig. 12.2, two infants were identified as genetically poor metabolizers, but the genotypic effect was not apparent until 15 weeks of age when the CYP2C19 enzyme was sufficiently expressed. The development of the enzyme allows the uncovering of pharmacogenetic differences. Optimal treatment with proton pump inhibitors in the first weeks of life may not

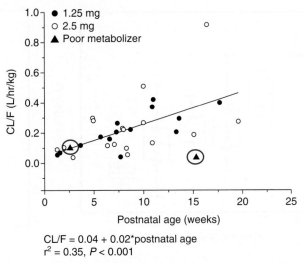

$$CL/F = 0.04 + 0.02\text{*}postnatal\ age$$
$$r^2 = 0.35,\ P < 0.001$$

Figure 12.2 Poor metabolizer status for pantoprazole clearance does not become apparent until 15 weeks of age, when the CYP2C19 enzyme is sufficiently expressed. Y-axis is weight-adjusted clearance and X-axis is postnatal age. (Figure modified from Figure 3 in Ward et al.: Single-dose, multi-dose, and population pharmacokinetics of pantoprazole in infants and preterm infants with a clinical diagnosis of gastroesophageal reflux disease [GERD]. *Eur J Clin Pharmacol* 2010;66:555–561.)

require knowledge of infant genotype, but by 3 months, knowing the poor metabolizer genotype would be important to prevent accumulation of the drug.

Even in young infants, effects of genetic variation in drug metabolism can be observed. Tramadol is a μ-opiate antagonist used in some NICUs for analgesia and serves as a model drug for the study of pharmacogenetics in infants. Tramadol is demethylated to its primary metabolite by CYP2D6. CYP2D6 activity can be classified into varying activity scores by translating the allelic genotype into a phenotypic metabolizing capacity in adults. Looking at ratios of parent drug to metabolite in the plasma and urine gives insight into catalytic activity of CYP2D6. As can be seen in Fig. 12.3, among an entire cohort of 82 infants with postmenstrual age (PMA) 25 to 62 weeks, the metabolism of tramadol increases with *CYP2D6* activity score.[13] It can also be seen that even within the same activity score, infants of older PMA have increased metabolic activity (lower parent drug to metabolite ratios). In drugs with a narrow therapeutic index, these genetic variations could have significant clinical effect. For example, a 42-week infant with a *CYP2D6* activity score of 0.5 would be at risk for more significant respiratory depression than a similarly aged infant with a *CYP2D6* activity score of 3. This is because in the poor metabolizer infant, parent drug could accumulate more easily with a continuous infusion or repeat dosing. In fact, this risk of respiratory depression with *CYP2D6* poor metabolizer status is included in the Food and Drug Administration drug label.

Alternatively, a predrug dosed in the neonatal period may not be effective because the infant lacks the enzyme required for activation of the drug to its active form. Oseltamivir for influenza is an example of a drug that requires this hepatic activation. Using liver samples from multiple infant age groups, Shi and colleagues showed that hydrolytic activity (prodrug to active drug) increased by four- to sevenfold between birth and 70 days of age. Liver samples from infants aged 1 to 31 days have 10% the mRNA expression and drug hydrolysis capacity of adults.[14] Thus oseltamivir dosed in the first few days of life will have very limited efficacy because little of the compound will be transformed to the active compound. But because the activating enzyme matures rapidly after birth, the postnatal surge in CES1 allows for effective use of oseltamivir in young infants.

The rapidly challenging developmental landscape of neonatal and pediatric pharmacology has important implications for research. First, we must not limit

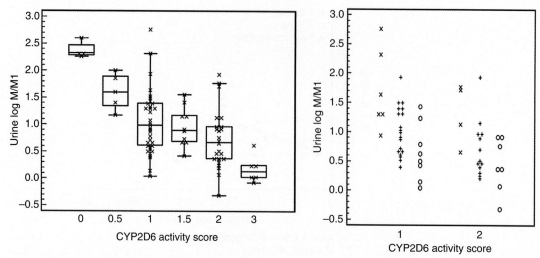

Figure 12.3 *(Left)* In infants, the ratio of parent drug (M = tramadol) to primary metabolite (M1 = *O*-demethyl tramadol) increases with increasing CYP2D6 activity score, based on genotype. *(Right)* Even among infants of the same genetic activity score for CYP2D6, the metabolism of tramadol increases with increasing postmenstrual age. (X) = <37 weeks, (+) = 37 to 41 weeks, (O) = >41 weeks. (Figure edited from Figures 2 and 5 in Allegaert et al.: Postmenstrual age and CYP2D6 polymorphisms determine tramadol O-demethylation in critically ill infants. *Pediatr Res* 2008;63[6]:674–679.)

ourselves to only studying genetic alterations that have been identified in adult populations. These alterations may not be pertinent to infants, and there may be novel alleles more important to the neonatal population. Second, before we can fully understand the importance of genetic factors, we must more clearly understand the ontogeny of DMEs, transporters, and drug targets so that the individual effects of development and genetics can be identified.

Pharmacogenetics of the Dose → Exposure → Response Paradigm

When a child is given a dose of a drug and does not respond as expected, there are multiple potential explanations. The first explanation is that the dose did not result in an adequate drug exposure, meaning there was never enough active drug in the system to have the wanted effect. There are examples in neonatology where drugs are likely ineffective because the exposure is insufficient. Ibuprofen is metabolized by CYP2C8 and CYP2C9, the expression of which increase in the postnatal period. When giving the same weight-based dose (i.e., 10 mg/kg for patent ductus arteriosus [PDA] closure), the drug exposure is much less in a 4-week-old infant than in a 1-week-old infant. Thus the "inefficacy" of ibuprofen for closure of the PDA as infants age is likely complicated by insufficient drug exposure.[15] This developmental dose–exposure variability can be confounded by genetic contributions to the dose–exposure paradigm (Fig. 12.4). For the same drug, ibuprofen, adults with a variant allele *CYP2C9*3* have decreased metabolism, leading to a 30% increase in drug exposure. *CYP2C8*3* has a 20% increase in ibuprofen clearance compared with the wild type, leading to a decreased exposure, and carriers of this polymorphism have fewer adverse events with ibuprofen therapy.[16] Although this has never been studied in infants, genetic variants in DMEs likely contribute to variability in the dose–exposure relationship.

Ontogeny and genetic variation in the drug target may also lead to variability in drug response by altering the exposure–response relationship. For example, if a receptor, ion channel, or other target of drug action is not present at a particular developmental stage or as a consequence of genetic variation, it is unlikely that the anticipated therapeutic response will be observed. Although human studies on the development

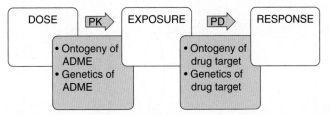

Figure 12.4 Both ontogeny and genetics can affect the relationship between dose and exposure (pharmacokinetics) and between exposure and response (pharmacodynamics). *ADME,* absorption, distribution, metabolism, and excretion; *PD,* pharmacodynamics; *PK,* pharmacokinetics. (Adapted from Lewis T. Precision therapeutics in the NICU: why are we missing the mark? *J Perinatol.* 2018. doi: 10.1038/s41372-018-0052-8.)

12

of drug targets are lacking, there are indirect examples of how development can affect the drug exposure–response relationship. In preterm infants treated with erythropoietin, later-gestation infants have a larger clinical response,[17] likely because erythropoiesis is more firmly established in the bone marrow and the erythroid progenitor cells have increased sensitivity to both exogenous and endogenous erythropoietin.

Examples of Pharmacogenetics Relevant to Neonatology

Maternal SNPs and Drug Effects During Pregnancy and Lactation

Maternal prenatal acetaminophen use has been associated with increased risk of childhood asthma, although the mechanisms are not clear. In a longitudinal study of >4000 mothers and >5000 children, maternal antioxidant genotype was correlated with risk of childhood asthma among women who took acetaminophen during pregnancy.[18] Polymorphisms in two important antioxidant genes, nuclear erythroid 2 p45-related factor 2 (*NRF2*) and glutathione s-transferase (*GST*), were assessed. The risk of asthma and wheezing with early-gestation acetaminophen exposure was increased with maternal minor allele of *NRF2*. Additionally, maternal SNPs in *GSTMI* increased risk of wheezing in childhood with late-gestation exposure, and these effects were amplified when *GSTMI* variants were also present in the child.

Efavirenz is an anti-HIV drug with known pharmacogenetic variation in metabolism. Maternal plasma concentrations vary with *CYP2B6* metabolizer status, with a common SNP 516G>T conferring decreased efavirenz metabolism in an allele-dependent fashion, with TT carriers having the slowest metabolism. A study of 134 breastfeeding women investigated the effects of *CYP2B6* genetics on breast milk and infant plasma concentrations of the drug. As can be seen in Fig. 12.5, infants with poor metabolizer mothers had higher levels of efavirenz in breast milk and in neonatal plasma compared with infants of wild-type mothers. As can be seen in Panel B, the allelic genotype at this locus does not explain all elevated plasma concentrations, as there was an infant of a wild-type mother who also had an elevated plasma concentration. The transfer of drug in breast milk is important for many reasons. First, the Panel on Antiretroviral Therapy and Medical Management of HIV-Infected Children (the Panel) recommends that efavirenz generally not be used in children aged 3 months to <3 years. Second, this low-dose exposure can lead to HIV resistance in the rare cases of failure of prevention of maternal-neonatal transmission of HIV.

Codeine is bioactivated to the active compound, morphine, by CYP2D6. There are reports both in children[19] and adults[20] of death from respiratory depression from typical doses in patients who carry an increased copy number of *CYP2D6*, and are thus ultra-rapid metabolizers (UMs). These UMs have rapid and complete conversion of codeine to morphine, leading to dangerously high plasma and CNS concentrations. Codeine has been discouraged in nursing mothers because there is highly variable conversion to morphine based on genotypic metabolic capacity of CYP2D6. In nursing

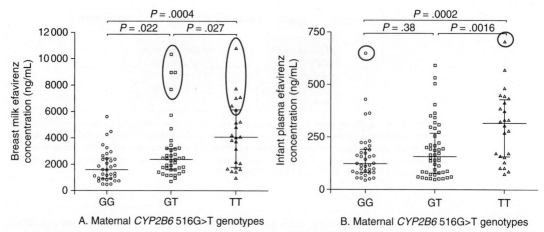

Figure 12.5 Infants who are breastfed by mothers who carry the GT and TT allele of CYP2B6 (decreased metabolism) have elevated levels of efavirenz in their milk (BM) and plasma compared with infants of wild-type mothers. Therapeutic plasma concentrations as low as 1000 ng/mL have been reported, so the infants circled in red have near-therapeutic concentrations from breast milk exposure. (Figure is edited from Figure 2 in Olagunju et al: Breast milk pharmacokinetics of efavirenz and breastfed infants' exposure in genetically defined subgroups of mother-infant pairs: an observational study. *Clin Infect Dis* 2015;61[3]:453–463.)

mothers, the ultra-rapid conversion of codeine to morphine can result in high and unsafe concentrations of morphine in breastfed infants. A 13-day-old infant died of a morphine overdose during a time when the mother was taking less than the prescribed dose of codeine for postpartum pain, and genetic testing of the mother proved that she was a UM.[21] The danger to the newborn is magnified because they have decreased glucuronidation capacity. If clinicians are going to use codeine in nursing women, a risk model has been published that combines maternal *CYP2D6* and *ABCB1* genotype and clinical factors. *CYP2D6* and *ABCB1* genetic polymorphisms were associated with an increased odds of CNS depression in breastfed infants (OR 2.68, 95% CI 1.61–4.48). This model can predict 87% of infant CNS depression with 80% sensitivity and 87% specificity.[22]

Thus knowing maternal genotype in key genes can help obstetricians and neonatologists understand the true risk of medications used during pregnancy and lactation. For drugs with high potential for neonatal and developmental side effects (pain medications, antidepressants, seizure medications), further pharmacogenetic studies are needed to identify the mother–infant pairs at the highest risk for poor outcomes.

Pharmacogenetics of Pain Medications

Because pain is a common symptom among medically ill patients, there is a growing literature about analgesic medications and appropriate dosing and titration in adults and older pediatric populations. Large interpatient variability is observed in the clinical response to pain medications, both with wanted efficacy and unwanted side effects such as sedation and respiratory depression. Multiple researchers have investigated the potential genetic underpinnings of these unpredictable responses, and the knowledge gained from this literature lays the groundwork for future pharmacogenetic studies in the neonatal population.

Morphine is the most commonly used opiate in the NICU for pain control. Large amounts of interindividual variation in response to morphine therapy have prompted groups to investigate the genetic underpinnings of variable response. The pharmacogenetics of morphine for postoperative pain have been investigated in older pediatric populations, and the results have potential implications in the neonatal setting. Morphine is transported into the liver by OCT1 and metabolized primarily by UGT2B7 to morphine-3-glucuronide (M3G, inactive metabolite) and morphine-6-glucuronide (M6G, active metabolite). In 146 children undergoing post-tonsillectomy

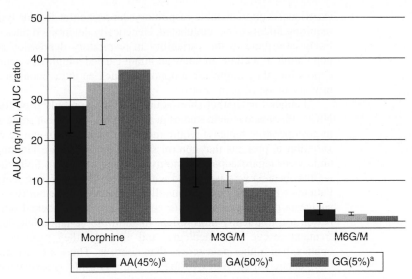

Figure 12.6   Carriers of the UGT2B7 −840G allele have decreased morphine glucuronidation in adult patients with sickle cell disease. In homozygous −840G patients, AUC of parent drug morphine is increased, and ratios of metabolite to parent drug are decreased. (Figure 1 from Darbari et al.: UGT2B7 promoter variant −840G>A contributes to the variability in hepatic clearance of morphine in patients with sickle cell disease. *Am J Hematology* 2008;83:200–202.)

pain control with morphine, loss of function variants in *OCT1* led to 20% less morphine clearance than in wild-type and heterozygous subjects.[23] The variant allele, *OCT1*3*, is present in 26% of Caucasians and 13% of African Americans, so observed interracial difference in morphine response may be due in part to differential clearance. Children with loss-of-function alleles in this hepatic transporter would be predicted to have better pain control with less morphine, because they are clearing the parent drug more slowly.

Once the morphine is transported into the hepatocyte, UGT2B7 catalytic activity determines the rate of metabolism. In 86 adults, homozygous carriers of a loss-of-function haplotype (−161C/T in promoter and 802C/T in Exon 2) had reduced M6G-to-morphine ratios compared with noncarriers of these alleles.[24] Because M6G is a more potent analgesic than the parent drug morphine, decreased levels of this metabolite can contribute to variable pain resolution. In 20 adult patients with sickle cell disease, carriers and patients homozygous for the *UGT2B7* −840G>A SNP showed decreased morphine glucuronidation compared with wild-type patients[25] (Fig. 12.6). The variant allele was present in 70% of this sample, making this *UGT2B7* potentially relevant to a significant portion of the population. A child's genetic potential for morphine metabolism will determine morphine clearance, and the ratio of parent drug to active and inactive metabolites can affect response to treatment for pain control and also the risk of respiratory depression with drug accumulation. Knowing whether an infant is a carrier of these common SNPs could potentially guide initial dose selection and drip titration, so future studies of pain control in infants should consider these genetic variables.

In addition to morphine transport into liver and hepatic metabolism, the rate of morphine efflux from the CNS compartment is an important variable in clinical response. Among 263 children who underwent tonsillectomy, the genotype of *ABCB1* (also known as P-glycoprotein or P-gp) was investigated for correlations with respiratory depression. Children with GG and GA genotypes at *ABCB1* rs9282564 have an increased risk of respiratory depression leading to prolonged postanesthesia care unit stays. Each additional copy of the minor allele conferred an increased odds by 4.7-fold.[26] Clinicians who use morphine to treat postoperative pain in infants have experienced unpredictable respiratory depression at low or typical doses, at times requiring infants to be reintubated. Genetically determined rates of CNS opiate efflux likely contribute to the variability in respiratory depression seen in the neonatal population. If a clinician knew an infant carried a high-risk genotype for respiratory depression, they might use a nonopiate such as intravenous acetaminophen for the primary mode of pain control.

Fentanyl is another short-acting opiate commonly used for pain control in the NICU. Pharmacogenetic studies in adults have shown that some amount of variability in postoperative fentanyl requirements for pain control can be explained by genetic variation in proteins that control sensory mechanotransduction. In 350 adults who underwent laparoscopic colectomy, carriage of variant SNPs in *LAMB3* (encoding laminin beta-3) was associated with 24-hour postoperative fentanyl requirements.[27] Patients who carried the variant allele demanded more boluses of patient-controlled analgesia doses compared with controls and were "locked out" from pressing the button too frequently more often. In addition, variant allele carriers required more frequent rescue pain medicine, and although they received more postoperative opiates, had higher pain scores than controls. There are also adult studies showing that genetic variation in *OPRM1*[28,29] and *CYP3A4*[30] is associated with postoperative opiate requirements in various populations.

Methadone is increasingly used in the neonatal and infant population for the treatment of neonatal abstinence syndrome (NAS), both after in utero opiate exposure and prolonged medical opiate exposure in the NICU. There is extensive evidence in adults that genetic variation in *CYP2B6* has a significant impact on methadone pharmacokinetics. As discussed in a review article on genetic predictors of placental opiate transfer,[31] a study of 336 patients undergoing methadone maintenance therapy showed an association between *CYP2B6* haplotypes containing both intronic and exonic SNPs and plasma concentrations of methadone and the concentration-to-dose ratio.[32] A re-analysis of extreme patient dose requirements in a different cohort of methadone maintenance patients has shown that certain *CYP2B6* SNPs are more or less common in patients with high and low methadone concentrations, strengthening the etiologic link between genetic changes in the metabolizing enzyme and differences in methadone plasma concentrations.[33] A systematic review shows that patients homozygous for the *CYP2B6*6* allele have higher methadone plasma concentrations, suggesting that methadone metabolism is significantly slower in *6* homozygous carriers.[34]

Although pain and sedation medications are historically titrated to effect, proponents of personalized medicine would argue that we can do better for our patients. If an infant has a clear genetic predictor of increased risk of adverse event (respiratory depression) or decreased effectiveness (will be in pain for hours while opiate dose is increased from the "standard" starting dose), then it is incumbent on the physician to use all of the tools possible to provide optimal care. Granted, the clinical impact of many of these genetic changes is not clear in infants, but it seems beyond time to increase the number of pharmacogenetic studies in the field of neonatal analgesia and sedation.

Pharmacogenetics of Neonatal Abstinence Syndrome

In addition to the prior discussed genetic influences on opiate transport into the liver and hepatic opiate metabolism, an important predictor of clinical response to opiate treatment for NAS is the drug target at the effector site. *OPRM1* encodes the μ-opioid receptor 1, which is the main receptor target for methadone and morphine therapy in NAS. The *OPRM1* 118A>G SNP is associated with reduced need for pharmacologic intervention and shorter length of treatment in infants with in utero–acquired NAS.[35] Increased methylation of the *OPRM1* promoter, hypothesized to lead to gene silencing, is associated with worse NAS outcomes (more likely to require ≥2 medications to control NAS) in a cohort of 86 infants.[36] In addition to the μ-opiate receptor, SNPs in the catecholamine O-methyltransferase (*COMT*) gene have been associated with decreased need for postnatal treatment and shorter length of stay in NAS infants.[37] The COMT protein is responsible for dopamine metabolism, so the hypothesis is

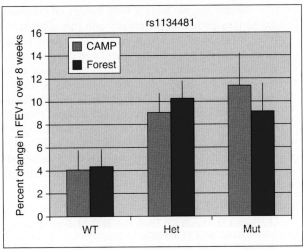

Figure 12.7   Percent change in FEV$_1$ after 8 weeks of inhaled corticosteroid treatment by T gene rs1134481 genotype in two study populations. (Reprinted with permission of the American Thoracic Society. Copyright © 2018 American Thoracic Society. From Tantisira et al. Genone-wide association identifies the T Gene as a novel asthma pharmacogenetic locus. *Am J Respir Cit Care Med* 2012;185:1286–1291. The American Journal of Respiratory and Critical Care Medicine is an official journal of the American Thoracic Society.)

that loss-of-function SNPs in this enzyme lead to higher endogenous dopamine levels and decreased NAS severity.

Pharmacogenetics of Steroid Treatment for Bronchospasm

Inhaled and systemic steroids are commonly used in patients with asthma, with a resultant wide range in clinical response. Recognizing that this interindividual variability could be genetic in origin, asthma researchers have performed various studies to identify genetic predictors of steroid response. SNPs in steroid metabolism and response genes have shown significant and clinically meaningful associations with inhaled steroid response phenotype. For example, children who carry *CYP3A4*22* demonstrate a significantly greater improvement in asthma control when treated with fluticasone compared with children who do not carry the allele.[38] A genome-wide association study of inhaled steroid response has identified the T gene as a pharmacogenetic locus. In two large asthma study cohorts, the SNP rs1134481 is associated with change in FEV$_1$ after 8 weeks of treatment (Fig. 12.7).[39] Although we do not treat asthma in the NICU, infants with bronchopulmonary dysplasia (BPD) present with a similar physiology of inflammation, bronchospasm, and air trapping and are thus commonly treated with inhaled and systemic steroids. As in asthma, there is a wide range of clinical response to steroids in the BPD population. Borrowing from and building upon the pharmacogenetic knowledge in asthma can allow BPD researchers to identify important pharmacogenetic loci in this neonatal and infant population, leading to more personalized steroid therapy.

Conclusion

There are challenges to implementing pharmacogenetics in the NICU. The ontogeny of drug biotransformation and distribution are far better understood than the ontogeny of drug targets, making it hard to know an exact "therapeutic concentration" to aim for with many of our drug therapies. As a profession, we still have much to learn about how organ dysfunction and metabolism-altering interventions (i.e., therapeutic hypothermia) affect drug pharmacokinetics and pharmacodynamics before genetics are even taken into consideration. Until recently, there were no readily available genotyping assays with a rapid enough turnaround time to be useful in the acute care setting, making integration of pharmacogenetics into ICU care impossible.

Neonatologists have a long history of "titration to effect" medicine, but there are serious patient implications with this approach. For example, how long does it take to titrate to an effect when the system is rapidly changing, while both the clearance of the drug and the drug target are potentially developing? Once the clearance mechanism and drug target are fully expressed, do genetics determine which infants respond to the drug right away, which do in a delayed fashion, and which infants do not respond at all? The promise of personalized medicine suggests that we can improve patient care by taking into account patient-specific variables beyond basic covariates such as weight and age. Pharmacogenetics, if studied adequately and implemented correctly, has the potential to identify individual patients most likely to deviate substantially from dosing requirements and outcomes designed for "populations" and thereby improve neonatal pharmaceutical therapy.

REFERENCES

1. Hsieh EM, Hornik CP, Clark RH, et al. Medication use in the neonatal intensive care unit. *Am J Perinatol*. 2014;31:811–821.
2. Sato H, Uchida T, Toyota K, et al. Association of neonatal hyperbilirubinemia in breast-fed infants with ugt1a1 or slcos polymorphisms. *J Hum Genet*. 2015;60:35–40.
3. Ergin H, Bican M, Atalay OE. A causal relationship between udp-glucuronosyltransferase 1a1 promoter polymorphism and idiopathic hyperbilirubinemia in turkish newborns. *Turk J Pediatr*. 2010;52:28–34.
4. Schelleman H, Chen J, Chen Z, et al. Dosing algorithms to predict warfarin maintenance dose in caucasians and african americans. *Clin Pharmacol Ther*. 2008;84:332–339.
5. Perera MA, Gamazon E, Cavallari LH, et al. The missing association: Sequencing-based discovery of novel snps in vkorc1 and cyp2c9 that affect warfarin dose in african americans. *Clin Pharmacol Ther*. 2011;89:408–415.
6. Blake MJ, Castro L, Leeder JS, et al. Ontogeny of drug metabolizing enzymes in the neonate. *Semin Fetal Neonatal Med*. 2005;10:123–138.
7. Chen YT, Trzoss L, Yang D, et al. Ontogenic expression of human carboxylesterase-2 and cytochrome p450 3a4 in liver and duodenum: Postnatal surge and organ-dependent regulation. *Toxicology*. 2015;330:55–61.
8. Stevens JC, Hines RN, Gu C, et al. Developmental expression of the major human hepatic cyp3a enzymes. *J Pharmacol Exp Ther*. 2003;307:573–582.
9. Peeters MY, Prins SA, Knibbe CA, et al. Pharmacokinetics and pharmacodynamics of midazolam and metabolites in nonventilated infants after craniofacial surgery. *Anesthesiology*. 2006;105:1135–1146.
10. Ince I, de Wildt SN, Wang C, et al. A novel maturation function for clearance of the cytochrome p450 3a substrate midazolam from preterm neonates to adults. *Clin Pharmacokinet*. 2013;52:555–565.
11. Mukherjee A, Dombi T, Wittke B, et al. Population pharmacokinetics of sildenafil in term neonates: Evidence of rapid maturation of metabolic clearance in the early postnatal period. *Clin Pharmacol Ther*. 2009;85:56–63.
12. Ward RM, Kearns GL, Tammara B, et al. A multicenter, randomized, open-label, pharmacokinetics and safety study of pantoprazole tablets in children and adolescents aged 6 through 16 years with gastroesophageal reflux disease. *J Clin Pharmacol*. 2011;51:876–887.
13. Allegaert K, van Schaik RH, Vermeersch S, et al. Postmenstrual age and cyp2d6 polymorphisms determine tramadol o-demethylation in critically ill neonates and infants. *Pediatr Res*. 2008;63:674–679.
14. Shi D, Yang D, Prinssen EP, et al. Surge in expression of carboxylesterase 1 during the post-neonatal stage enables a rapid gain of the capacity to activate the anti-influenza prodrug oseltamivir. *J Infect Dis*. 2011;203:937–942.
15. Hirt D, Van Overmeire B, Treluyer JM, et al. An optimized ibuprofen dosing scheme for preterm neonates with patent ductus arteriosus, based on a population pharmacokinetic and pharmacodynamic study. *Br J Clin Pharmacol*. 2008;65:629–636.
16. Lopez-Rodriguez R, Novalbos J, Gallego-Sandin S, et al. Influence of cyp2c8 and cyp2c9 polymorphisms on pharmacokinetic and pharmacodynamic parameters of racemic and enantiomeric forms of ibuprofen in healthy volunteers. *Pharmacol Res*. 2008;58:77–84.
17. Saleh MI, Nalbant D, Widness JA, et al. Population pharmacodynamic analysis of erythropoiesis in preterm infants for determining the anemia treatment potential of erythropoietin. *Am J Physiol Regul Integr Comp Physiol*. 2013;304:R772–R781.
18. Shaheen SO, Newson RB, Ring SM, et al. Prenatal and infant acetaminophen exposure, antioxidant gene polymorphisms, and childhood asthma. *J Allergy Clin Immunol*. 2010;126:1141–1148 e1147.
19. Ciszkowski C, Madadi P, Phillips MS, et al. Codeine, ultrarapid-metabolism genotype, and postoperative death. *N Engl J Med*. 2009;361:827–828.
20. Gasche Y, Daali Y, Fathi M, et al. Codeine intoxication associated with ultrarapid cyp2d6 metabolism. *N Engl J Med*. 2004;351:2827–2831.
21. Koren G, Cairns J, Chitayat D, et al. Pharmacogenetics of morphine poisoning in a breastfed neonate of a codeine-prescribed mother. *Lancet*. 2006;368:704.
22. Sistonen J, Madadi P, Ross CJ, et al. Prediction of codeine toxicity in infants and their mothers using a novel combination of maternal genetic markers. *Clin Pharmacol Ther*. 2012;91:692–699.

23. Fukuda T, Chidambaran V, Mizuno T, et al. Oct1 genetic variants influence the pharmacokinetics of morphine in children. *Pharmacogenomics*. 2013;14:1141–1151.
24. Sawyer MB, Innocenti F, Das S, et al. A pharmacogenetic study of uridine diphosphate-glucuronosyltransferase 2b7 in patients receiving morphine. *Clin Pharmacol Ther*. 2003;73:566–574.
25. Darbari DS, van Schaik RH, Capparelli EV, et al. Ugt2b7 promoter variant -840g>a contributes to the variability in hepatic clearance of morphine in patients with sickle cell disease. *Am J Hematol*. 2008;83:200–202.
26. Sadhasivam S, Chidambaran V, Zhang X, et al. Opioid-induced respiratory depression: Abcb1 transporter pharmacogenetics. *Pharmacogenomics J*. 2015;15:119–126.
27. Mieda T, Nishizawa D, Nakagawa H, et al. Genome-wide association study identifies candidate loci associated with postoperative fentanyl requirements after laparoscopic-assisted colectomy. *Pharmacogenomics*. 2016;17:133–145.
28. Fukuda K, Hayashida M, Ide S, et al. Association between oprm1 gene polymorphisms and fentanyl sensitivity in patients undergoing painful cosmetic surgery. *Pain*. 2009;147:194–201.
29. Landau R, Kern C, Columb MO, et al. Genetic variability of the mu-opioid receptor influences intrathecal fentanyl analgesia requirements in laboring women. *Pain*. 2008;139:5–14.
30. Zhang W, Chang YZ, Kan QC, et al. Cyp3a4*1g genetic polymorphism influences cyp3a activity and response to fentanyl in chinese gynecologic patients. *Eur J Clin Pharmacol*. 2010;66:61–66.
31. Lewis T, Dinh J, Leeder JS. Genetic determinants of fetal opiate exposure and risk of neonatal abstinence syndrome: Knowledge deficits and prospects for future research. *Clin Pharmacol Ther*. 2015;98:309–320.
32. Wang SC, Ho IK, Tsou HH, et al. Cyp2b6 polymorphisms influence the plasma concentration and clearance of the methadone s-enantiomer. *J Clin Psychopharmacol*. 2011;31:463–469.
33. Dobrinas M, Crettol S, Oneda B, et al. Contribution of cyp2b6 alleles in explaining extreme (s)-methadone plasma levels: A cyp2b6 gene resequencing study. *Pharmacogenet Genomics*. 2013;23:84–93.
34. Dennis BB, Bawor M, Thabane L, et al. Impact of abcb1 and cyp2b6 genetic polymorphisms on methadone metabolism, dose and treatment response in patients with opioid addiction: A systematic review and meta-analysis. *PLoS ONE*. 2014;9:e86114.
35. Wachman EM, Hayes MJ, Brown MS, et al. Association of oprm1 and comt single-nucleotide polymorphisms with hospital length of stay and treatment of neonatal abstinence syndrome. *JAMA*. 2013;309:1821–1827.
36. Wachman EM, Hayes MJ, Lester BM, et al. Epigenetic variation in the mu-opioid receptor gene in infants with neonatal abstinence syndrome. *J Pediatr*. 2014;165:472–478.
37. Wachman EM, Hayes MJ, Sherva R, et al. Variations in opioid receptor genes in neonatal abstinence syndrome. *Drug Alcohol Depend*. 2015;155:253–259.
38. Stockmann C, Fassl B, Gaedigk R, et al. Fluticasone propionate pharmacogenetics: Cyp3a4*22 polymorphism and pediatric asthma control. *J Pediatr*. 2013;162:1222–1227, 1227 e1221–1222.
39. Tantisira KG, Damask A, Szefler SJ, et al. Genome-wide association identifies the t gene as a novel asthma pharmacogenetic locus. *Am J Respir Crit Care Med*. 2012;185:1286–1291.

12

CHAPTER 13

Antibiotic Considerations for Necrotizing Enterocolitis

Marie-Eve Rochon, MD, MSc, FRCPC, Ahmed Moussa, MD, MMed, FRCPC, Julie Autmizguine, MD, MHS, FRCPC

13

- NEC results in an intraabdominal infection, and treatment includes antimicrobial therapy, bowel rest, and surgery if clinically or radiologically indicated.
- In the absence of evidence-based guidelines, many antibiotic combinations are used for NEC treatment in current practice.
- Ampicillin and gentamicin are probably adequate for treatment of mild to moderate NEC.
- For moderate to severe NEC, antimicrobial treatment should include anaerobic coverage.

Necrotizing enterocolitis (NEC) is a common and devastating disease in infants with an incidence of approximately 1 for 1000 live births.[1] Prematurity is an important risk factor with 5% to 10% of very-low-birth-weight (VLBW; <1500 g) infants affected.[2] Despite treatment, the overall mortality from NEC varies from 15% to 50% in VLBW infants.[3] Complications include delayed enteral feeding (and poor nutrition), prolonged parenteral nutrition, intestinal strictures, short bowel syndrome, and developmental delay.[4-6] Spontaneous intestinal perforation, sometimes confused with NEC, is a different clinical entity, occurring in the first week of life in very premature infants,[7] and will not be discussed in this chapter. The etiology of NEC is multifactorial, and its treatment includes gut rest, antibiotics, and in specific situations, surgery. In this chapter, we will discuss the different modalities concerning the antimicrobial therapy of NEC.

Pathogenesis of Necrotizing Enterocolitis

The pathogenesis of NEC involves intestinal mucosal injury caused by intestinal inflammation, ischemia, and bacterial overgrowth taking place in a highly vulnerable gastrointestinal tract.[8] NEC is strongly related to prematurity, with over 90% of infants with NEC born prematurely.[9] Premature infants have impaired gastrointestinal motility, absorption, and microcirculatory regulation, as well as immature epithelial barrier function.[10] They are also at risk for hypoxia, infection, and repeated fasting periods, which increase their risk of developing NEC.[11]

NEC is associated with an inappropriate inflammatory host response to external stimuli such as bacterial enteric colonization or enteral feedings.[12] Immature enterocytes have increased production of proinflammatory mediators and toll-like receptor 4 expression, which induce recruitment of proinflammatory lymphocytes in the intestinal epithelium and contribute to development of NEC.[13,14] Although hypotheses of genetic predisposition have been raised, no specific genes have been identified.[15] Human milk is somewhat protective against NEC, especially when breastfeeding is exclusive and started early.[16,17] Breast milk provides immunoglobulins, lactoferrin, lysozymes, growth factors, and healthy bacteria to promote development of a favorable intestinal microbiota.[18,19] Hypoxic-ischemic events, which are potentiated by perinatal asphyxia, congenital heart disease, and a hemodynamically significant patent ductus arteriosus

(PDA), may also be associated with NEC.[20,21] Intrauterine growth restriction from placental insufficiency increases the risk of NEC because of redistribution of blood flow to the brain and other vital organs secondarily leading to reduced intestinal perfusion.[22,23] Finally, recent evidence showed that NEC is associated with a disturbed and poorly diversified intestinal flora, leading to disproportionate proliferation of pathogenic bacteria.[24–27] Imbalanced intestinal microbiota may result from antibiotic exposure for other infections, including urinary tract infections, which have been associated with increased risk of NEC within 7 days.[28] Premature infants are especially at high risk of imbalanced intestinal microbiota given their frequent exposure to antibiotics and their prolonged hospitalization.[10,29,30]

In summary, although multiple factors are involved in its pathophysiology, NEC ultimately results in bacterial overgrowth, mimicking a complicated intraabdominal infection, and is characterized by bowel inflammation with mucosal edema, ulcerations, hemorrhages and coagulation necrosis, localized or diffused peritonitis, and, in some cases, bowel perforation.[8,9]

Clinical Presentation and Diagnosis of Necrotizing Enterocolitis

Age of onset is typically inversely proportional to gestational age (GA). Term and late preterm infants usually develop NEC in the first week of life and very preterm

Table 13.1 MODIFIED BELL STAGING FOR NEC[111,125]

Bell Stages	Abdominal Signs and Symptoms	Systemic Signs and Symptoms	Radiologic Features	Treatment
I Suspected NEC				
IA	Feeding intolerance, mild abdominal distention, occult blood in stools	Mild systemic symptoms (apnea and bradycardia, temperature instability)	Nonspecific: normal or signs of ileus, mild intestinal dilatation	Close clinical observation NPO Consider antibiotics without anaerobic coverage
IB	Stage IA plus grossly bloody stools			
II Proven NEC				
IIA mild	Prominent abdominal distension,	Mild systemic symptoms (as stage I)	Intestinal dilatation, *pneumatosis intestinalis,* portal venous gas	Close clinical, laboratory, and radiologic observation NPO, gastric decompression, intravenous fluids and antibiotics with or without anaerobic coverage
IIB moderate	abdominal tenderness and wall edema, grossly bloody stools	Moderate systemic symptoms (stage I plus thrombocytopenia, metabolic acidosis)		
III Advanced NEC				
IIIA	As stage II plus signs of peritonitis	Severe systemic symptoms (stage II plus need for mechanical ventilation, hypotension and	Stage II plus fixed bowel loops, severe ascites	Same as stage II, including anaerobic coverage plus Consider surgical intervention
IIIB		shock, severe metabolic and respiratory acidosis, disseminated intravascular coagulation)	Stage IIIB plus pneumoperitoneum	Same as stage III plus Exploratory laparotomy and resection of necrotic bowel or peritoneal drainage

NEC, Necrotizing enterocolitis; NPO, nil per os.
Adapted from Walsh MC, Kliegman RM. Necrotizing enterocolitis: treatment based on staging criteria. *Pediatr Clin North Am.* 1986;33(1):179–201 and Hall NJ, Eaton S, Pierro A. Royal Australasia of Surgeons Guest Lecture. Necrotizing enterocolitis: prevention, treatment, and outcome. *J Pediatr Surg.* 2013;48(12):2359–2367.

infants after the second or third week of life.[31] NEC presents with both digestive and systemic manifestations. Infants generally have abdominal distention and/or tenderness, feeding intolerance, and occult or grossly bloody stools. Nonspecific systemic signs include apnea and bradycardia, lethargy, poor perfusion, and respiratory distress. The disease can be mild with only feeding intolerance or sudden and fulminant with multiorgan failure.[32]

Laboratory studies supporting the diagnosis of NEC include abnormal complete blood count with neutropenia or thrombocytopenia, hyponatremia, and high C-reactive protein concentrations. Coagulopathy and metabolic acidosis are suggestive of a severe disease.[9] Radiologic studies are used to confirm the diagnosis of NEC and stage disease severity according to Bell criteria (Table 13.1).[32] Plain abdominal radiography may reveal distended, fixed bowel loops; air fluid levels; *pneumatosis intestinalis* (intramural gas); portal venous gas; or pneumoperitoneum in the case of intestinal perforation.[33] Serial radiographs are useful to follow the progression of the disease in the first few days of NEC. Doppler ultrasonography is a highly sensitive exam for portal venous gas when diagnosis is uncertain. It may also be a sensitive way to identify infants with bowel necrosis, who may benefit from surgery prior to bowel perforation.[34]

Management of Necrotizing Enterocolitis

When NEC is suspected or confirmed, patients are given bowel rest and medical supportive care, which may include volume expansion, vasopressors, ventilation, and blood product transfusions. Clinical and radiologic evolution determine the need for surgery for the most severe cases.[10] Moreover, given the similarities between NEC and intraabdominal infections in children and adults, management typically includes broad-spectrum antibiotics.

Antimicrobial Therapy

Although many pathogens have been associated with NEC, no specific microorganism has consistently been linked to this condition. Blood culture is positive in 20% to 30% of cases,[35,36] and there is an associated meningitis in 0.5% to 1% of infants with NEC.[37,38] However, for most infants with NEC, no microorganism is identified and a polymicrobial infection may be assumed. Enterobacteriaceae (e.g., *Escherichia coli, Klebsiella* species), anaerobic bacteria (e.g., *Bacteroides* sp., *Clostridium* sp.), and aerobic gram-positive bacteria (e.g., *Enterococcus* sp.) are among the main potentially pathogenic bacteria colonizing the intestine of infants with NEC.[39,40] More rarely, *Candida* sp. and viruses (e.g., *Cytomegalovirus, Rotavirus,* and *Norovirus*) have also been associated with NEC.[41–43] Multiple combinations of antimicrobial agents may be used to cover these pathogens (Table 13.2).

Ampicillin

Ampicillin is a beta-lactam routinely used for empiric treatment of early- and late-onset neonatal sepsis. It is active against most *Enterococcal* species, *Streptococcal* species, and *E. coli* isolates. Ampicillin has good cerebrospinal fluid (CSF) penetration through inflamed meninges.[44,45] It is generally well tolerated in infants, but has been associated with an increased risk of seizures in infants given very high doses.[46,47] Ampicillin is poorly bound to plasma protein (10%) and has a half-life of 2 to 4 hours; its elimination is predominantly renal (90%).[48,49] A prospective multicenter pharmacokinetics (PK) study in 73 infants (GA range: 24–41 weeks) suggested a strong correlation between ampicillin clearance and postmenstrual age (PMA) and serum creatinine.[50]

Cefotaxime

Cefotaxime is a third-generation cephalosporin active against *Streptococcal* sp. and most gram-negative rods. It has good CSF penetration and is recommended for treatment of suspected meningitis.[44,45] Cefotaxime has minimal toxicity and a favorable safety profile in infants.[51,52] However, use of cefotaxime has been associated with development of resistance to gram-negative bacteria[52,53] and with an increased

Table 13.2 INTRAVENOUS ANTIMICROBIAL THERAPY FOR TREATMENT OF NEC IN INFANTS[126,127]

Antibiotics	Dosage			
Ampicillin (IV / IM)[50]	GA at birth ≤ 34 weeks			GA at birth > 34 weeks and PNA ≤ 28 days
	PNA < 7 days	PNA ≥ 8 and ≤ 28 days		
	50 mg/kg q12h	75 mg/kg q12h		50 mg/kg q8h
Clindamycin (IV)[81]	PMA ≤ 32 weeks	PMA > 32 and ≤ 40 weeks		PMA > 40 and ≤ 60 weeks
	5 mg/kg q8h	7 mg/kg q8h		9 mg/kg q8h
Piperacillin-Tazobactam (IV)[64]	PMA ≤ 30 weeks	PMA 30–35 weeks		PMA 35–49 weeks
	100 mg/kg q8h	80 mg/kg q6h		80 mg/kg q4h
Meropenem (IV)[67,70]	GA at birth < 32 weeks		GA at birth ≥ 32 weeks	
	PNA < 14 days	PNA ≥ 14 days	PNA < 14 days	PNA ≥ 14 days
	20 mg/kg q12h	20 mg/kg q8h	20 mg/kg q8h	30 mg/kg q8h
Metronidazole (IV)[88]		PMA < 34 weeks	PMA 34–40 weeks	PMA > 40 weeks
	Loading dose	Maintenance dose		
	15 mg/kg	7.5 mg/kg q12h	7.5 mg/kg q8h	7.5 mg/kg q6h
Cefotaxime (IV/ IM)[109]	Body weight ≤ 2 kg		Body weight ≥ 2 kg	
	≤ 7 days of age	≥ 7 days of age	≤ 7 days of age	≥ 7 days of age
	50 mg/kg q12 h	50 mg/kg q8-12 h	50 mg/kg q12 h	50 mg/kg q8 h
Gentamicin or Tobramycin (IV / IM)[73,109]	Body weight ≤ 2 kg		Body weight ≥ 2 kg	
	≤ 7 days of age	≥ 7 days of age	≤ 7 days of age	≥ 7 days of age
	5 mg/kg q48 h	4-5 mg/kg q24–48 h	4 mg/kg q 24h	4 mg/kg q12–24 h
Antifungals	**Dosage**			
Fluconazole (IV)[96,127,128]	12 mg/kg/day q24h Consider loading dose 25 mg/kg			

IV, intravenous; *IM*, intramuscular; *GA*, gestational age; *PNA*, postnatal age; *PMA*, postmenstrual age.
Adapted from Pineda LC, Watt KM. New antibiotic dosing in infants. *Clin Perinatol.* 2015;42(1):167–176, ix–x and Autmizguine J, et al. Pharmacokinetics and pharmacodynamics of antifungals in children: clinical implications. *Drugs.* 2014;74(8):891–909.

risk of fungal infection in preterm infants because of its very broad spectrum.[54,55] Approximately half of cefotaxime is excreted unchanged in urine and 20% is converted into an active metabolite by the liver.[56] Consistent with renal maturation, cefotaxime clearance increases with GA with a half-life of 1.9 to 7 hours in preterm infants.[57]

Piperacillin-Tazobactam

Piperacillin-tazobactam is a combination of an ureidopenicillin and a beta-lactam inhibitor preventing bacterial cell wall synthesis of gram-positive and gram-negative bacteria, including anaerobic bacteria. Some gram-negative bacteria may develop piperacillin-tazobactam resistance through extended-spectrum beta-lactamases.[58] Piperacillin-tazobactam is inadequate for treatment of meningitis because of suboptimal CSF penetration of tazobactam.[59] This antibiotic has a good safety profile in infants and children.[60,61] However, its use may increase the risk of invasive candidiasis because of its very broad spectrum of action. Dosing is usually based on the piperacillin component.

Piperacillin is mainly excreted by the kidneys[62] with a half-life of 1.5 to 9 hours in premature infants. Clearance is correlated with PMA and birth weight (BW).[63,64]

Meropenem

Meropenem, from the carbapenem class, is effective against most gram-positive, gram-negative, anaerobic, and even extended beta-lactamase–producing bacteria and has good CSF penetration.[65] It is well tolerated in infants with no drug-attributable major adverse events as demonstrated in a safety and efficacy study involving 200 infants <3 months of age.[66,67] In a retrospective study of over 5000 infants, meropenem was associated with a lower risk of seizures or death compared with imipenem/cilastatin.[68] Meropenem is poorly bound to proteins (2%) and primarily excreted by the kidneys with 70% excreted unchanged in urine.[69] In infants, the half-life of meropenem is approximately 2.5 hours with clearance increasing with PMA and inversely related to serum creatinine.[70] However, similarly to cefotaxime and piperacillin-tazobactam, meropenem may be associated with an increased risk of invasive candidiasis because of its very broad spectrum of action.

Gentamicin

Gentamicin is an aminoglycoside known to inhibit bacterial protein synthesis through its liaison to the 30S ribosomal subunit. It is particularly active against aerobic gram-negative bacteria, but also acts synergistically against gram-positive organisms. Of note, gentamicin has no effect against anaerobic bacteria. It is highly hydrophilic and has reduced CSF penetration.[71] Gentamicin is associated with adverse nephrotoxic and ototoxic effects that are enhanced when combined with third-generation cephalosporins or diuretics.[72] Monitoring of both peak (6–10 μg/mL) and trough (0.5–2 μg/mL) blood concentrations of this medication and renal function is important to achieve a level of efficiency and prevent toxicity, respectively. Furthermore, hearing testing should be performed in all infants after a prolonged course of gentamicin. It is mainly eliminated via the kidneys with a half-life ranging from 3 to 12 hours in term and preterm infants, respectively.[73,74]

Clindamycin

Clindamycin is a lincosamide antibiotic with bacteriostatic properties against several obligate anaerobes. Binding of clindamycin to the 50S ribosomal subunit inhibits bacterial protein synthesis. The rate of colonization or infection with clindamycin-resistant bacteria in premature infants is unknown, but its use is now discouraged for the treatment of complicated intraabdominal infections in older children and adults because of increasing resistance to clindamycin.[75] Although its CSF penetration is considered poor, it can reach therapeutic concentrations when high doses are used in adults.[76] In a safety study involving 62 preterm and term infants, clindamycin was not associated with adverse events deemed related to the study drug.[77] However, three preterm infants who had clindamycin exposure in the upper range presented with seizures. Further data on clindamycin safety and efficacy in NEC is expected with an ongoing randomized controlled trial (RCT) of different antibiotic regimens (SCAMP trial; NCT01994993). Clindamycin is predominantly metabolized by the liver CYP450 3A4 enzyme and is excreted through urine and feces.[78–80] Clindamycin clearance is correlated with BW and PMA with a half-life of 2.5 to 10 hours in infants and a clearance of about 50% of adult values at a PMA of 39.5 weeks.[81]

Metronidazole

Metronidazole is active against most obligate anaerobes. It causes a loss of helical DNA with subsequent inhibition of bacterial protein synthesis.[82] Metronidazole has good CSF penetration.[83] Safety studies in premature infants suggest an acceptable safety profile with no significant adverse events reported.[84,85] Metronidazole is partly metabolized by the liver CYP450 2A6 enzyme[86] and mostly eliminated by the kidney.[87] In preterm infants, its clearance increases with BW and PMA with a half-life of approximately 20 hours compared with 8 hours in adults.[88]

Fluconazole

Fluconazole is effective against most *Candida* species, especially *C. albicans*,[89] and has good CSF penetration.[90] Safety studies in premature infants have shown good tolerance, with the only reported adverse events being a reversible elevation of liver enzymes and direct bilirubin not considered clinically significant.[91–96] Fluconazole does not undergo significant metabolism and is predominantly excreted unchanged in urine.[97] PK studies have demonstrated that fluconazole clearance increases with advancing GA and postnatal age (PNA).[98]

Antimicrobial Regimens

To date, studies have failed to demonstrate the optimal antimicrobial treatment for NEC.[75,99] The only guideline addressing this issue was published by the Surgical Infection Society and the Infectious Diseases Society of America in 2010. Even though these guidelines mainly discuss the treatment of complicated intraabdominal infections in adults and older children, they recommend broad-spectrum antibiotics, including ampicillin, gentamicin, and metronidazole; ampicillin, cefotaxime, and metronidazole; or meropenem for NEC. They also specify that clindamycin should not be routinely used in older children and adults because of emergent resistance of *Bacteroides fragilis*, but there are insufficient data in infants with NEC to make similar recommendations. Finally, therapeutic fluconazole or amphotericin B should only be added if cultures are consistent with fungal infection.[75] Due to lack of an evidence-based guideline, multiple antibiotic combinations are used for the treatment of NEC in current practice.

One of the first observational studies on antimicrobial regimens involved 90 infants (<2500 g BW) and compared the combination of cefotaxime and vancomycin with ampicillin and gentamicin for the treatment of NEC.[100] The cefotaxime and vancomycin regimen was associated with decreased mortality and less peritoneal-positive bacterial culture, but this study was limited by its observational design and small sample size. Furthermore, some pathogens isolated were *Staphylococcus* sp., which are not typically involved in the pathogenesis of NEC and were not covered by ampicillin or gentamicin.

There has been debate over the need to include anaerobic antimicrobial therapy for NEC. It is unclear whether anaerobic bacteria play a pathogenic or a protective role in the pathogenesis of NEC. Disruption of the intestinal mucosa with subsequent intramural invasion by anaerobic bacteria causes *pneumatosis intestinalis*.[101] But anaerobic bacteria are also known to produce short-chain fatty acids potentially regulating the intestinal inflammatory response.[102] Moreover, gram-negative rods, as opposed to anaerobic bacteria, have been shown to be predominant in the stools of VLBW infants who developed NEC compared with those who did not.[30]

Three studies have addressed the issue of anaerobic antimicrobial therapy in NEC; two in premature infants and one in late-preterm and term infants.[103–105] First, in premature infants, the largest study involved a retrospective cohort of 2780 VLBW infants with NEC in which outcomes were compared between those with and without anaerobic antimicrobial therapy on the first day of NEC.[103] Results suggest that for infants with medical NEC, anaerobic coverage was not associated with lower mortality, but with small increased risk of intestinal strictures. However, among infants with surgical NEC, anaerobic antimicrobial therapy was associated with lower mortality. These results suggest that anaerobic coverage is beneficial in cases of severe and perforated (stage III) NEC. Given the retrospective design of this study, the use of anaerobic antimicrobial therapy may have been confounded by disease severity. Therefore, the higher rate of strictures observed in infants treated with anaerobic antimicrobial therapy could be explained by more severe disease rather than as a consequence of the antimicrobial treatment.

The other important study in premature infants is an RCT comparing ampicillin-gentamicin to ampicillin-gentamicin-clindamycin for the treatment of NEC in 42 premature infants.[104] This RCT showed no beneficial effect on mortality or intestinal perforation with addition of clindamycin to the initial regimen, but a significant longer time to successful reinstitution of enteral feeding and a higher incidence of late stricture formation in the clindamycin group (5/15 with clindamycin versus 1/18 without, $P = 0.022$). Of note, infants were excluded if intestinal perforation occurred <12 hours after randomization and therefore are most comparable to the medical NEC subgroup of infants from the observational study described earlier.

Finally, in late-preterm and term infants with radiologic NEC (GA ≥34 weeks, n = 229), an observational study showed that the addition of metronidazole for ≥4 consecutive days was not associated with better outcomes.[105] As opposed to the study in VLBW infants described earlier, mortality of infants with stage III NEC was not significantly lower with metronidazole treatment (9% with metronidazole versus 33% without, total of 17 patients). However, this lack of statistical difference may be explained by the limited sample size or baseline differences in the two populations.

In summary, empiric antimicrobial treatment of NEC should be effective against most pathogenic bacteria present in the intestinal flora (e.g., *E. faecalis* and gram-negative bacilli). For surgical NEC, there is some evidence that anaerobic coverage is beneficial by reducing mortality.[103] For medical NEC, there are insufficient data to recommend anaerobic coverage for all infants because studies have not shown any benefit regarding survival or other clinical outcomes. There is probably no indication for anaerobic coverage in mild NEC (stage I and IIA), but experts generally agree that it should be considered in the management of moderate NEC (stage IIB). Piperacillin-tazobactam, with or without gentamicin, and the combination of ampicillin, gentamicin, and metronidazole are two reasonable options. If meningitis is suspected, meropenem or cefotaxime should be included in the empirical antimicrobial treatment. Local resistance patterns should also be considered in the choice of the antibiotic regimen. Moreover, it is important to adapt the antimicrobial spectrum if a pathogen has been identified in blood, peritoneal liquid, or surgical specimen cultures. For example, if a coagulase-negative *Staphylococcus* is identified, vancomycin should be added to the initial treatment. Finally, fluconazole should be considered in infants with a clinical deterioration while receiving broad-spectrum antibiotics. An ongoing multicenter RCT is currently looking at safety and efficacy of antimicrobial regimens in infants with complicated intraabdominal infections with the aim of determining the optimal empiric antimicrobial therapy for NEC (SCAMP trial; NCT01994993).

Duration of Medical Treatment

There is no evidence supporting the optimal duration of antimicrobial therapy for NEC. For a complicated intraabdominal infection in children and adults, antimicrobial therapy is limited to 4 to 7 days unless there are signs of an uncontrolled infection.[75] As sometimes seen in clinical practice, antimicrobial therapy may be discontinued after 5 to 10 days in stage I or IIA NEC if there is resolution of symptoms.[75,106–108] If NEC is associated with bacteremia or sepsis, duration of the antimicrobial therapy should be 10 to 14 days; a 14-day treatment course is recommended when there is a positive blood culture for gram-negative bacilli.[109] In summary, even in the absence of evidence-based guidelines, experts agree that antimicrobial therapy should last 5 to 14 days, depending on the evolution of the disease.[75,108] If an intraabdominal abscess has been identified, antibiotics should be continued until clinical and radiologic response is established. Recurrence of NEC after a first course of antimicrobial or surgical treatment is approximately 5% and does not appear to be reduced by extending duration of the initial treatment.[110] However, a prolonged broad-spectrum antibiotic course potentially increases the risk of subsequent colonization and sepsis with resistant bacteria and fungi because of disturbances in the microbiome; thus treatment duration should be limited to the minimal effective duration.

Bowel Rest and Supportive Care

To prevent further bowel injury, infants are placed *nil per os* (NPO) and gastric decompression is provided with intermittent low nasogastric/orogastric suction. Supportive care is continued for a variable period depending on severity and course of the disease. Serial abdominal examinations, blood chemistry, hematologic studies, and radiographs are used to follow evolution of NEC and response to treatment.[111]

Surgical Intervention

Bowel perforation with pneumoperitoneum is the only absolute indication for surgical intervention in NEC. Severe disease with cardiovascular instability and disease progression despite optimal medical treatment should be considered as relative indications for surgery.[111] Up to 40% of infants with NEC require a surgical intervention.[112] Studies have tried to determine the best surgical technique between explorative laparotomy and peritoneal drainage, but none of these have shown superiority in terms of mortality or morbidity.[113,114] A large RCT (NEST trial) by the National Institute of Child Health and Human Development Neonatal Research Network is in progress to determine the best surgical approach. During exploratory laparotomy, surgeons perform resection of necrotic or perforated bowel with subsequent primary anastomosis, stoma creation, or "clip and drop back" technique. Other approaches include peritoneal drainage allowing abdominal decompression and enteric content evacuation.[115] Intraoperative Gram stains and cultures should be performed.[75]

Prevention of Necrotizing Enterocolitis

Because NEC can be a devastating disease for premature infants, it is important to adopt available preventive strategies. For example, anti-H_2 medication and prolonged antibiotic therapy have been identified as risk factors for NEC.[26,116] Consequently, prolonged use of anti-H_2 medication and broad-spectrum antibiotics without a documented infection should be avoided in this population. Early use of nonsteroidal antiinflammatory drugs to close a PDA has not been shown to decrease the risk of NEC.[21,117] Some preventive interventions, however, have been shown to reduce the incidence of NEC. First, early initiation of enteral feeding with human milk has been shown to reduce the incidence of NEC in premature infants.[118] Furthermore, prophylactic administration of probiotics to premature infants >1000 grams has been shown to reduce the incidence of severe NEC and mortality.[119,120] However, bacteremia or contamination of probiotic preparations with pathogenic bacteria is a possible risk of probiotic use in very premature neonates.[121,122] There is no evidence for prophylactic oral immunoglobulin administration for prevention of NEC.[123] Finally, enteral prophylactic antibiotic treatment has been considered, but the cost/benefit ratio was not favorable because of associated emergence of resistant bacteria.[124]

Conclusion

In summary, NEC is a multifactorial disease resulting in a complicated intraabdominal infection with potentially devastating complications, including intestinal strictures, short-bowel syndrome, and death. There is currently no evidence to recommend a specific antimicrobial regimen for NEC treatment, but broad-spectrum antibiotics should cover *Enterococci* and most enteric gram-negative bacilli. Anaerobic antimicrobial therapy should also be considered in the regimen in case of moderate to severe NEC. Clinicians should take local resistance patterns and culture results into account in their choice of antibiotic therapy.

REFERENCES

1. Holman RC, Stoll BJ, Curns AT, et al. Necrotising enterocolitis hospitalisations among neonates in the United States. *Paediatr Perinat Epidemiol.* 2006;20:498–506.
2. Fanaroff AA, et al. Trends in neonatal morbidity and mortality for very low birthweight infants. *Am J Obstet Gynecol.* 2007;196(2):147.e1–147.e8.
3. Fitzgibbons SC, et al. Mortality of necrotizing enterocolitis expressed by birth weight categories. *J Pediatr Surg.* 2009;44(6):1072–1075, discussion 1075–6.
4. Hintz SR, et al. Neurodevelopmental and growth outcomes of extremely low birth weight infants after necrotizing enterocolitis. *Pediatrics.* 2005;115(3):696–703.
5. Rees CM, Pierro A, Eaton S. Neurodevelopmental outcomes of neonates with medically and surgically treated necrotizing enterocolitis. *Arch Dis Child Fetal Neonatal Ed.* 2007;92(3):F193–F198.
6. Murthy K, et al. Short-term outcomes for preterm infants with surgical necrotizing enterocolitis. *J Perinatol.* 2014;34(10):736–740.

7. Meyer CL, Payne NR, Roback SA. Spontaneous, isolated intestinal perforations in neonates with birth weight less than 1,000 g not associated with necrotizing enterocolitis. *J Pediatr Surg*. 1991; 26(6):714–717.
8. Ballance WA, et al. Pathology of neonatal necrotizing enterocolitis: a ten-year experience. *J Pediatr*. 1990;117(1 Pt 2):S6–S13.
9. Hsueh W, et al. Neonatal necrotizing enterocolitis: clinical considerations and pathogenetic concepts. *Pediatr Dev Pathol*. 2003;6(1):6–23.
10. Lin PW, Stoll BJ. Necrotising enterocolitis. *Lancet*. 2006;368(9543):1271–1283.
11. Terrin G, Scipione A, De Curtis M. Update in pathogenesis and prospective in treatment of necrotizing enterocolitis. *Biomed Res Int*. 2014;2014:543765.
12. Nanthakumar NN, et al. Inflammation in the developing human intestine: A possible pathophysiologic contribution to necrotizing enterocolitis. *Proc Natl Acad Sci USA*. 2000;97(11):6043–6048.
13. Caplan MS, Simon D, Jilling T. The role of PAF, TLR, and the inflammatory response in neonatal necrotizing enterocolitis. *Semin Pediatr Surg*. 2005;14(3):145–151.
14. Tremblay E, et al. Gene expression profiling in necrotizing enterocolitis reveals pathways common to those reported in Crohn's disease. *BMC Med Genomics*. 2016;9:6.
15. Bhandari V, et al. Familial and genetic susceptibility to major neonatal morbidities in preterm twins. *Pediatrics*. 2006;117(6):1901–1906.
16. Murgas Torrazza R, Neu J. The developing intestinal microbiome and its relationship to health and disease in the neonate. *J Perinatol*. 2011;31(suppl 1):S29–S34.
17. Kimak KS, et al. Influence of Enteral Nutrition on Occurrences of Necrotizing Enterocolitis in Very-Low-Birth-Weight Infants. *J Pediatr Gastroenterol Nutr*. 2015;61(4):445–450.
18. Harmsen HJ, et al. Analysis of intestinal flora development in breast-fed and formula-fed infants by using molecular identification and detection methods. *J Pediatr Gastroenterol Nutr*. 2000;30(1): 61–67.
19. Hanson LA, Korotkova M, Telemo E. Breast-feeding, infant formulas, and the immune system. *Ann Allergy Asthma Immunol*. 2003;90(6 suppl 3):59–63.
20. Christensen RD, et al. Necrotizing enterocolitis in term infants. *Clin Perinatol*. 2013;40(1):69–78.
21. Dollberg S, Lusky A, Reichman B. Patent ductus arteriosus, indomethacin and necrotizing enterocolitis in very low birth weight infants: a population-based study. *J Pediatr Gastroenterol Nutr*. 2005;40(2): 184–188.
22. Engineer N, Kumar S. Perinatal variables and neonatal outcomes in severely growth restricted preterm fetuses. *Acta Obstet Gynecol Scand*. 2010;89(9):1174–1181.
23. Sharma D, Shastri S, Sharma P. Intrauterine Growth Restriction: Antenatal and Postnatal Aspects. *Clin Med Insights Pediatr*. 2016;10:67–83.
24. Morrow AL, et al. Early microbial and metabolomic signatures predict later onset of necrotizing enterocolitis in preterm infants. *Microbiome*. 2013;1(1):13.
25. de la Cochetiere MF, et al. Early intestinal bacterial colonization and necrotizing enterocolitis in premature infants: the putative role of Clostridium. *Pediatr Res*. 2004;56(3):366–370.
26. Warner BB, et al. Gut bacteria dysbiosis and necrotising enterocolitis in very low birthweight infants: a prospective case-control study. *Lancet*. 2016;387(10031):1928–1936.
27. Zhou Y, et al. Longitudinal analysis of the premature infant intestinal microbiome prior to necrotizing enterocolitis: a case-control study. *PLoS ONE*. 2015;10(3):e0118632.
28. Pidena LC, et al. Association between positive urine cultures and necrotizing enterocolitis in a large cohort of hospitalized infants. *Early Hum Dev*. 2015;91(10):583–586.
29. Alexander VN, Northrup V, Bizzarro MJ. Antibiotic exposure in the newborn intensive care unit and the risk of necrotizing enterocolitis. *J Pediatr*. 2011;159(3):392–397.
30. Freedberg DE, Lebwohl B, Abrams JA. The impact of proton pump inhibitors on the human gastrointestinal microbiome. *Clin Lab Med*. 2014;34(4):771–785.
31. Wilson R, et al. Age at onset of necrotizing enterocolitis: an epidemiologic analysis. *Pediatr Res*. 1982;16(1):82–85.
32. Bell MJ, et al. Neonatal necrotizing enterocolitis. Therapeutic decisions based upon clinical staging. *Ann Surg*. 1978;187(1):1–7.
33. Zani A, Pierro A. Necrotizing enterocolitis: controversies and challenges. *F1000Res*. 2015;4:1373.
34. Yikilmaz A, et al. Prospective evaluation of the impact of sonography on the management and surgical intervention of neonates with necrotizing enterocolitis. *Pediatr Surg Int*. 2014;30(12):1231–1240.
35. Uauy RD, et al. Necrotizing enterocolitis in very low birth weight infants: biodemographic and clinical correlates. National Institute of Child Health and Human Development Neonatal Research Network. *J Pediatr*. 1991;119(4):630–638.
36. Beeby PJ, Jeffery H. Risk factors for necrotising enterocolitis: the influence of gestational age. *Arch Dis Child*. 1992;67(4 Spec No):432–435.
37. Kliegman RM, Walsh MC. The incidence of meningitis in neonates with necrotizing enterocolitis. *Am J Perinatol*. 1987;4(3):245–248.
38. Chan KL. A study of pre-antibiotic bacteriology in 125 patients with necrotizing enterocolitis. *Acta Paediatr Suppl*. 1994;396:45–48.
39. Elgin TG, Kern SL, McElroy SJ. Development of the neonatal intestinal microbiome and its association with necrotizing enterocolitis. *Clin Ther*. 2016;38(4):706–715.
40. Brower-Sinning R, et al. Mucosa-associated bacterial diversity in necrotizing enterocolitis. *PLoS ONE*. 2014;9(9):e105046.
41. Parra-Herran CE, et al. Intestinal candidiasis: an uncommon cause of necrotizing enterocolitis (NEC) in neonates. *Fetal Pediatr Pathol*. 2010;29(3):172–180.

13

42. Brook I. Microbiology and management of neonatal necrotizing enterocolitis. *Am J Perinatol*. 2008; 25(2):111–118.

43. Rotbart HA, et al. An outbreak of rotavirus-associated neonatal necrotizing enterocolitis. *J Pediatr*. 1983;103(3):454–459.

44. Peltola H, Anttila M, Renkonen OV. Randomised comparison of chloramphenicol, ampicillin, cefotaxime, and ceftriaxone for childhood bacterial meningitis. Finnish Study Group. *Lancet*. 1989;1(8650):1281–1287.

45. Tunkel AR, et al. Practice guidelines for the management of bacterial meningitis. *Clin Infect Dis*. 2004;39(9):1267–1284.

46. Shaffer CL, et al. Ampicillin-induced neurotoxicity in very-low-birth-weight neonates. *Ann Pharmacother*. 1998;32(4):482–484.

47. Hornik CP, et al. Electronic health records and pharmacokinetic modeling to assess the relationship between ampicillin exposure and seizure risk in neonates. *J Pediatr*. 2016;178:125–129.e1.

48. Hermans J, et al. Pharmacokinetic analysis of ampicillin concentration in neonates: comparison of two pharmacokinetic models and of two numerical methods. *Arzneimittelforschung*. 1975;25(6): 947–949.

49. Colburn WA, et al. Pharmacokinetic model for serum concentrations of ampicillin in the newborn infant. *J Infect Dis*. 1976;134(1):67–69.

50. Tremoulet A, et al. Characterization of the population pharmacokinetics of ampicillin in neonates using an opportunistic study design. *Antimicrob Agents Chemother*. 2014;58(6):3013–3020.

51. de Louvois J, Mulhall A, Hurley R. The safety and pharmacokinetics of cefotaxime in the treatment of neonates. *Pediatr Pharmacol (New York)*. 1982;2(4):275–284.

52. Spritzer R, et al. Five years of cefotaxime use in a neonatal intensive care unit. *Pediatr Infect Dis J*. 1990;9(2):92–96.

53. Nordmann P, Guibert M. Extended-spectrum beta-lactamases in Pseudomonas aeruginosa. *J Antimicrob Chemother*. 1998;42(2):128–131.

54. Saiman L, et al. Risk factors for Candida species colonization of neonatal intensive care unit patients. *Pediatr Infect Dis J*. 2001;20(12):1119–1124.

55. Benjamin DK Jr, et al. Neonatal candidiasis among extremely low birth weight infants: risk factors, mortality rates, and neurodevelopmental outcomes at 18 to 22 months. *Pediatrics*. 2006;117(1): 84–92.

56. Kearns GL, et al. Cefotaxime and desacetylcefotaxime pharmacokinetics in very low birth weight neonates. *J Pediatr*. 1989;114(3):461–467.

57. Gouyon JB, et al. Pharmacokinetics of cefotaxime in preterm infants. *Dev Pharmacol Ther*. 1990; 14(1):29–34.

58. D'Angelo RG, et al. Treatment options for extended-spectrum beta-lactamase (ESBL) and AmpC-producing bacteria. *Expert Opin Pharmacother*. 2016;17(7):953–967.

59. Nau R, et al. Kinetics of piperacillin and tazobactam in ventricular cerebrospinal fluid of hydrocephalic patients. *Antimicrob Agents Chemother*. 1997;41(5):987–991.

60. Pillay T, et al. Piperacillin/tazobactam in the treatment of Klebsiella pneumoniae infections in neonates. *Am J Perinatol*. 1998;15(1):47–51.

61. Reed MD, et al. Single-dose pharmacokinetics of piperacillin and tazobactam in infants and children. *Antimicrob Agents Chemother*. 1994;38(12):2817–2826.

62. Sorgel F, Kinzig M. The chemistry, pharmacokinetics and tissue distribution of piperacillin/tazobactam. *J Antimicrob Chemother*. 1993;31(supplA):39–60.

63. Cohen-Wolkowiez M, et al. Population pharmacokinetics of piperacillin using scavenged samples from preterm infants. *Ther Drug Monit*. 2012;34(3):312–319.

64. Cohen-Wolkowiez M, et al. Developmental pharmacokinetics of piperacillin and tazobactam using plasma and dried blood spots from infants. *Antimicrob Agents Chemother*. 2014;58(5):2856–2865.

65. Odio CM, et al. Prospective, randomized, investigator-blinded study of the efficacy and safety of meropenem vs. cefotaxime therapy in bacterial meningitis in children. Meropenem Meningitis Study Group. *Pediatr Infect Dis J*. 1999;18(7):581–590.

66. Cohen-Wolkowiez M, et al. Safety and effectiveness of meropenem in infants with suspected or complicated intra-abdominal infections. *Clin Infect Dis*. 2012;55(11):1495–1502.

67. Bradley JS, et al. Meropenem pharmacokinetics, pharmacodynamics, and Monte Carlo simulation in the neonate. *Pediatr Infect Dis J*. 2008;27(9):794–799.

68. Hornik CP, et al. Adverse events associated with meropenem versus imipenem/cilastatin therapy in a large retrospective cohort of hospitalized infants. *Pediatr Infect Dis J*. 2013;32(7):748–753.

69. Ljungberg B, Nilsson-Ehle I. Pharmacokinetics of meropenem and its metabolite in young and elderly healthy men. *Antimicrob Agents Chemother*. 1992;36(7):1437–1440.

70. Smith PB, et al. Population pharmacokinetics of meropenem in plasma and cerebrospinal fluid of infants with suspected or complicated intra-abdominal infections. *Pediatr Infect Dis J*. 2011;30(10): 844–849.

71. Sullins AK, Abdel-Rahman SM. Pharmacokinetics of antibacterial agents in the CSF of children and adolescents. *Paediatr Drugs*. 2013;15(2):93–117.

72. Cross CP, et al. Effect of sepsis and systemic inflammatory response syndrome on neonatal hearing screening outcomes following gentamicin exposure. *Int J Pediatr Otorhinolaryngol*. 2015;79(11): 1915–1919.

73. Reimche LD, et al. An evaluation of gentamicin dosing according to renal function in neonates with suspected sepsis. *Am J Perinatol*. 1987;4(3):262–265.

74. Pacifici GM. Clinical pharmacokinetics of penicillins, cephalosporins and aminoglycosides in the neonate: a review. *Pharmaceuticals (Basel)*. 2010;3(8):2568–2591.
75. Solomkin JS, et al. Diagnosis and management of complicated intra-abdominal infection in adults and children: guidelines by the Surgical Infection Society and the Infectious Diseases Society of America. *Clin Infect Dis*. 2010;50(2):133–164.
76. Gatti G, Malena M, Casazza R, et al. Penetration of clindamycin and its metabolite N-demethylclindamycin into cerebrospinal fluid following intravenous infusion of clindamycin phosphate in patients with AIDS. *Antimicrob Agents Chemother*. 1998;42:3014–3017.
77. Gonzalez D, et al. Clindamycin pharmacokinetics and safety in preterm and term infants. *Antimicrob Agents Chemother*. 2016;60(5):2888–2894.
78. DeHaan RM, et al. Pharmacokinetic studies of clindamycin hydrochloride in humans. *Int J Clin Pharmacol*. 1972;6(2):105–119.
79. DeHaan RM, et al. Pharmacokinetic studies of clindamycin phosphate. *J Clin Pharmacol*. 1973;13(5): 190–209.
80. Wynalda MA, et al. In vitro metabolism of clindamycin in human liver and intestinal microsomes. *Drug Metab Dispos*. 2003;31(7):878–887.
81. Gonzalez D, et al. Use of opportunistic clinical data and a population pharmacokinetic model to support dosing of clindamycin for premature infants to adolescents. *Clin Pharmacol Ther*. 2014; 96(4):429–437.
82. Knight RC, Skolimowski IM, Edwards DI. The interaction of reduced metronidazole with DNA. *Biochem Pharmacol*. 1978;27(17):2089–2093.
83. Warner JF, Perkins RL, Cordero L. Metronidazole therapy of anaerobic bacteremia, meningitis, and brain abscess. *Arch Intern Med*. 1979;139(2):167–169.
84. Upadhyaya P, Bhatnagar V, Basu N. Pharmacokinetics of intravenous metronidazole in neonates. *J Pediatr Surg*. 1988;23(3):263–265.
85. Suyagh M, et al. Metronidazole population pharmacokinetics in preterm neonates using dried blood-spot sampling. *Pediatrics*. 2011;127(2):e367–e374.
86. Pearce RE, et al. The role of human cytochrome P450 enzymes in the formation of 2-hydroxymetronidazole: CYP2A6 is the high affinity (low Km) catalyst. *Drug Metab Dispos*. 2013;41(9):1686–1694.
87. Jager-Roman E, et al. Pharmacokinetics and tissue distribution of metronidazole in the newborn infant. *J Pediatr*. 1982;100(4):651–654.
88. Cohen-Wolkowiez M, et al. Population pharmacokinetics of metronidazole evaluated using scavenged samples from preterm infants. *Antimicrob Agents Chemother*. 2012;56(4):1828–1837.
89. Kaufman DA. Challenging issues in neonatal candidiasis. *Curr Med Res Opin*. 2010;26(7):1769–1778.
90. Mian UK, et al. Comparison of fluconazole pharmacokinetics in serum, aqueous humor, vitreous humor, and cerebrospinal fluid following a single dose and at steady state. *J Ocul Pharmacol Ther*. 1998;14(5):459–471.
91. Kaufman D, et al. Fluconazole prophylaxis against fungal colonization and infection in preterm infants. *N Engl J Med*. 2001;345(23):1660–1666.
92. Kicklighter SD, et al. Fluconazole for prophylaxis against candidal rectal colonization in the very low birth weight infant. *Pediatrics*. 2001;107(2):293–298.
93. Manzoni P, et al. Prophylactic fluconazole is effective in preventing fungal colonization and fungal systemic infections in preterm neonates: a single-center, 6-year, retrospective cohort study. *Pediatrics*. 2006;117(1):e22–e32.
94. Aghai ZH, et al. Fluconazole prophylaxis in extremely low birth weight infants: association with cholestasis. *J Perinatol*. 2006;26(9):550–555.
95. Parikh TB, et al. Fluconazole prophylaxis against fungal colonization and invasive fungal infection in very low birth weight infants. *Indian Pediatr*. 2007;44(11):830–837.
96. Turner K, et al. Fluconazole pharmacokinetics and safety in premature infants. *Curr Med Chem*. 2012;19(27):4617–4620.
97. Label F. DIFLUCAN (Fluconazole). 2011. **Reference ID: 2956251**.
98. Wade KC, et al. Population pharmacokinetics of fluconazole in young infants. *Antimicrob Agents Chemother*. 2008;52(11):4043–4049.
99. Shah D, Sinn JK. Antibiotic regimens for the empirical treatment of newborn infants with necrotising enterocolitis. *Cochrane Database Syst Rev*. 2012;(8):CD007448.
100. Scheifele DW, et al. Comparison of two antibiotic regimens for neonatal necrotizing enterocolitis. *J Antimicrob Chemother*. 1987;20(3):421–429.
101. Pear BL. Pneumatosis intestinalis: a review. *Radiology*. 1998;207(1):13–19.
102. Smith PM, et al. The microbial metabolites, short-chain fatty acids, regulate colonic Treg cell homeostasis. *Science*. 2013;341(6145):569–573.
103. Autmizguine J, et al. Anaerobic antimicrobial therapy after necrotizing enterocolitis in VLBW infants. *Pediatrics*. 2015;135(1):e117–e125.
104. Luo LJ, et al. Broad-spectrum antibiotic plus metronidazole may not prevent the deterioration of necrotizing enterocolitis from stage ii to iii in full-term and near-term infants: a propensity score-matched cohort study. *Medicine (Baltimore)*. 2015;94(42):e1862.
105. Faix RG, Polley TZ, Grasela TH. A randomized, controlled trial of parenteral clindamycin in neonatal necrotizing enterocolitis. *J Pediatr*. 1988;112:271–277.
106. World Health Organization. Guidelines on maternal, newborn, child and adolescent health approved by the WHO Guidelines review comittee: Recommandations on newborn health.

107. Gleason CA, Devaskar SU. *Avery's Diseases of the Newborn*. 9th ed. Elsevier Inc; 2012.
108. Zani A, et al. International survey on the management of necrotizing enterocolitis. *Eur J Pediatr Surg*. 2015;25(1):27–33.
109. American Academy of Pediatrics, Kimberlin DW, Brady MT, Jackson MA, et al, Red Book 2015 Report of the Committee on Infectious Disease; 2015.
110. Stringer MD, et al. Recurrent necrotizing enterocolitis. *J Pediatr Surg*. 1993;28(8):979–981.
111. Hall NJ, Eaton S, Pierro A. Royal Australasia of Surgeons Guest Lecture. Necrotizing enterocolitis: prevention, treatment, and outcome. *J Pediatr Surg*. 2013;48(12):2359–2367.
112. Henry MC, Moss RL. Necrotizing enterocolitis. *Annu Rev Med*. 2009;60:111–124.
113. Moss RLD, et al. Laparotomy versus peritoneal drainage for necrotizing enterocolitis and perforation. *N Engl J Med*. 2006;354(21):2225–2234.
114. Rao SC, et al. Peritoneal drainage versus laparotomy as initial surgical treatment for perforated necrotizing enterocolitis or spontaneous intestinal perforation in preterm low birth weight infants. *Cochrane Database Syst Rev*. 2011;(6):CD006182.
115. Papillon S, et al. Necrotizing enterocolitis: contemporary management and outcomes. *Adv Pediatr*. 2013;60(1):263–279.
116. Zvizdic Z, et al. Contributing factors for development of necrotizing enterocolitis in preterm infants in the neonatal intensive care unit. *Mater Sociomed*. 2016;28(1):53–56.
117. Kort EJ. Patent ductus arteriosus in the preterm infant: an update on morbidity and mortality. *Curr Pediatr Rev*. 2016;12(2):98–105.
118. Quigley M, McGuire W. Formula versus donor breast milk for feeding preterm or low birth weight infants. *Cochrane Database Syst Rev*. 2014;(4):CD002971.
119. Aceti A, et al. Probiotics for prevention of necrotizing enterocolitis in preterm infants: systematic review and meta-analysis. *Ital J Pediatr*. 2015;41:89.
120. Olsen R, et al. Prophylactic probiotics for preterm infants: a systematic review and meta-analysis of observational studies. *Neonatology*. 2016;109(2):105–112.
121. Bertelli C, et al. Bifidobacterium longum bacteremia in preterm infants receiving probiotics. *Clin Infect Dis*. 2015;60:924–927.
122. Jenke A, et al. Bifidobacterium septicaemia in an extremely low-birthweight infant under probiotic therapy. *Arch Dis Child Fetal Neonatal Ed*. 2012;97:F217–F218.
123. Foster JP, Seth R, Cole MJ. Oral immunoglobulin for preventing necrotizing enterocolitis in preterm and low birth weight neonates. *Cochrane Database Syst Rev*. 2016;(4):CD001816.
124. Torikai M, et al. Prophylactic efficacy of enteral miconazole administration for neonatal intestinal perforation and its potential mechanism. *Pediatr Surg Int*. 2016;32(10):953–957.
125. Walsh MC, Kliegman RM. Necrotizing enterocolitis: treatment based on staging criteria. *Pediatr Clin North Am*. 1986;33(1):179–201.
126. Pineda LC, Watt KM. New antibiotic dosing in infants. *Clin Perinatol*. 2015;42(1):167–176, ix–x.
127. Autmizguine J, et al. Pharmacokinetics and pharmacodynamics of antifungals in children: clinical implications. *Drugs*. 2014;74(8):891–909.
128. Piper L, et al. Fluconazole loading dose pharmacokinetics and safety in infants. *Pediatr Infect Dis J*. 2011;30(5):375–378.

CHAPTER 14

Antibiotic Dosing Considerations for Term and Preterm Infants

Samantha Dallefeld, MD, Chi Dang Hornik, PharmD, BCPS,
Kanecia Zimmerman, MD, MPH, Michael Cohen-Wolkowiez, MD, PhD

14

- Immature drug metabolism and clearance in infants mandate careful consideration to appropriately dose antibiotics.
- Use of age-based surrogates for dosing in infants should account for prenatal and postnatal changes in renal and hepatic growth and maturation.
- Dosing of renally eliminated antibiotics should consider both physiologic changes and the potential for acute kidney injury.
- Modification of dose frequency and duration may lead to more optimal bacterial killing while minimizing side effects; however, more studies are needed in infants.
- ECMO and therapeutic hypothermia alter drug disposition, often necessitating dose modification and drug monitoring.

Introduction

Each year, severe infections in infants account for more than 1 million deaths worldwide.[1] Early and appropriate antibiotic therapy for these infections can be lifesaving; therefore appropriate dosing of antibiotics is essential.[2] Unfortunately, antibiotic dosing is particularly challenging in infants. Infants differ physiologically compared with older children and adults, and these differences alter drug absorption, distribution, metabolism, and elimination.[3]

Compared with older children and adults, infants have variable absorption of oral drugs due to increased gastric pH, delayed gastric emptying time, decreased intestinal motility, and increased intestinal permeability.[4-6] Limited muscle mass and a high body surface area to weight ratio can lead to high intramuscular and percutaneous drug absorption and altered drug distribution for these formulations.[4,7] In addition, infants have a higher proportion of total body water per body mass and a greater percentage of water in the extracellular compartment, leading to higher volume of distribution (Vd) for water-soluble drugs.[4] The low percentage of fat and muscle per neonatal body mass can lead to high plasma concentrations of lipophilic drugs.[4]

Infants also have lower plasma concentrations of protein and lower drug protein-binding affinity compared with older children and adults.[5] These properties lead to higher concentrations of unbound drug that readily cross membranes and can result in greater drug effect.[4,8] For drugs that target the central nervous system (CNS), increased permeability of the blood–brain barrier and a higher ratio of cerebral to systemic blood flow can lead to increased efficacy at a lower effective drug dose and more frequent or severe CNS side effects in infants.[5,9] Protein-binding properties in infants may also affect drug metabolism and clearance (CL). Lower protein binding in infants compared with older children and adults may lead to unexpectedly high hepatic metabolism and renal clearance for some drugs.[5,8,9] However, lower expression

167

of hepatic enzymes, lower glomerular filtration rate (GFR) normalized to body size, and immature tubular secretion and tubular reabsorption in infants most often result in lower drug metabolism and clearance per body mass relative to older children and adults.[4,5,10,11]

Physiologic differences in infants compared with older children and adults require careful consideration to appropriately scale antibiotic dosing from studies conducted in older populations. In addition, interindividual variability in drug disposition is pronounced, which can lead to substantial differences in exposure in infants of similar sizes and ages. Therefore dosing in infants requires direct study and special consideration of drug pharmacokinetics (PK) and pharmacodynamics (PD).[12]

PK modeling and simulation techniques can be used to overcome many of the challenges associated with dosing in infants.[13,14] These methods incorporate neonatal characteristics that affect drug disposition to derive neonatal-specific dosing regimens. Characteristics commonly incorporated include age, weight, and markers of illness severity. However, the variables on which dosing recommendations for specific drugs are based often depend on data availability and the number of infants in the study population. These efforts have sometimes resulted in disparate recommendations for dosing certain antibiotic therapies.

To identify areas of disparate recommendations, we performed a literature search in PubMed for articles published between 1990 and 2016 using the following terms: *infant, antibiotic, population, pharmacokinetics, postmenstrual, postnatal, gestational age, renal, hepatic, maturation, continuous infusion, prolonged infusion, prophylaxis, CNS penetration, blood brain barrier, ECMO,* and *hypothermia*. Here, we detail our opinion on the existing controversies for dosing of antibiotics in infants.

Antibiotic Dosing Based on Markers of Neonatal Growth and Maturation

Drug disposition in infants not only differs from that in older children and adults but also changes throughout the neonatal period. Physiologic systems responsible for drug metabolism and clearance, primarily the hepatic and renal systems, grow and mature over time. Specific stages of hepatic and renal growth and maturation must be considered for appropriate dosing of antibiotic therapy in infants.

Hepatic metabolism and clearance of drugs primarily depend on the activity of drug-metabolizing enzymes and alterations in hepatic blood flow.[11] Hepatic morphogenesis occurs during the first 10 weeks of gestation, followed by hyperplasia and hypertrophy that continue into adulthood.[10] As the fetal liver matures anatomically, it gains functional maturity characterized by increasing enzyme activity and metabolic capacity.[10,15] Cytochrome P450 (CYP) isoenzymes, which facilitate phase I reactions and enhance drug elimination, are expressed in the fetal liver at 30% to 60% of adult values and most often demonstrate increased activity over time during the neonatal period.[3,11] However, isoenzyme-specific ontogeny varies widely among individuals and precludes generalization of CYP development.[3,11] For example, CYP3A7 activity is greatest at birth and decreases over the first month after birth. Activity of CYP3A4 and CYP2D6 is limited over the first months to years after birth, but these isoenzymes are two of the greatest contributors to drug metabolism in children and adults.[3,8,11]

Enzymes that facilitate phase II conjugation reactions also have variable enzyme levels and metabolic activity at birth.[11] Some pathways, such as sulfate conjugation, exhibit higher enzyme activity at birth compared with adult levels; others, including UDP-glucuronosyltransferase isoenzymes, exhibit lower activity levels at birth and reach adult levels months to years after birth.[15] Limited enzyme expression and activity can result in toxic drug levels, whereas high enzyme activity can lead to enhanced first-pass metabolism, reduced bioavailability, improved clearance, and drug concentrations inadequate for optimal drug efficacy.[3,16]

Hepatic metabolism and drug clearance also depend on hepatic blood flow, which undergoes dramatic changes after birth.[15] At birth, umbilical blood flow ceases, resulting in a fourfold decrease in hepatic blood flow and a threefold decrease in oxygen delivery to the liver.[15] Because hepatic blood flow governs hepatic clearance of drugs with high hepatic extraction ratios, reduced hepatic blood flow after birth has the potential to reduce clearance of these drugs.[15] Alternatively, hepatic clearance of drugs with low extraction ratios is likely to be most limited by the immaturity of drug-metabolizing enzymes in the neonatal period.[15]

Most antimicrobials are primarily eliminated via the kidneys. Optimal clearance depends on full formation of nephrons, the functional unit of the kidney, and adequate hemodynamic milieu for nephron function.[17] Nephrogenesis begins at 5 to 6 weeks gestational age (GA) and is complete by approximately 35 weeks GA.[18] Fetal urine production and glomerular filtration begin at 9 to 10 weeks GA, and tubular absorption at 12 to 14 weeks GA.[17] Before birth, fluid homeostasis is regulated by maternal and placental exchange.[17] After birth, glomerular and tubular homeostatic regulation transition from the placenta to the neonatal kidney.[17] The glomerulus filters cells, proteins, and other large molecules from the blood, leaving an ultrafiltrate that can undergo solute and water reabsorption and secretion by the tubules.[19] During the process of birth, blood flow also transitions from maternal to neonatal control and results in increased cardiac output and circulation to the kidneys, decreased renal vascular resistance, and high renal perfusion pressure.[17,18] These changes provide the optimal hemodynamic condition for neonatal renal function.[17,20] However, despite these maturational changes, neonatal kidney function is impaired compared with that of adults.[17]

GFR, the flow rate of filtered fluid through the kidney, provides evidence of impaired kidney function in infants relative to adults, as well as fluctuations in renal function over time. GFR is very low at birth, even in a full-term infant, but rapidly increases during the first postnatal week to reach a body surface area–adjusted value approximately 25% of that of a typical adult.[17] Subsequently, GFR (expressed in mL/minute/1.73 m^2) increases rapidly to reach approximately 50% of adult values at 48 weeks postmenstrual age (PMA) and approach adult values between 6 months and 1 year of age.[8,21] Although preterm infants also experience an increase in GFR after birth, the GFR is lower in this population[17] and increases more slowly compared with term infants.[20] Tubular function matures later than glomerular function, but also reaches adult values by about 1 year of age.[16]

Because we cannot directly account for neonatal hepatic and renal growth and maturation when determining antibiotic dosing, we must use surrogates. Postnatal age (PNA), PMA, birth weight, and GA are commonly used surrogates, and each has advantages and disadvantages.

Postnatal Age

PNA, the number of days or weeks after birth, is usually an accurate and known value that is easily obtained for PK studies. For drugs with renal clearance through glomerular filtration, investigators have demonstrated that drug clearance increases rapidly in term infants between days 3 and 10 after birth.[16,20] Although studies differ on the presence of these rapid postnatal changes in very young preterm infants, daily changes in drug clearance during the early neonatal period suggest that PNA-based dosing can help ensure adequate antimicrobial concentrations for maximal bacterial killing.[16]

Common sources for antiinfective dosing, such as the Red Book, include recommendations for PNA-based dosing for cefotaxime, clindamycin, metronidazole, nafcillin, and piperacillin-tazobactam (Table 14.1).[22] However, PNA-based dosing recommendations exist within the US Food and Drug Administration (FDA) product labels for only a few antibiotics administered to infants, including cefotaxime and linezolid. Potential reasons for limited recommendations in product labels include the inability of PNA to account for hepatic and renal growth and functional activity that begins before term birth. Differences in maturation of hepatic and renal function between preterm and full-term infants is an increasingly important consideration given the increased survival of infants as young as 22 weeks GA.[20] In addition, CYP isoenzymes have variable expression and activity throughout gestation that should be taken into account.[23] For example, although CYP2D6 matures rapidly after birth,

Text continued on p. 174

Table 14.1 REPRESENTATIVE INTRAVENOUS DOSING RECOMMENDATIONS FOR COMMONLY USED ANTIBIOTICS IN INFANTS

Antibiotic	FDA Label	AAP/Red Book[22] or Nelson's Pediatric Antimicrobial Therapy[66,95]	PK Studies	ECMO and Hypothermia
Ampicillin	Septicemia: 150–200 mg/kg/day (no interval provided) Meningitis: 150–200 mg/kg/day div q3–4h	Non-meningitis: ≤2 kg: PNA ≤7 days: 50 mg/kg/dose q12h PNA 8–28 days: 50 mg/kg/dose q8h >2 kg: PNA ≤7 days: 50 mg/kg/dose q12h PNA 8–28 days: 50 mg/kg/dose q6h Meningitis: ≤7 days: 100 mg/kg/dose q8h >7 days: 75 mg/kg/dose q6h Surgical prophylaxis: 50 mg/kg single dose	**Tremoulet et al., 2014[96]** GA ≤34 wk and PNA ≤7 days: 50 mg/kg/dose q12h GA ≤34 wk and PNA ≥8 and ≤28 days: 75 mg/kg/dose q12h GA >34 wk and PNA ≤28 days: 50 mg/kg/dose q8h **Kaplan et al., 1974[73]** Preterm infants: 33.3 mg/kg/dose q8h PNA <7 days: 25 mg/kg/dose q12h PNA 7–28 days: 50 mg/kg/dose q8h Meningitis: **Tunkel et al., 2004[68]** PNA ≤7 days: 50 mg/kg/dose q8h PNA 8–28 days: 50 mg/kg/dose q6h or 66.6 mg/kg/dose q8h	
Cefazolin	25–50 mg/kg/day div q6–8h (up to 100 mg/kg/day for severe infections)	≤2 kg: 25 mg/kg/dose q12h >2 kg: PNA ≤7 days: 25 mg/kg/dose q12h PNA 8–28 days: 25 mg/kg/dose q8h	**De Cock et al., 2014[79]** ≤2 kg: PNA ≤7 days: 25 mg/kg/dose q12h PNA 8–28 days: 25 mg/kg/dose q8h >2 kg: PNA ≤7 days: 50 mg/kg/dose q12h PNA 8–28 days: 50 mg/kg/dose q8h	
Cefepime	Not labeled <2 mo of age	≤2 kg: PNA ≤7 days: 50 mg/kg/dose q12h PNA 8–28 days: 50 mg/kg/dose q8h >2 kg: 50 mg/kg/dose q8h	**Capparelli et al., 2005[97]** PNA <14 days: 30 mg/kg/dose q12h PNA >14 days: 50 mg/kg/dose q8h	

Drug	Dosing		Meningitis / Other	ECMO / Special
Cefotaxime	0–1 wk: 50 mg/kg/dose q12h 1–4 wk: 50 mg/kg/dose q8h >4 wk: 50–180 mg/kg/day divided q4–6h	≤2 kg: PNA ≤7 days: 50 mg/kg/dose q12h PNA 8–28 days: 50 mg/kg/dose q8–12h >2 kg: PNA ≤7 days: 50 mg/kg/dose q12h PNA 8–28 days: 50 mg/kg/dose q8h	Meningitis: Tunkel et al., 2004[68] PNA ≤7 days: 100–150 mg/kg/day div q8–12h PNA 8–28 days: 150–200 mg/kg/day div q6–8h	ECMO: Ahsman et al., 2010[98] Standard dosing per FDA label
Ceftazidime	0–4 wk: 30 mg/kg/dose q12h	≤2 kg: PNA ≤7 days: 50 mg/kg/dose q12h PNA 8–28 days: 50 mg/kg/dose q8h >2 kg: PNA ≤7 days: 50 mg/kg/dose q12h PNA 8–28 days: 50 mg/kg/dose q8h	Meningitis: Tunkel et al., 2004[68] PNA ≤7 days: 100–150 mg/kg/day div q8–12h PNA 8–28 days: 150 mg/kg/day div q8h	
Clindamycin	<1 mo of age: 15–20 mg/kg/day div q6–8h	≤2 kg: PNA ≤7 days: 5 mg/kg/dose q12h PNA 8–28 days: 5 mg/kg/dose q8h >2 kg: PNA ≤7 days: 5 mg/kg/dose q8h PNA 8–28 days: 5 mg/kg/dose q6h	Gonzalez et al., 2014[25] PMA ≤32 wk: 5 mg/kg q8h PMA >32–40 wks: 7 mg/kg q8h PMA >40–60 wks: 9 mg/kg q8h	
Gentamicin	≤1 wk: 2.5 mg/kg/dose q12h >1 wk: 2.5 mg/kg/dose q8h	≤2 kg: PNA ≤7 days: 5 mg/kg/dose q48h PNA 8–28 days: 5 mg/kg/dose q36h >2 kg: PNA ≤7 days: 4 mg/kg/dose q24h PNA 8–28 days: 4–5 mg/kg/dose q24h Surgical prophylaxis: 2.5 mg/kg single dose	Fuchs et al., 2014[65] GA ≤29 wks: 5 mg/kg/dose q48h GA >29 and ≤34 wks: 4 mg/kg q24h Mohamed et al., 2012[63] Dosing interval of q36–48h as effective as q24h dosing interval Meningitis: Tunkel et al., 2004[68] ≤7 days: 5 mg/kg/day div q12h 8–28 days: 7.5 mg/kg/day div q8h	ECMO: Sherwin et al., 2016[87] <3 mo: 4–5 mg/kg/dose once, then check 2 h and 8–12 h concentrations 3 mo–2 yrs: 9.5 mg/kg/dose once, then check 2 h and 8–12 h concentrations Hypothermia: Frymoyer et al., 2013[94] 4–5 mg/kg/dose q36h
Linezolid	<7 days: 10 mg/kg/dose q12h >7 days: 10 mg/kg/dose q8h	≤2 kg: PNA ≤7 days: 10 mg/kg/dose q12h PNA 8–28 days: 10 mg/kg/dose q8h >2 kg: 10 mg/kg/dose q8h	Kearns et al., 2003[32] 10 mg/kg/dose q8h	

14

Continued

Table 14.1   REPRESENTATIVE INTRAVENOUS DOSING RECOMMENDATIONS FOR COMMONLY USED ANTIBIOTICS IN INFANTS—cont'd

Antibiotic	FDA Label	AAP/Red Book[22] or Nelson's Pediatric Antimicrobial Therapy[66,95]	PK Studies	ECMO and Hypothermia
Meropenem	Not labeled <3 mo of age	≤2 kg: PNA ≤14 days: 20 mg/kg/dose q12h PNA 15–28 days: 20 mg/kg/dose q8h >2 kg: PNA ≤14 days: 20 mg/kg/dose q8h PNA 15–28 days: 30 mg/kg/dose q8h	Smith et al., 2011[31] GA <32 wk and PNA <14 days: 20 mg/kg/dose q12h GA <32 wk and ≥14 days: 20 mg/kg/dose q8h GA ≥32 wk and <14 days: 20 mg/kg/dose q8h GA ≥32 wk and ≥14 days: 30 mg/kg/dose q8h van den Anker et al., 2009[33] GA >30 wk: 40 mg/kg/dose q8h, 4h infusion if MIC 4–8 µg/mL or meningitis	ECMO: Sherwin et al., 2016[87] Loading dose: 40 mg/kg Maintenance: 200 mg/kg/day continuous infusion or 33.3 mg/kg over 3h q4h
Metronidazole	Not labeled for pediatrics	≤2 kg: 7.5 mg/kg/dose q12h >2 kg: Loading dose: 15 mg/kg Maintenance dose: PNA ≤7 days: 7.5 mg/kg/dose q8h PNA 8–28 days: 7.5 mg/kg/dose q6h	Cohen-Wolkowiez et al., 2012, 2013[26a,26b] Loading dose: 15 mg/kg PMA <34 wk: 7.5 mg/kg/dose q12h PMA 34–40 wk: 7.5 mg/kg/dose q8h PMA >40 wk: 7.5 mg/kg/dose q6h Surgical prophylaxis: Bratzler et al., 2013[77] <1.2 kg: 7.5 mg/kg as a single dose 30–60 min before procedure ≥1.2 kg: 15 mg/kg as a single dose 30–60 min before procedure	
Nafcillin	Not labeled for pediatrics	<2 kg: PNA ≤7 days: 25 mg/kg/dose q12h PNA 8–28 days: 25 mg/kg/dose q8h >2 kg: PNA ≤7 days: 25 mg/kg/dose q8h PNA 8–28 days: 25 mg/kg/dose q6h	Banner et al., 1980[29] LBW infants: <7 days: 50 mg/kg/dose q12h >7 days: 33 mg/kg/dose q8h Meningitis: Tunkel et al., 2004[68] PNA ≤7 days: 75 mg/kg/day div q8–12h PNA 8–28 days: 100–150 mg/kg/day div q6–8h	

Penicillin G crystalline	Septicemia: 150,000–300,000 units/kg/day div q4–6h Meningitis: 250,000 units/kg/day div q4h *Appropriate reductions should be made in newborns	≤2 kg: PNA ≤7 days: 25,000–50,000 units/kg/dose q12h PNA 8–28 days: 25,000–50,000 units/kg/dose q8h >2 kg: PNA ≤7 days: 25,000–50,000 units/kg/dose q12h PNA 8–28 days: 25,000–50,000 units/kg/dose q8h Meningitis: PNA ≤7 days: 250,000–450,000 units/kg/day div q8h PNA 8–28 days: 450,000–500,000 units/kg/day div q6h	**Metsvaht et al., 2007**[100] VLBW infants: 25,000 units/kg/dose q12h **McCracken et al., 1973**[101] 25,000 units/kg/dose q12h
Piperacillin-tazobactam	Not labeled for <2 mo of age	<2 kg and ≤7 days: 100 mg piperacillin/kg/dose q8h <2 kg and 8–28 days: 80 mg piperacillin/kg/dose q6h ≥2 kg: 80 mg piperacillin/kg/dose q6h	**Cohen-Wolkowiez et al., 2014**[24] PMA ≤30 wk: 100 mg/kg/dose q8h PMA 30–35 wk: 80 mg/kg/dose q6h PMA 35–49 wk: 80 mg/kg/dose q4h **Li et al., 2013**[99] Birth weight 1 kg and PNA 3 days: 10 mg/kg/dose q8h Birth weight 4.5 kg and PNA 7 days: 100 mg/kg/dose q6h
Vancomycin	Loading dose: 15 mg/kg/dose Maintenance: ≤1 wk: 10 mg/kg/dose q12h >1 wk: 10 mg/kg/dose q8h	**Bradley et al., 2016**[66] PNA ≤60 days: GA ≤28 wk (Scr in mg/dL): Scr <0.5: 15 mg/kg/dose q12h Scr 0.5–0.7: 20 mg/kg/dose q24h Scr 0.8–1: 15 mg/kg/dose q24h Scr 1.1–1.4: 10 mg/kg/dose q24h Scr >1.4: 15 mg/kg/dose q48h GA >28 wk (Scr in mg/dL): Scr <0.7: 15 mg/kg/dose q12h Scr 0.7–0.9: 20 mg/kg/dose q24h Scr 1–1.2: 15 mg/kg/dose q24h Scr 1.3–1.6: 10 mg/kg/dose q24h Scr >1.6: 15 mg/kg/dose q48h PNA >60 days: 45–60 mg/kg/day div q8h	Meningitis: **Tunkel et al., 2004**[68] PNA ≤7 days: 20–30 mg/kg/day div q8–12h PNA 8–28 days: 30–45 mg/kg/day div q6–8h ECMO: **Sherwin et al., 2016**[87] 20 mg/kg once, then check 2 h and 8–12 h concentrations

14

AAP, American Academy of Pediatrics; *div*, divided; *ECMO*, extracorporeal membrane oxygenation; *FDA*, US Food and Drug Administration; *GA*, gestational age; *LBW*, low birth weight; *PK*, pharmacokinetic; *PMA*, postmenstrual age; *PNA*, postnatal age; *Scr*, serum creatinine.

this isoenzyme is detectable in some fetal livers at less than 30 weeks GA.[23] Dosing based on PNA alone would not account for the presence of CYP2D6 activity in some preterm infants.

Postmenstrual Age

PMA, the sum of PNA (in weeks) and GA, has been used as a surrogate for preterm and term hepatic and renal growth and maturation.[6] Because of an in-depth understanding of the relationship between PMA and GFR in both preterm and term infants, PMA may be particularly helpful for dosing drugs that are eliminated through the kidneys by glomerular filtration.[6] When PMA-based dosing was used for piperacillin-tazobactam in preterm and term infants, the predefined therapeutic target was achieved in >90% of infants (see Table 14.1).[24] PMA-based dosing has also been recommended for drugs such as clindamycin and metronidazole.[25,26] Importantly, accurate PMA may be difficult to ascertain because the value for GA relies on maternal report of last menstrual period, imaging-based estimates, or clinical scoring systems.

Birth Weight and Postnatal Age

Birth weight and PNA are surrogates that, when used together for dosing, account for some degree of preterm maturation, and the values are often more readily available than GA. Use of birth weight may have added benefit in small for GA infants, who have smaller kidney volumes, higher serum creatinine (Scr) levels at 1 day of age, and decreased urine output during the first week after birth compared with those whose growth is appropriate for GA.[27] Dosing based on combined parameters of birth weight and PNA may adequately account for decreased renal clearance and therefore reduce toxicity in this population.[27] This strategy has been recommended for amikacin and nafcillin.[28,29]

Postnatal Age and Gestational Age

A final approach for dosing based on surrogates of organ maturation is to consider both PNA and GA as independent markers of maturation. GA (in weeks) correlates well with prebirth maturation of organ function, whereas PNA (in days) identifies the rapid increases in GFR that occur in the days after birth.[30] Unfortunately, identification of GA and PNA as statistically significant covariates for neonatal PK models is often more difficult than using the combined measure of PMA. Each additional covariate requires an increase in study sample size, and sample size is often lacking in neonatal studies. Nonetheless, PNA- and GA-based dosing strategies have been recommended for linezolid, meropenem, and penicillin.[31–34]

Antibiotic Dosing Based on Indicators of Renal Dysfunction

Critical illness in hospitalized infants can further complicate changes in renal function after birth.[35] Hypoxia, stress, and nephrotoxic medications can limit adaptive properties and lead to acute kidney injury (AKI).[35] AKI, defined as a sudden decline in kidney function, results in derangements in fluid balance, electrolytes, and waste products.[35] Therefore AKI can result in drug toxicity if dosing does not adequately account for it.

The most appropriate marker for defining AKI has been a subject of great debate. Although change in Scr is most commonly used to define AKI, collaborative efforts by the Acute Kidney Injury Network, the Kidney Disease: Improving Global Outcomes (KDIGO) group, and others have led to the development of more standardized definitions based on Scr, estimated creatinine clearance (CrCL), or urine output.[36,37] The neonatal modification of the KDIGO criteria defines AKI based on a rise in Scr or decrease in urine output but has not yet been validated in large multicenter studies.[35] Thus there is still controversy regarding a standardized definition for AKI. Scr, CrCL, estimated GFR, cystatin-C (cys-c), urine neutrophil gelatinase–associated lipocalin (NGAL), and kidney injury molecule 1 (KIM-1) have each been used to determine renal function in infants, with variable incorporation in dosing recommendations (Table 14.2).

Serum Creatinine

Many PK studies in infants use Scr for drug dosing because it is an easily obtained laboratory value and does not require calculation. Creatinine is a measured byproduct of muscle metabolism that is primarily filtered by the glomerulus and excreted unchanged by the kidneys. In a review of 61 articles using pediatric pharmacometric modeling and simulation to optimize dosing of renally eliminated antibiotics, Scr affected drug CL in 46% of reported models.[38] Vancomycin is an example of an antibiotic primarily eliminated by glomerular filtration, where adequate dosing based on renal function is essential to avoid drug toxicity.[39] Accordingly, investigators have identified an independent association between Scr and vancomycin clearance in infants; an increase in Scr from 0.2 to 1 mg/dL resulted in nearly 80% decrease in vancomycin clearance.[39] Simulated dosing based on Scr in infants <60 days of age resulted in a 40% greater likelihood of achieving consistent serum vancomycin concentrations compared with previously published age-based dosing strategies.[39]

However, others feel that Scr-based dosing is an unreliable variable in infants. Primarily, Scr reflects maternal-derived creatinine in the first few days after birth.[20] Further, Scr values differ in term and preterm infants. In preterm infants, Scr reflects the process of nephrogenesis until its completion at 35 weeks, and values may not approach those of a term infant for 1 to 3 months after birth.[17] In very low birth weight (VLBW) infants, Scr levels initially increase due to transient reabsorption across immature tubules and return to baseline by the second week after birth as glomerular filtration and tubular function mature.[40] Between weeks 3 and 7 after birth, Scr rapidly decreases, reaching an equilibrium between creatinine production and excretion by approximately 8 weeks of age.[40] In addition to these changes, Scr values can vary depending on the bioanalytical assay and assay interference by neonatal protein and bilirubin levels.[41] Finally, Scr values fail to reflect small changes in urine output and GFR. Scr requires time for accumulation that often lags behind clinical deterioration.[42] Reliance on Scr for dosing can inappropriately delay dosing adjustments required to maintain appropriate drug exposure.[42]

Glomerular Filtration Rate

Accurate measurement of GFR requires conducting a nuclear medicine study in which a radiopharmaceutical tracer is administered and GFR is calculated based on the presence of radiotracer in the blood at varying time intervals.[43] The gold-standard evaluation of GFR in children requires an infusion of inulin, a substance freely filtered by the glomerulus and not secreted, metabolized, or reabsorbed by the renal tubules, with serial urine sample collection.[44] Such studies are not available at most medical centers and are impractical for clinical use to monitor changing renal function.

As a result of the complexities of actual GFR measurement, GFR is often estimated using formulas to calculate an approximation to CrCL.[44] One method for calculating estimated CrCL is the Schwartz equation:

$$\text{GFR } (mL/min \text{ per } 1.73 \ m^2) = k \times \text{height } (cm)/\text{Scr } (mg/dL),$$

where k depends upon age and sex. However, this approach overestimates GFR by 20% to 40%, attributed to a change in creatinine assay methods since the development of the formula.[44] An alternative approach is the updated Schwartz equation:

$$\text{GFR } (mL/min \text{ per } 1.73 \ m^2) = 0.413 \times \text{height } (cm)/\text{Scr } (mg/dL),$$

which is considered to be one of the best methods for estimating GFR in children, although it is not specific to infants.[44] Both of these CrCL calculations depend on an accurate height measurement, which may be difficult to obtain in critically ill infants.[44,45]

Investigators have used CrCL as determined by the original Schwartz equation to determine vancomycin dosing for treatment of late-onset staphylococcal sepsis in preterm and term infants. Based on CrCL measurements, infants received a median

Table 14.2 ADVANTAGES AND DISADVANTAGES OF ANTIBIOTIC DOSING BASED ON INDICATORS OF RENAL FUNCTION

	Serum Creatinine	Estimated Glomerular Filtration Rate	Cystatin-C	Urinary Neutrophil Gelatinase–Associated Lipocalin	Kidney Injury Molecule 1
Advantages	• Frequently obtained laboratory value • Results obtained rapidly • Complex calculations not required • Commonly used to identify renal dysfunction	• Accounts for Scr • Incorporates variations in renal function by age and sex	• Serum concentrations depend only on GFR • Rises more rapidly than Scr when GFR decreases • Estimates GFR independent of age, sex, weight, or height • Unable to cross the placenta; should not reflect maternal renal function	• Easily measured • Rises early after renal injury	• Detected in the urine only with AKI • Correlates with mortality from renal dysfunction in VLBW infants
Disadvantages	• Reflects maternal creatinine in the first week after birth • Changes often, based on age and clinical condition • Values may not reflect small changes in urine output or GFR • Values vary based on assay used to run the test and neonatal protein and bilirubin levels	• May be calculated by a variety of methods • Schwartz equation overestimates true GFR • Calculation depends on an accurate height measurement	• Costly • Limited availability • Lacks robust evidence and clinical trials	• No trials evaluating its use in antibiotic dosing	• No trials evaluating its use in antibiotic dosing

AKI, Acute kidney injury; *GFR*, glomerular filtration rate; *Scr*, serum creatinine; *VLBW*, very low birth weight.

dose of 30 mg/kg/day (interquartile range 21–42), and approximately 54% of patients achieved the goal PD target of area under the concentration time curve (AUC) from 0 to 24 hours/minimum inhibitory concentration (MIC) ≥400 μg•hr/mL.[46]

Cystatin-C

Cys-c is a cysteine protease inhibitor that is synthesized by all nucleated cells, filtered by the glomeruli, and metabolized by the proximal renal tubule cells.[47,48] Unlike creatinine, which is primarily filtered by the glomerulus but also secreted by the proximal tubule and extrarenally eliminated, serum concentrations of cys-c depend only on GFR and rise more rapidly than Scr when GFR decreases.[47] Therefore cys-c is potentially a more accurate indicator of renal function than Scr or CrCL.[47,48] Cys-c concentrations are also elevated in premature infants, reflecting immaturity of the kidneys, and concentrations reflect maturation in renal function over time, reaching adult values by approximately 1 year of age.[47] Further, preliminary evidence suggests cys-c does not cross the placenta; therefore measurements of cys-c in the first days after birth should not reflect maternal levels.[49] In one study comparing serum cys-c to Scr in term infants, cys-c was a better marker of vancomycin clearance with more reliable predictions of serum vancomycin concentrations.[48] Despite these potential advantages, cys-c measurement is costly, availability is limited, and few studies have evaluated cys-c as a covariate in neonatal PK models.[17,49]

Other Potential Biomarkers

NGAL and KIM-1 represent other potential markers of renal function. NGAL, expressed in neutrophils, monocytes, and macrophages, is an innate mediator of immune response.[42,50] Urinary excretion of NGAL may represent early stages of AKI when few clinical signs and symptoms are evident.[50] A less well-studied marker of renal function is KIM-1, a transmembrane glycoprotein not detected in the urine under normal conditions.[42,50] In animal models, AKI is evident when KIM-1 concentrations are increased in proximal tubule cells and secreted in the urine.[50] Investigators have shown that KIM-1 correlates with mortality in VLBW infants, suggesting the contribution of renal dysfunction to mortality in this population.[50] To our knowledge, neither NGAL nor KIM-1 has been used in PK modeling and simulation studies to determine dosing of antibiotics in infants.

Continuous, Prolonged, and Extended Infusion Dosing Regimens

Bactericidal effects of antibiotics are either time or concentration dependent. Time-dependent effects are characteristic of beta-lactams, erythromycin, and linezolid.[51] Such effects are optimal when drug concentrations are maintained above MIC, the lowest drug concentration that prevents visible bacterial growth for an extended period.[52] Concentration-dependent bactericidal action, characteristic of aminoglycosides and metronidazole, requires both a high maximum concentration and AUC, the total drug exposure over time, relative to the MIC.[51,52] Although intermittent-infusion antibiotic dosing regimens are the standard of clinical practice worldwide in children and adults, investigators have explored alternative dosing regimens, including continuous infusions, prolonged infusions, and extended-interval dosing to capitalize on time- or concentration-dependent properties of antibiotics in these populations.[51,53]

Continuous infusions, intravenous (IV) administration of a drug without interruption, prolong the time that an antibiotic concentration is maintained above MIC.[51,53] Prolonged infusions involve intermittent dosing with drug administration over an extended period, allowing for reduction in overall daily dose.[51] In older children and adults, continuous and prolonged infusions are thought to lead to increased efficacy of antibiotics that exhibit time-dependent bactericidal action because they lead to earlier attainment and maintenance of target concentrations.[53,54] Extended-interval dosing maximizes concentration-dependent killing by targeting high peak concentrations and enables more time for drug clearance between doses.[55,56]

Investigators have extrapolated studies from adult populations to support these alternative dosing regimens in infants.[57] In theory, maintenance of target concentrations over a longer duration may more optimally treat infants infected with multidrug-resistant bacteria or microorganisms with low susceptibility.[51,53] However, potential benefits and toxicities of alternative dosing regimens are not well defined in infants.

Continuous Infusion

In addition to the potential PD advantages for time-dependent antimicrobials, use of continuous infusions may lead to a reduced need to access an IV line for drug administration and elimination of therapeutic drug monitoring.[53,58] Certainly in infants, repeated access of IV lines is associated with catheter-associated bloodstream infection, and therapeutic drug monitoring is complicated by the limited blood volume and technical difficulties associated with phlebotomy.[59] In a Dutch study in infants >34 weeks GA at high clinical or obstetric risk of neonatal infection immediately after birth, administration of IV amoxicillin as a loading dose (33 mg/kg) followed by continuous infusion (100 mg/kg/day) achieved therapeutic drug concentrations within 1 day and maintained therapeutic concentrations at 3 days in 96% of the subjects.[54]

Although continuous infusions may provide therapeutic benefit, sparse data limit widespread adoption of this dosing strategy. Investigators have not yet evaluated the effect of continuous dosing on clinical and microbiologic outcomes.[51,53] Further, because infants have reduced CL and maintain concentrations above MIC for longer periods compared with older children and adults, continuous infusions may expose infants to an unnecessary risk of toxicity. Additional limitations include reduced line availability when infants are also administered incompatible medications, other therapeutic infusions, or total parenteral nutrition.[53]

Prolonged Infusions

Prolonged infusions are an alternative to continuous infusions and may partially relieve the burden of IV access issues while maximizing drug exposure for antibiotics with time-dependent killing.[58] This strategy has been used in dosing simulations for meropenem; infants >30 weeks GA had therapeutic target attainment in >90% of cases when administered 40 mg/kg every 8 hours as a prolonged 4-hour infusion.[33]

Compared with older preterm and term infants, prolonged infusion of meropenem in critically ill VLBW infants may not offer benefit. In a study comparing a standard 30-minute infusion of meropenem versus a 4-hour prolonged infusion in VLBW infants, prolonged infusion did not improve the percentage of time for which drug levels exceeded MIC.[60] This absence of an apparent benefit from prolonged infusion in VLBW infants might be due to lower meropenem clearance in these infants compared with older preterm and term infants.

More studies are needed to evaluate the efficacy and toxicity of prolonged antibiotic infusions in preterm and term infants. Until then, prolonged infusion recommendations in adults should not be extrapolated to infants.

Extended Interval

In older children and adults, extended-interval dosing is used for antibiotics subject to adaptive resistance (a phenomenon resulting in a reduced bacterial killing effect with subsequent doses of the drug) and those with concentration-dependent killing.[61] Proponents of extended-interval dosing suggest that this method allows adaptive resistance time to resolve, thereby resulting in improved drug efficacy.[58]

Investigators have evaluated the safety and efficacy of a high-dose, extended-interval regimen for aminoglycosides in infants.[62] Gentamicin, an aminoglycoside, is a prototypical drug for extended-interval dosing because it exerts concentration-dependent bacterial killing.[62] A standard treatment for suspected neonatal sepsis, gentamicin is FDA approved in this population at doses of 2.5 mg/kg IV every 8 hours for infants >1 week of age and 2.5 mg/kg every 12 hours for premature or term infants ≤1 week of age. In a dosing simulation study of preterm infants with

Escherichia coli, higher-than-labeled doses of gentamicin administered every 36 to 48 hours had similar efficacy and AUC compared with more frequent dosing.[63] This regimen also resulted in decreased adaptive resistance, which can occur within 36 hours of standard drug administration. Further, extended dosing of gentamicin may lead to lower risk for drug accumulation in the renal tubules and inner ear, leading to decreased nephrotoxicity and ototoxicity.[62,63]

Extended-interval dosing may be of particular benefit in premature infants who have decreased GFR.[64] In an age-based dosing study of gentamicin in 1449 preterm and term infants, infants >34 weeks GA were expected to reach target concentrations with 4 mg/kg IV every 24 hours. However, most infants ≤29 weeks GA had supra-therapeutic trough levels with this dosing interval.[65] A dosing regimen of 5 mg/kg every 48 hours was required to achieve target peak concentrations, presumably secondary to a larger Vd and lower GFR compared with older preterm and term infants.[65] Several studies and the American Academy of Pediatrics recommend gentamicin dosing by GA and PNA ranging from 4 to 5 mg/kg IV every 24 to 48 hours despite the FDA label recommending lower doses and less frequent intervals in infants.[66]

Dosing Targeting the Central Nervous System

Neonatal bacterial meningitis is a devastating disease with high mortality and morbidity that warrants prompt diagnosis and effective treatment.[67] Clinical signs of bacterial meningitis are often subtle, and confirmatory testing by cerebrospinal fluid (CSF) cultures is not always available.[67,68] Because meningitis can exist in the absence of other obvious sources for infection, antibiotic dosing for infants with any suspected infection must allow adequate penetration of the blood–brain barrier while limiting toxicity.[69]

Optimal antibiotic penetration into the CSF occurs when meninges are inflamed and the administered drug is a small (<400 KDa), lipophilic, and minimally protein-bound molecule.[70] However, available literature to further guide antibiotic dosing is limited, and determining the extent of CNS penetration is difficult. CNS drug penetration is most accurately described as a ratio of drug AUC in CSF to drug AUC in plasma.[16] However, this method requires serial invasive sampling of the CSF, which is not feasible in critically ill infants. CSF sampling by ventricular drain may be easier to perform; however, adult studies have shown much lower drug concentrations in ventricular versus lumbar CSF samples.[71] To our knowledge, no pediatric studies compare drug concentrations obtained by various CSF sampling methods. Such challenges have resulted in single paired CSF and plasma samples from infants in existing studies, which limit the ability to evaluate PK or develop generalizable information regarding CNS drug penetration.[72]

Ampicillin is one of the most widely accepted antibiotics used empirically for the treatment of neonatal bacterial meningitis.[68] In a study of preterm and term infants, doses of 40 to 70 mg/kg resulted in CSF concentrations of 11% to 65% of paired plasma concentrations, prompting investigators to recommend higher total daily doses and more frequent dosing intervals for treatment of meningitis compared with septicemia (see Table 14.1).[73] Current FDA guidelines for ampicillin as treatment for bacterial meningitis are not specific to infants; however, the Red Book recommends 300 mg/kg/day divided q8h for infants ≤7 days PNA and q6h for infants >7 days PNA.[22]

Others argue that high interindividual variability observed with ampicillin dosing and increased permeability of the blood–brain barrier in the setting of meningitis may lead to high ampicillin concentrations in the CSF and neurotoxicity, particularly in VLBW infants with reduced drug CL.[74] A retrospective observational study of 131,723 infants with median GA of 35 weeks (twenty-fifth, seventy-fifth percentile: 32, 38) demonstrated a relationship between increased odds of seizures and both higher simulated maximum ampicillin concentration at steady state (C_{maxss}, mg/mL) and AUC from 0 to 24 hours (AUC_{24}, mg*h/dL) derived from a one-compartment PK model.[75] The odds of seizures were not related to ampicillin doses, however.

Dosing to Prevent Surgical Site Infections

Surgical site infections occur frequently in VLBW infants, in infants after gastroschisis closure, and in infants undergoing cardiac surgery.[76] Although consensus guidelines provide standardized dosing recommendations for the prevention of surgical site infections in all age groups, these guidelines do not account for the unique physiology of preterm and term infants undergoing surgical procedures.[77,78] Therefore controversy exists regarding the most appropriate perioperative dosing amounts and schedules to prevent surgical site infections in infants.

In children and adults with normal renal function, the recommended frequency of intraoperative antibiotic dosing is two times the half-life of the antibiotic.[77] For example, for infants with gastroschisis who are commonly administered piperacillin-tazobactam, current guidelines recommend intraoperative dosing every 2 hours based on piperacillin-tazobactam half-life in adults.[77] However, in a study evaluating term and preterm infants <61 days of age, the half-life of piperacillin-tazobactam was 2.5 and 5.3 hours, respectively.[26] Therefore less frequent intraoperative dosing should be considered for younger infants undergoing surgery.

Cefazolin is the most common perioperative antibiotic administered for patients of all ages to prevent surgical site infections, including infants.[77] Existing guidelines recommend redosing every 4 hours intraoperatively; however, this recommendation does not account for altered disposition due to immature renal function or body composition of infants compared with older children and adults.[77] Based on the differences in neonatal physiology, PK modeling and simulation predict that a dosing regimen of every 8 to 12 hours will reach efficacy targets of unbound cefazolin concentrations >8 mg/L (PD target) for 60% of the dosing interval in >90% of infants (see Table 14.1).[79] More studies are needed to characterize the effects of surgery on perioperative antibiotic distribution and clearance. Existing evidence suggests that current dosing recommendations are inadequate and that the interval between repeat doses is too short in infants.[77]

Dosing in Severe Illness

Optimization of antibiotic dosing can have added challenges when therapeutic modalities such as extracorporeal membrane oxygenation (ECMO) or hypothermia alter drug disposition.

Extracorporeal Membrane Oxygenation

In the setting of ECMO, antibiotic Vd is generally increased; the volume of pump prime (200–250 mL) results in a 50% to 100% increase in neonatal circulating blood volume and leads to dilution of the added drug.[80] In addition, the membrane oxygenator and tubing materials can adsorb drugs, particularly those that are lipophilic.[80] Adsorption of drug by circuit components may depend on the age of the circuit and number and duration of drugs to which the circuit is exposed; however, data are inconsistent, with one study identifying higher loss (40%) in a more aged circuit (1 day of support) compared with a newly primed circuit (20%).[81,82] Generally, a higher Vd on ECMO requires higher loading doses of antibiotic therapy to achieve therapeutic benefit.[80]

In addition to high Vd, patients supported with ECMO often have decreased drug clearance. Decreased clearance often results from organ dysfunction associated with critical illness, but may also be exacerbated by ECMO.[80] For example, venoarterial ECMO is associated with nonphysiologic, nonpulsatile blood flow to the kidneys, which may contribute to renal dysfunction.[80] Using criteria based on a change in Scr, the reported incidence of AKI in infants on ECMO is >60% with only 46% of infants showing some degree of renal recovery during the ECMO course.[83] Nonpulsatile flow may similarly contribute to reduced hepatic function and metabolism by 20% to 50%.[84] Decreased clearance may also represent reversible adsorption or increased plasma concentrations as drug previously adsorbed by the ECMO circuit reenters circulation.[85] However, this process has not been well studied. Rarely, investigators have demonstrated an increased clearance on ECMO, which may reflect improving organ function over time.[86]

Given the increase in Vd and decreased CL of drugs on ECMO, therapeutic drug monitoring may be particularly helpful to optimize dosing in that setting.[87] PK modeling and simulation studies are increasingly performed in this population, and dosing recommendations have been published for cefotaxime, gentamicin, meropenem, and vancomycin in infants.[87]

Hypothermia

Critically ill infants with birth depression are often treated with therapeutic hypothermia, defined as a core temperature <35°C.[88] As a result of hypoxic injury incurred in utero or at birth, infants undergoing therapeutic hypothermia often have liver and kidney dysfunction.[89,90] Although neonatal studies are limited, hypothermia has been shown to further decrease hepatic function and drug clearance. Enzymatic kinetic energy is decreased in hypothermia, resulting in fewer drug–enzyme collisions and reduced enzyme activity.[91] Clearance of drugs metabolized by cytochrome P450 enzymes is reduced by 7% to 22% per °C below 37°C.[88,92] In contrast, glomerular filtration is a passive transport system and requires no energy.[93] Nonetheless, a decrease in GFR of up to 50% has been demonstrated in a hypothermic animal model and is expected in vivo due to decreased cardiac output, increased blood viscosity, and cold-induced vasoconstriction.[91,93]

Accordingly, antibiotic doses in hypothermic infants should be decreased for drugs with hepatic metabolism or renal clearance to maintain efficacy and avoid potential toxicity.[92,94] In term infants undergoing therapeutic hypothermia, decreased frequency of gentamicin dosing of 4 to 5 mg/kg every 36 hours (as opposed to the standard interval of every 24 hours) achieved target peak and trough concentrations in >90% of infants.[94]

Conclusion

Optimal antibiotic dosing is essential to decrease morbidity and mortality in infants. New study designs have improved the acceptability and ease of performing clinical trials in this vulnerable population, and PK modeling and simulation techniques have enabled investigators to make antibiotic dosing recommendations based on neonatal physiology. However, many questions regarding dosing of antibiotics in infants remain. In addition to continued conduct of PK antibiotic trials in infants, investigators should seek to identify the most appropriate measure of organ growth and maturation during the neonatal period and the ideal marker of renal impairment. Future studies should also establish appropriate antibiotic dosing regimens to maximize bacterial killing and ensure adequate CNS penetration while minimizing toxicity, define guidelines for perioperative antibiotic management that are specific to preterm and term infants, and identify adequate dosing for critically ill infants on ECMO or receiving therapeutic hypothermia.

REFERENCES

1. Tzialla C, Borghesi A, Serra G, et al. Antimicrobial therapy in neonatal intensive care unit. *Ital J Pediatr*. 2015;41:27.
2. Cantey JB, Wozniak PS, Sanchez PJ. Prospective surveillance of antibiotic use in the neonatal intensive care unit: results from the SCOUT study. *Pediatr Infect Dis J*. 2015;34:267–272.
3. Allegaert K, Verbesselt R, Naulaers G, et al. Developmental pharmacology: neonates are not just small adults.... *Acta Clin Belg*. 2008;63:16–24.
4. O'Hara K, Wright IM, Schneider JJ, et al. Pharmacokinetics in neonatal prescribing: evidence base, paradigms and the future. *Br J Clin Pharmacol*. 2015;80:1281–1288.
5. Ku LC, Smith PB. Dosing in neonates: special considerations in physiology and trial design. *Pediatr Res*. 2015;77:2–9.
6. Anderson BJ, Holford NH. Understanding dosing: children are small adults, neonates are immature children. *Arch Dis Child*. 2013;98:737–744.
7. Tom-Revzon C. Erratic absorption of intramuscular antimicrobial delivery in infants and children. *Expert Opin Drug Metab Toxicol*. 2007;3:733–740.
8. Kearns GL, Abdel-Rahman SM, Alander SW, et al. Developmental pharmacology–drug disposition, action, and therapy in infants and children. *N Engl J Med*. 2003;349:1157–1167.

9. Seyberth HW, Kauffman RE. Basics and dynamics of neonatal and pediatric pharmacology. *Handb Exp Pharmacol*. 2011;205:3–49.
10. Blake MJ, Castro L, Leeder JS, et al. Ontogeny of drug metabolizing enzymes in the neonate. *Semin Fetal Neonatal Med*. 2005;10:123–138.
11. Hines RN. Developmental expression of drug metabolizing enzymes: impact on disposition in neonates and young children. *Int J Pharm*. 2013;452:3–7.
12. Laughon MM, Avant D, Tripathi N, et al. Drug labeling and exposure in neonates. *JAMA Pediatr*. 2014;168:130–136.
13. Zhao P, Zhang L, Grillo JA, et al. Applications of physiologically based pharmacokinetic (PBPK) modeling and simulation during regulatory review. *Clin Pharmacol Ther*. 2011;89:259–267.
14. Autmizguine J, Benjamin DK Jr, Smith PB, et al. Pharmacokinetic studies in infants using minimal-risk study designs. *Curr Clin Pharmacol*. 2014;9:350–358.
15. Alcorn J, McNamara PJ. Ontogeny of hepatic and renal systemic clearance pathways in infants: part I. *Clin Pharmacokinet*. 2002;41:959–998.
16. Yaffe SJ, Aranda JV. *Neonatal and Pediatric Pharmacology: Therapeutic Principles in Practice*. Philadelphia: Lippincott Williams & Wilkins; 2005.
17. Botwinski CA, Falco GA. Transition to postnatal renal function. *J Perinat Neonatal Nurs*. 2014;28: 150–154.
18. Rodieux F, Wilbaux M, van den Anker JN, et al. Effect of kidney function on drug kinetics and dosing in neonates, infants, and children. *Clin Pharmacokinet*. 2015;54:1183–1204.
19. Gattineni J, Baum M. Developmental changes in renal tubular transport-an overview. *Pediatr Nephrol*. 2015;30:2085–2098.
20. Rhodin MM, Anderson BJ, Peters AM, et al. Human renal function maturation: a quantitative description using weight and postmenstrual age. *Pediatr Nephrol*. 2009;24:67–76.
21. Holford N, Heo YA, Anderson B. A pharmacokinetic standard for babies and adults. *J Pharm Sci*. 2013;102:2941–2952.
22. Brady MT, Jackson MA, Kimberlin DW, et al, eds. *Red Book 2015: 2015 Report of the Committee on Infectious Diseases*. Elk Grove Village, Illinois: American Academy of Pediatrics; 2015.
23. Hines RN, McCarver DG. The ontogeny of human drug-metabolizing enzymes: phase i oxidative enzymes. *J Pharmacol Exp Ther*. 2002;300:355.
24. Cohen-Wolkowiez M, Watt KM, Zhou C, et al. Developmental pharmacokinetics of piperacillin and tazobactam using plasma and dried blood spots from infants. *Antimicrob Agents Chemother*. 2014;58:2856–2865.
25. Gonzalez D, Melloni C, Yogev R, et al. Use of opportunistic clinical data and a population pharmacokinetic model to support dosing of clindamycin for premature infants to adolescents. *Clin Pharmacol Ther*. 2014;96:429–437.
26a. Cohen-Wolkowiez M, Ouellet D, Smith PB. Population pharmacokinetics of metronidazole evaluated using scavenged samples from preterm infants. *Antimicrob Agents Chemother*. 2012;56: 1828–1837.
26b. Cohen-Wolkowiez M, Sampson M, Bloom BT, et al. Determining population and developmental pharmacokinetics of metronidazole using plasma and dried blood spot samples from premature infants. *Pediatr Infect Dis J*. 2013;32:956–961.
27. Aly H, Davies J, El-Dib M, et al. Renal function is impaired in small for gestational age premature infants. *J Matern Fetal Neonatal Med*. 2013;26:388–391.
28. De Cock RF, Allegaert K, Schreuder MF, et al. Maturation of the glomerular filtration rate in neonates, as reflected by amikacin clearance. *Clin Pharmacokinet*. 2012;51:105–117.
29. Banner W Jr, Gooch WM 3rd, Burckart G, et al. Pharmacokinetics of nafcillin in infants with low birth weights. *Antimicrob Agents Chemother*. 1980;17:691–694.
30. Ette EI, Williams PJ, eds. *Pharmacometrics: The Science of Quantitative Pharmacology*. Hoboken, N.J.: John Wiley & Sons; 2007.
31. Smith PB, Cohen-Wolkowiez M, Castro LM, et al. Population pharmacokinetics of meropenem in plasma and cerebrospinal fluid of infants with suspected or complicated intra-abdominal infections. *Pediatr Infect Dis J*. 2011;30:844–849.
32. Kearns GL, Jungbluth GL, Abdel-Rahman SM, et al. Impact of ontogeny on linezolid disposition in neonates and infants. *Clin Pharmacol Ther*. 2003;74:413–422.
33. van den Anker JN, Pokorna P, Kinzig-Schippers M, et al. Meropenem pharmacokinetics in the newborn. *Antimicrob Agents Chemother*. 2009;53:3871–3879.
34. Bradley JS, Peacock G, Krug SE, et al. Pediatric anthrax clinical management. *Pediatrics*. 2014;133: e1411–e1436.
35. Selewski DT, Charlton JR, Jetton JG, et al. Neonatal acute kidney injury. *Pediatrics*. 2015;136:e463.
36. Mehta RL, Kellum JA, Shah SV, et al. Acute Kidney Injury Network: report of an initiative to improve outcomes in acute kidney injury. *Crit Care*. 2007;11:R31–R.
37. National Guideline Clearinghouse. KDIGO 2012 clinical practice guideline for the evaluation and management of chronic kidney disease. In Rockville MD: Agency for Healthcare Research and Quality (AHRQ); 2013. Available from: https://www.guideline.gov/summaries/summary/46510/kdigo -2012-clinical-practice-guideline-for-the-evaluation-and-management-of-chronic-kidney-disease.
38. Wilbaux M, Fuchs A, Samardzic J, et al. Pharmacometric approaches to personalize use of primarily renally eliminated antibiotics in preterm and term neonates. *J Clin Pharmacol*. 2016;56: 909–935.
39. Capparelli EV, Lane JR, Romanowski GL, et al. The influences of renal function and maturation on vancomycin elimination in newborns and infants. *J Clin Pharmacol*. 2001;41:927–934.

40. Bateman DA, Thomas W, Parravicini E, et al. Serum creatinine concentration in very-low-birth-weight infants from birth to 34–36 wk postmenstrual age. *Pediatr Res.* 2015;77:696–702.
41. Peake M, Whiting M. Measurement of serum creatinine–current status and future goals. *Clin Biochem Rev.* 2006;27:173–184.
42. Argyri I, Xanthos T, Varsami M, et al. The role of novel biomarkers in early diagnosis and prognosis of acute kidney injury in newborns. *Am J Perinatol.* 2013;30:347–352.
43. Murray AW, Barnfield MC, Waller ML, et al. Assessment of glomerular filtration rate measurement with plasma sampling: a technical review. *J Nucl Med Technol.* 2013;41:67–75.
44. Schwartz GJ, Munoz A, Schneider MF, et al. New equations to estimate GFR in children with CKD. *J Am Soc Nephrol.* 2009;20:629–637.
45. Schwartz GJ, Work DF. Measurement and estimation of GFR in children and adolescents. *Clin J Am Soc Nephrol.* 2009;4:1832–1843.
46. Bhongsatiern J, Stockmann C, Roberts JK, et al. Evaluation of vancomycin use in late-onset neonatal sepsis using the area under the concentration-time curve to the minimum inhibitory concentration >/=400 target. *Ther Drug Monit.* 2015;37:756–765.
47. Finney H, Newman DJ, Thakkar H, et al. Reference ranges for plasma cystatin C and creatinine measurements in premature infants, neonates, and older children. *Arch Dis Child.* 2000;82:71–75.
48. Shin JE, Lee SM, Eun HS, et al. Usefulness of serum cystatin C to determine the dose of vancomycin in neonate. *Korean J Pediatr.* 2015;58:421–426.
49. Filler G, Guerrero-Kanan R, Alvarez-Elias AC. Assessment of glomerular filtration rate in the neonate: Is creatinine the best tool? *Curr Opin Pediatr.* 2016;28:173–179.
50. Krawczeski CD, Woo JG, Wang Y, et al. Neutrophil gelatinase-associated lipocalin concentrations predict development of acute kidney injury in neonates and children after cardiopulmonary bypass. *J Pediatr.* 2011;158(6):1009–1015.e1. doi:10.1016/j.jpeds.2010.12.057.
51. Kasiakou SK, Sermaides GJ, Michalopoulos A, et al. Continuous versus intermittent intravenous administration of antibiotics: a meta-analysis of randomised controlled trials. *Lancet Infect Dis.* 2005;5:581–589.
52. de Hoog M, Mouton JW, van den Anker JN. New dosing strategies for antibacterial agents in the neonate. *Semin Fetal Neonatal Med.* 2005;10:185–194.
53. Lee H. Prolonged or continuous infusion of IV antibiotics as initial treatment strategy. *Infect Chemother.* 2016;48:140–142.
54. van Boekholt A, Fleuren H, Mouton J, et al. Serum concentrations of amoxicillin in neonates during continuous intravenous infusion. *Eur J Clin Microbiol Infect Dis.* 2016;35:1007–1012.
55. Bertels RA, Semmekrot BA, Gerrits GP, et al. Serum concentrations of cefotaxime and its metabolite desacetyl-cefotaxime in infants and children during continuous infusion. *Infection.* 2008;36:415–420.
56. Salehifar E, Rafati MR. Extended-interval dosing of aminoglycosides in pediatrics: a narrative review. *J Pediatr Rev.* 2015;3:e2652.
57. Walker MC, Lam WM, Manasco KB. Continuous and extended infusions of beta-lactam antibiotics in the pediatric population. *Ann Pharmacother.* 2012;46:1537–1546.
58. Zhao W, Lopez E, Biran V, et al. Vancomycin continuous infusion in neonates: dosing optimisation and therapeutic drug monitoring. *Arch Dis Child.* 2013;98:449–453.
59. Lee JH. Catheter-related bloodstream infections in neonatal intensive care units. *Korean J Pediatr.* 2011;54:363–367.
60. Padari H, Metsvaht T, Korgvee LT, et al. Short versus long infusion of meropenem in very-low-birth-weight neonates. *Antimicrob Agents Chemother.* 2012;56:4760–4764.
61. Bailey TC, Little JR, Littenberg B, et al. A meta-analysis of extended-interval dosing versus multiple daily dosing of aminoglycosides. *Clin Infect Dis.* 1997;24:786–795.
62. Contopoulos-Ioannidis DG, Giotis ND, Baliatsa DV, et al. Extended-interval aminoglycoside administration for children: a meta-analysis. *Pediatrics.* 2004;114:e111–e118.
63. Mohamed AF, Nielsen EI, Cars O, et al. Pharmacokinetic-pharmacodynamic model for gentamicin and its adaptive resistance with predictions of dosing schedules in newborn infants. *Antimicrob Agents Chemother.* 2012;56:179–188.
64. Freeman CD, Nicolau DP, Belliveau PP, et al. Once-daily dosing of aminoglycosides: review and recommendations for clinical practice. *J Antimicrob Chemother.* 1997;39:677–686.
65. Fuchs A, Guidi M, Giannoni E, et al. Population pharmacokinetic study of gentamicin in a large cohort of premature and term neonates. *Br J Clin Pharmacol.* 2014;78:1090–1101.
66. Bradley JS, Nelson JD, Cantey JB, et al. *2016 Nelson's Pediatric Antimicrobial Therapy.* Elk Grove Village, Illinois: American Academy of Pediatrics; 2016.
67. Ku LC, Boggess KA, Cohen-Wolkowiez M. Bacterial meningitis in infants. *Clin Perinatol.* 2015;42:29–45, vii–viii.
68. Tunkel AR, Hartman BJ, Kaplan SL, et al. Practice guidelines for the management of bacterial meningitis. *Clin Infect Dis.* 2004;39:1267–1284.
69. Phares CR, Lynfield R, Farley MM, et al. Epidemiology of invasive group B streptococcal disease in the United States, 1999-2005. *JAMA.* 2008;299:2056–2065.
70. Levison ME, Levison JH. Pharmacokinetics and pharmacodynamics of antibacterial agents. *Infect Dis Clin North Am.* 2009;23:791–815.
71. Nau R, Sorgel F, Prange HW. Pharmacokinetic optimisation of the treatment of bacterial central nervous system infections. *Clin Pharmacokinet.* 1998;35:223–246.
72. Nau R, Sörgel F, Eiffert H. Penetration of drugs through the blood-cerebrospinal fluid/blood-brain barrier for treatment of central nervous system infections. *Clin Microbiol Rev.* 2010;23:858–883.

73. Kaplan JM, McCracken GH Jr, Horton LJ, et al. Pharmacologic studies in neonates given large dosages of ampicillin. *J Pediatr*. 1974;84:571–577.

74. Shaffer CL, Davey AM, Ransom JL, et al. Ampicillin-induced neurotoxicity in very-low-birth-weight neonates. *Ann Pharmacother*. 1998;32:482–484.

75. Hornik CP, Benjamin DK Jr, Smith PB, et al. Electronic health records and pharmacokinetic modeling to assess the relationship between ampicillin exposure and seizure risk in neonates. *J Pediatr*. 2016; 178:125–129.

76. Murray MT, Corda R, Turcotte R, et al. Implementing a standardized perioperative antibiotic prophylaxis protocol for neonates undergoing cardiac surgery. *Ann Thorac Surg*. 2014;98:927–933.

77. Bratzler DW, Dellinger EP, Olsen KM, et al. Clinical practice guidelines for antimicrobial prophylaxis in surgery. *Am J Health Syst Pharm*. 2013;70:195–283.

78. Stevens DL, Bisno AL, Chambers HF, et al. Practice guidelines for the diagnosis and management of skin and soft tissue infections: 2014 update by the Infectious Diseases Society of America. *Clin Infect Dis*. 2014;59:e10–e52.

79. De Cock RF, Smits A, Allegaert K, et al. Population pharmacokinetic modelling of total and unbound cefazolin plasma concentrations as a guide for dosing in preterm and term neonates. *J Antimicrob Chemother*. 2014;69:1330–1338.

80. Wildschut ED, Ahsman MJ, Allegaert K, et al. Determinants of drug absorption in different ECMO circuits. *Intensive Care Med*. 2010;36:2109–2116.

81. Dagan O, Klein J, Gruenwald C, et al. Preliminary studies of the effects of extracorporeal membrane oxygenator on the disposition of common pediatric drugs. *Ther Drug Monit*. 1993;15:263–266.

82. Bhatt-Meht V, Annich G. Sedative clearance during extracorporeal membrane oxygenation. *Perfusion*. 2005;20:309–315.

83. Zwiers AJ, de Wildt SN, Hop WC, et al. Acute kidney injury is a frequent complication in critically ill neonates receiving extracorporeal membrane oxygenation: a 14-year cohort study. *Crit Care*. 2013;17:R151.

84. Mori A, Watanabe K, Onoe M, et al. Regional blood flow in the liver, pancreas and kidney during pulsatile and nonpulsatile perfusion under profound hypothermia. *Jpn Circ J*. 1988;52:219–227.

85. Mulla H, Lawson G, von Anrep C, et al. *In vitro* evaluation of sedative drug losses during extracorporeal membrane oxygenation. *Perfusion*. 2000;15:21–26.

86. Ahsman MJ, Hanekamp M, Wildschut ED, et al. Population pharmacokinetics of midazolam and its metabolites during venoarterial extracorporeal membrane oxygenation in neonates. *Clin Pharmacokinet*. 2010;49:407–419.

87. Sherwin J, Heath T, Watt K. Pharmacokinetics and dosing of anti-infective drugs in patients on extracorporeal membrane oxygenation: a review of the current literature. *Clin Ther*. 2016;38:1976–1994.

88. de Haan TR, Bijleveld YA, van der Lee JH, et al. Pharmacokinetics and pharmacodynamics of medication in asphyxiated newborns during controlled hypothermia. The PharmaCool multicenter study. *BMC Pediatr*. 2012;12:45.

89. Gupta C, Massaro AN, Ray PE. A new approach to define acute kidney injury in term newborns with hypoxic ischemic encephalopathy. *Pediatr Nephrol*. 2016;31:1167–1178.

90. Choudhary M, Sharma D, Dabi D, et al. Hepatic dysfunction in asphyxiated neonates: prospective case-controlled study. *Clin Med Insights Pediatr*. 2015;9:1–6.

91. van den Broek MP, Groenendaal F, Egberts AC, et al. Effects of hypothermia on pharmacokinetics and pharmacodynamics: a systematic review of preclinical and clinical studies. *Clin Pharmacokinet*. 2010;49:277–294.

92. Tortorici MA, Kochanek PM, Poloyac SM. Effects of hypothermia on drug disposition, metabolism, and response: a focus of hypothermia-mediated alterations on the cytochrome P450 enzyme system. *Crit Care Med*. 2007;35:2196–2204.

93. Guignard JP, Gillieron P. Effect of modest hypothermia on the immature kidney. *Acta Paediatr*. 1997;86:1040–1041.

94. Frymoyer A, Meng L, Bonifacio SL, et al. Gentamicin pharmacokinetics and dosing in neonates with hypoxic ischemic encephalopathy receiving hypothermia. *Pharmacotherapy*. 2013;33:718–726.

95. Bradley JS, Kimberlin DW, Nelson JD. *2014 Nelson's Pediatric Antimicrobial Therapy*. Elk Grove Village, Illinois: American Academy of Pediatrics; 2014.

96. Tremoulet A, Le J, Poindexter B, et al. Characterization of the population pharmacokinetics of ampicillin in neonates using an opportunistic study design. *Antimicrob Agents Chemother*. 2014;58:3013–3020.

97. Capparelli E, Hochwald C, Rasmussen M, et al. Population pharmacokinetics of cefepime in the neonate. *Antimicrob Agents Chemother*. 2005;49:2760–2766.

98. Ahsman MJ, Wildschut ED, Tibboel D, et al. Pharmacokinetics of cefotaxime and desacetylcefotaxime in infants during extracorporeal membrane oxygenation. *Antimicrob Agents Chemother*. 2010;54: 1734–1741.

99. Li Z, Chen Y, Li Q, et al. Population pharmacokinetics of piperacillin/tazobactam in neonates and young infants. *Eur J Clin Pharmacol*. 2013;69:1223–1233.

100. Metsvaht T, Oselin K, Ilmoja M, et al. Pharmacokinetics of penicillin G in very-low-birth-weight neonates. *Antimicrob Agents Chemother*. 2007;51(6):1995–2000.

101. McCracken GH Jr, Ginsberg C, Chrane DF, et al. Clinical pharmacology of penicillin in newborn infants. *J Pediatr*. 1973;82(4):692–698.

CHAPTER 15

Antifungal Dosing Considerations for Term and Preterm Infants

Jodi Lestner, MBChB, MRes, MRCPCH, William Hope, BMBS, FRACP, FRCPA, PhD

- Invasive fungal disease (IFD) is associated with poor outcomes in high-risk infants. Prompt diagnosis and treatment is required.

- Infection due to non-*albicans* Candida spp. are common in the NICU and should be considered when selecting empiric antifungal regimens.

- The pharmacodynamics of IFD in infants are characterized by early and widespread seeding into deep tissue subcompartments. Drug penetration into tissue subcompartments is an important determinant of therapeutic success.

- Older antifungal drugs (fluconazole and amphotericin B deoxycholate) continue to be favored firstline agents in infants. Despite many decades of use, the evidence to support currently recommended doses of these drugs is limited.

- Recent data suggest higher therapeutic doses of fluconazole, including the use of a loading dose, may be required to treat IFD in infants. Safety data to support intensified dosing is required.

- Data to define safe and effective doses of newer antifungal drugs (second generation triazoles and echinocandins) in infants are needed.

Introduction

Invasive fungal disease (IFD) is a common and serious diagnosis in the neonatal intensive care unit (NICU). The incidence of IFD is highest in premature infants and in infants with risk factors that include the presence of indwelling vascular catheters, abdominal surgery, necrotizing enterocolitis, and exposure to broad-spectrum antibiotics. Mortality associated with IFD in premature infants is substantial (>30%), and neurodevelopmental sequelae among survivors are common; thus there is a clear clinical need for prompt diagnosis and aggressive treatment.[1,2]

The pharmacodynamics of IFD in the infant differ from older children and adults. Infection in this population often manifests with subtle, nonspecific features despite widespread organ involvement. The urinary tract and central nervous system (CNS) are the most clinically important sites of hematogenous seeding. Drug penetration into these tissue subcompartments is an important determinant of therapeutic success. Diffuse CNS involvement, in the form of hematogenous *Candida* meningoencephalitis (HCME), is a syndrome that appears to uniquely affect the premature infant and is associated with poor clinical outcomes.[3] Clinical data to specifically support dosing regimens in the setting of HCME are needed.

The majority of systemic antifungal drugs have not been licensed for use in infants (Table 15.1), and knowledge of the pharmacokinetics–pharmacodynamics (PK–PD) of these drugs has historically been extremely limited. This lack of evidence has resulted in clinical uncertainty and wide variation in prescribing practice.[4] More

Table 15.1 RECOMMENDED THERAPEUTIC REGIMENS FOR ANTIFUNGAL AGENTS
CURRENTLY AVAILABLE FOR USE IN INFANTS

Drug	Formulation	Infant Regimen	Infant Licensing
Amphotericin B	Deoxycholate IV injection	1 mg/kg every 24 h	Unlicensed in infants
Amphotericin B	Liposomal IV injection	3–5 mg/kg every 24 h	Unlicensed in infants
Amphotericin B	Lipid complex IV injection	3–5 mg/kg every 24 h	Unlicensed in infants
Fluconazole	Capsule, oral suspension, and IV injection	0–2 wk: 6–12 mg/kg every 72 h 2–4 wk: 6–12 mg/kg every 48 h 4 wk and over: 6–12 mg/kg every 24 h Consider a loading dose 25 mg/kg	Treatment of mucosal candidiasis (oropharyngeal, esophageal), invasive candidiasis, and the prophylaxis of candidal infections
Itraconazole	Capsule, oral cyclodextrin suspension, and IV cyclodextrin injection	5 mg/kg every 12 h	Unlicensed in infants
Voriconazole	Capsule, oral suspension, and IV cyclodextrin injection	Limited data 3.5–14.5 mg/kg every 24 h. Therapeutic drug monitoring recommended.	Unlicensed in infants
Posaconazole	Oral suspension	Limited data 6 mg/kg every 8 h	Unlicensed in infants
Caspofungin	IV injection	0–3 mo: 25 mg/m^2 every 24 h 3 mo and over: 50 mg/m^2 every 24 h	Unlicensed in infants
Micafungin	IV injection	4–10 mg/kg every 24 h 10 mg/kg every 24 h required for CNS infection	Treatment and prophylaxis of invasive candidiasis if other antifungals are not appropriate
Anidulafungin	IV injection	1.5 mg/kg every 24 h	Unlicensed in infants

CNS, central nervous system; IV, intravenous.

rational treatment strategies are beginning to evolve as new antifungal agents are developed and data amassed to support evidence-based regimens for the prevention and treatment of neonatal IFD.

Case Study

A male infant weighing 720 g was born at 24 weeks gestation following spontaneous preterm labor. The pregnancy was complicated by premature rupture of membranes 3 days before delivery. The mother received a course of antenatal steroids and two doses of systemic antibiotic therapy before delivery. At delivery, the infant was floppy with poor respiratory effort and required intubation and admission to the NICU. Antimicrobial therapy with ampicillin and gentamicin was initiated after an initial blood culture specimen was obtained. Umbilical venous and arterial lines were placed and satisfactory positioning confirmed radiologically. Antifungal prophylaxis with oral fluconazole 6 mg/kg every 72 hours was administered according to local guidelines. Initial blood cultures were negative at 48 hours, and antibiotic therapy was stopped.

The infant was extubated and commenced on continuous positive airway pressure on the tenth day of life and achieved full enteral feedings on the twentieth day. On the 25th day of life, however, the infant appeared lethargic, developed hyperglycemia, and exhibited increased episodes of apnea that resulted in reintubation and mechanical ventilation. A repeat blood culture specimen was obtained, and antimicrobial therapy with nafcillin and gentamicin was initiated. Blood culture yielded *Candida parapsilosis* after 36 hours. Amphotericin B deoxycholate 1 mg/kg/day was commenced. The infant continued to deteriorate and on day 32 of life required maximal ventilatory and inotropic support. A cranial ultrasound on day 33 demonstrated multiple small echogenic foci measuring 1 to 2 mm scattered throughout both cerebral hemispheres, consistent with diffuse HCME. An abdominal ultrasound demonstrated an echogenic mass measuring 1 cm in diameter in the left renal pelvis consistent with a fungal ball. Over the next 5 days the infant's clinical condition continued to deteriorate. On day 35 urine output dropped to <0.5 mL/kg/hr and there was biochemical evidence of worsening renal impairment. Amphotericin B deoxycholate was reduced to 0.5 mg/kg/day and micafungin 4 mg/kg/day added. The infant's condition continued to deteriorate, and the infant died on day 40 of life.

This clinical case highlights that despite the reduction in overall incidence, IFD remains a grave diagnosis in the NICU. An established diagnosis of proven IFD is frequently delayed or absent. The high incidence of non-*albicans* species in clinical isolates confounds decisions about drug selection. Older drugs are generally used as firstline agents, and there remains clinical uncertainty about dosing in most cases. Here we review the current evidence for available systematic antifungal drugs for use in neonatal IFD. We highlight areas of clinical uncertainty where questions and controversies remain.

Triazoles

Fluconazole is a firstline agent in the treatment and prevention of IFD in infants.[5,6] The use of fluconazole prophylaxis 3 to 6 mg/kg every 72 hours in infants at risk of IFD is supported by several comparative and observational studies demonstrating significant reduction in *Candida* colonization and a reduced incidence of invasive candidiasis in infants <1000 g birth weight.[7–12] Fluconazole has a relatively narrow spectrum of antifungal activity. This is of particular importance in the NICU where a significant proportion of clinical isolates are non–*C. albicans* spp. that exhibit reduced susceptibility to triazoles.[13–15] It is unclear whether the widespread use of fluconazole prophylaxis is a contributory factor in an apparent rise in triazole resistance. To date, surveillance data suggest no increase in the emergence of less susceptible or inherently resistant *Candida* species in the NICU.[16,17]

Therapeutic regimens of fluconazole in infants were initially based on limited pharmacokinetic (PK) data at the time of licensing. A regimen of 6 mg/kg given every 72 hours from 0 to 2 weeks, every 48 hours from 2 to 4 weeks, and daily thereafter was proposed and is still included in a number of published dosing references.[18,19] This recommendation was largely based on a small phase II study of 12 premature infants that described a prolonged half-life in the first 2 weeks of life. Population PK studies have subsequently demonstrated that higher doses (12 mg/kg/day) are required from birth to attain exposures comparable to adults.[20–22] Moreover, recent evidence suggests that a loading dose of 25 mg/kg results in more rapid attainment of therapeutic targets associated with clinical efficacy in adults.[23] Although significantly increased rates of toxicity are improbable, larger safety studies are needed to further define the tolerability of higher dosing regimens in infants.

The second-generation triazoles (voriconazole and posaconazole) have an extended spectrum of antifungal activity against molds and other filamentous fungi. These drugs have been widely used for the treatment and prevention of IFD in older children and adults. Neither voriconazole nor posaconazole is currently licensed for infants, and their administration in the NICU has, to date, been limited to a small number of cases of compassionate use.[24–26] The use of these agents in clinical practice is likely to increase in the coming decades, and clinical PK studies are required to clarify appropriate neonatal dosing regimens. Further, therapeutic drug monitoring (TDM) of voriconazole and posaconazole is recommended, and therapeutic targets require prospective validation in this setting.[27]

Polyenes (Conventional and Lipid-Preparation Amphotericin B)

Amphotericin B (AmB) is available as AmB deoxycholate (DAmB) and in various lipid preparations (liposomal AmB; AmB lipid complex, AmB-LC; AmB colloidal dispersion, AmB-CD). DAmB 1 mg/kg/day is recommended as a firstline treatment for IFD in infants. In adults and older children, AmB lipid preparations 3 to 5 mg/kg/day are favored as a firstline therapy in IFD. This is primarily due to their improved toxicity profile, and in particular the significantly lower incidence of nephrotoxicity. In contrast to adults and older children, DAmB generally is better tolerated with a low incidence of nephrotoxicity. All formulations of AmB achieve low concentrations in urine at recommended doses, and their use is cautioned in infants in whom urinary tract involvement is common. Despite decades of off-label clinical use in infants, the evidence base to support these recommendations is surprisingly limited.[28–32] The small number of comparative and observational studies available report therapeutic failure (death, persistent positive microbiologic cultures, or need for additional antifungal therapy) in over one third of infants receiving AmB.[29,30] Furthermore, 20% to 50% of infants receiving DAmB develop clinically significant toxicity necessitating dose reduction or a change in therapy.[31,32] Recently, a large US-based retrospective cohort study of infants treated for proven IFD (n = 730) identified therapeutic failure rates of 38%, 47%, and 40% in infants receiving DAmB, AmB lipid preparations, and fluconazole, respectively. Overall mortality appeared significantly higher in infants receiving AmB lipid preparations compared with DAmB or fluconazole.[28] Clinical data describing the dosing regimens administered were not reported in this study, and subtherapeutic exposures may account for the reduced efficacy of AmB lipid preparations.

PK data in infants are also limited for AmB. Daily doses of DAmB 1 mg/kg/day achieve mean drug exposures that are comparable to those observed in older children and adults; however, interindividual variability in exposure is significant, particularly at extreme prematurity.[33–35] TDM has been proposed, but is not routinely used. The PK of AmB lipid preparations are incompletely understood. There are no clinical PK studies of liposomal AmB in infants and only a single study of AmB-LC in 28 infants, which suggested a prolonged terminal half-life with doses of 2.5 to 5 mg/kg/day.[36]

Importantly, no clinical data are available to specifically inform dosing regimens for AmB in the setting of IFD with CNS involvement. Preclinical models suggest that all forms of AmB penetrate poorly into cerebrospinal fluid (CSF) but achieve appreciable exposures within the parenchyma of the brain.[37] Among the available preparations liposomal AmB appears to exhibit the highest penetration into the brain based on quantification from tissue homogenates. Data to further define the kinetics of AmB within brain tissue would be informative.

Echinocandins

The echinocandins (caspofungin, micafungin, and anidulafungin) are large semisynthetic lipopeptides with fungicidal activity against *Candida* spp. Echinocandins are increasingly used as firstline agents for the treatment of disseminated candidiasis in older children and adults.[38] The role of echinocandins in infants is less clear, although available evidence suggests they are safe and effective.[39] There are several considerations regarding the use of echinocandins in the NICU. First is the intrinsically reduced in vitro susceptibility of *C. parapsilosis* to the echinocandin class. In view of this finding, the echinocandins are generally not recommended as firstline agents in proven *C. parapsilosis* infection. Clinical trials in adults, however, suggest that outcomes in patients receiving an echinocandin as treatment of invasive candidiasis due to *C. parapsilosis* are comparable (numerically fewer, but not statistically inferior) to standard therapy.[40] Furthermore, successful treatment of *C. parapsilosis* infection with caspofungin has been reported in infants.[41] *C. parapsilosis* is, however, a common isolate in the NICU (>40% of proven IFD in many centers).[14,15] As such, it may be prudent to consider alternative antifungal agents in clinically unstable patients who require empirical therapy and for cases of proven *C. parapsilosis* infection.

Second, the echinocandins are generally thought to be ineffective for the treatment of CNS infection. This supposition is largely based on the poor penetration of echinocandins into CSF.[42–44] Preclinical data, however, suggest that the echinocandins exhibit tissue kinetics similar to AmB and penetrate brain parenchyma in a dose-dependent manner, achieving substantial antifungal activity in preclinical models of HCME.[45] Available clinical data also suggest that the echinocandins may be effective agents for the treatment of HCME.[46]

There are limited PK data to support dosing of the echinocandins in infants. Caspofungin 25 mg/m^2 daily results in exposures (defined in terms of peak and trough concentrations) comparable to those observed in adults receiving 50 mg daily.[47] Micafungin 4 mg/kg/day is licensed for the treatment of invasive candidiasis in infants. Premature infants, however, appear to exhibit a shorter half-life and more rapid rate of drug clearance compared with older children and adults and may require more frequent dosing.[48] Recent experimental and clinical pharmacokinetic data suggest that higher doses (10 mg/kg/day) are required to treat HCME.[44,49,50] Comparative trials to assess the safety and efficacy of high-dose micafungin regimens are currently underway. The echinocandins do not achieve therapeutic concentrations in urine and may not be effective agents for the treatment of candiduria.[51] Finally, there has been some debate regarding the potential of micafungin to induce hepatic tumors based on data from rats exposed to prolonged high-dose therapy.[52] To date, there are no clinical data to suggest an elevated risk hepatotoxicity of tumorigenesis in humans, despite extensive clinical usage in adults. Similar preclinical experiments with the other available echinocandins have not been performed.

The evidence supporting the use of anidulafungin in infants is limited. Anidulafungin 1.5 mg/kg/day appears to result in exposures in infants comparable with older children receiving the same weight-adjusted dosage and adults receiving 100 mg daily.[53–55] A PK–PD bridging study suggests that higher doses are required to treat HCME (e.g., 9 mg/kg loading dose followed by 4.5 mg/kg/day).[56] The safety of this higher dosage has not yet been determined.

Conclusion

The incidence of IFD in the neonatal population has reduced in recent years. Nevertheless, clinical outcomes in infants with proven and probable IFD remain poor. Clinical guidelines recommend well-established antifungal drugs (fluconazole and AmB) as firstline therapy in neonatal IFD. Although clinical experience with these agents is extensive, the underlying evidence to support dosing recommendations has historically been limited. Recent evidence has suggested that enhanced dosing of fluconazole is required to achieve exposures comparable to those in older children and adults. Studies to define optimized dosing regimens of AmB, particularly for lipid preparations, are needed. The role for newer antifungal agents (echinocandins and second-generation triazoles) in the NICU remains somewhat unclear. Preclinical and clinical PK are required to clarify dosing regimens and therapeutic targets for these agents to facilitate their use.

REFERENCES

1. Benjamin DK Jr, Stoll BJ, Fanaroff AA, et al. Neonatal candidiasis among extremely low birth weight infants: risk factors, mortality rates, and neurodevelopmental outcomes at 18 to 22 months. *Pediatrics.* 2006;117:84–92.
2. Stoll BJ, Hansen NI, Adams-Chapman I, et al. Neurodevelopmental and growth impairment among extremely low-birth-weight infants with neonatal infection. *JAMA.* 2004;292:2357–2365.
3. Cohen-Wolkowiez M, Smith PB, Mangum B, et al. Neonatal *Candida* meningitis: significance of cerebrospinal fluid parameters and blood cultures. *J Perinatol.* 2007;27:97–100.
4. Lestner JM, Versporten A, Doerholt K, et al. Systemic antifungal prescribing in neonates and children: outcomes from the Antibiotic Resistance and Prescribing in European Children (ARPEC) Study. *Antimicrob Agents Chemother.* 2015;59:782–789.
5. Hope WW, Castagnola E, Groll AH, et al. ESCMID* guideline for the diagnosis and management of *Candida* diseases 2012: prevention and management of invasive infections in neonates and children caused by *Candida* spp. *Clin Microbiol Infect.* 2012;18(7):38–52.
6. Pappas PG, Kauffman CA, Andes DR, et al. Clinical Practice Guideline for the Management of Candidiasis: 2016 Update by the Infectious Diseases Society of America. *Clin Infect Dis.* 2016;62: e1–e50.
7. Aydemir C, Oguz SS, Dizdar EA, et al. Randomised controlled trial of prophylactic fluconazole versus nystatin for the prevention of fungal colonisation and invasive fungal infection in very low birth weight infants. *Arch Dis Child Fetal Neonatal Ed.* 2011;96:F164–F168.

8. Clerihew L, Austin N, McGuire W. Systemic antifungal prophylaxis for very low birthweight infants: a systematic review. *Arch Dis Child Fetal Neonatal Ed.* 2008;93:F198–F200.

9. Kaufman D, Boyle R, Hazen KC, et al. Fluconazole prophylaxis against fungal colonization and infection in preterm infants. *N Engl J Med.* 2001;345:1660–1666.

10. Kaufman D, Boyle R, Hazen KC, et al. Twice weekly fluconazole prophylaxis for prevention of invasive *Candida* infection in high-risk infants of <1000 grams birth weight. *J Pediatr.* 2005;147:172–179.

11. Kicklighter SD, Springer SC, Cox T, et al. Fluconazole for prophylaxis against candidal rectal colonization in the very low birth weight infant. *Pediatrics.* 2001;107:293–298.

12. Manzoni P, Stolfi I, Pugni L, et al. A multicenter, randomized trial of prophylactic fluconazole in preterm neonates. *N Engl J Med.* 2007;356:2483–2495.

13. Goel N, Ranjan PK, Aggarwal R, et al. Emergence of nonalbicans Candida in neonatal septicemia and antifungal susceptibility: experience from a tertiary care center. *J Lab Physicians.* 2009;1:53–55.

14. Sarvikivi E, Lyytikainen O, Soll DR, et al. Emergence of fluconazole resistance in a *Candida parapsilosis* strain that caused infections in a neonatal intensive care unit. *J Clin Microbiol.* 2005;43:2729–2735.

15. Juyal D, Sharma M, Pal S, et al. Emergence of non-*albicans* Candida species in neonatal candidemia. *N Am J Med Sci.* 2013;5:541–545.

16. Healy CM, Campbell JR, Zaccaria E, et al. Fluconazole prophylaxis in extremely low birth weight neonates reduces invasive candidiasis mortality rates without emergence of fluconazole-resistant *Candida* species. *Pediatrics.* 2008;121:703–710.

17. Manzoni P, Leonessa M, Galletto P, et al. Routine use of fluconazole prophylaxis in a neonatal intensive care unit does not select natively fluconazole-resistant *Candida* subspecies. *Pediatr Infect Dis J.* 2008;27:731–737.

18. World Health Organization. World Health Organization Model Formulary for Children. Geneva, 2010.

19. Paediatric Formulary Committee. *British National Formulary for Children 2016-2017.* London: Pharmaceutical Press; 2016.

20. Wade KC, Benjamin DK Jr, Kaufman DA, et al. Fluconazole dosing for the prevention or treatment of invasive candidiasis in young infants. *Pediatr Infect Dis J.* 2009;28:717–723.

21. Wade KC, Wu D, Kaufman DA, et al. Population pharmacokinetics of fluconazole in young infants. *Antimicrob Agents Chemother.* 2008;52:4043–4049.

22. Schwarze R, Penk A, Pittrow L. Treatment of candidal infections with fluconazole in neonates and infants. *Eur J Med Res.* 2000;5:203–208.

23. Piper L, Smith PB, Hornik CP, et al. Fluconazole loading dose pharmacokinetics and safety in infants. *Pediatr Infect Dis J.* 2011;30:375–378.

24. Subudhi CPK CP, Settle P, Moise J, et al. Primary cutaneous aspergillosis in a preterm neonate: potential therapeutic role of posaconazole. In *Interscience Conference on Antimicrobial Agents and Chemotherapy (ICAAC),* 2008.

25. Celik IH, Demirel G, Oguz SS, et al. Compassionate use of voriconazole in newborn infants diagnosed with severe invasive fungal sepsis. *Eur Rev Med Pharmacol Sci.* 2013;17:729–734.

26. Kohli V, Taneja V, Sachdev P, et al. Voriconazole in newborns. *Indian Pediatr.* 2008;45:236–238.

27. Groll AH, Castagnola E, Cesaro S, et al. Fourth European Conference on Infections in Leukaemia (ECIL-4): guidelines for diagnosis, prevention, and treatment of invasive fungal diseases in paediatric patients with cancer or allogeneic haemopoietic stem-cell transplantation. *Lancet Oncol.* 2014;15:e327–e340.

28. Ascher SB, Smith PB, Watt K, et al. Antifungal therapy and outcomes in infants with invasive *Candida* infections. *Pediatr Infect Dis J.* 2012;31:439–443.

29. Driessen M, Ellis JB, Cooper PA, et al. Fluconazole vs. amphotericin B for the treatment of neonatal fungal septicemia: a prospective randomized trial. *Pediatr Infect Dis J.* 1996;15:1107–1112.

30. Linder N, Klinger G, Shalit I, et al. Treatment of candidaemia in premature infants: comparison of three amphotericin B preparations. *J Antimicrob Chemother.* 2003;52:663–667.

31. Jeon GW, Koo SH, Lee JH, et al. A comparison of AmBisome to amphotericin B for treatment of systemic candidiasis in very low birth weight infants. *Yonsei Med J.* 2007;48:619–626.

32. Lopez Sastre JB, Coto Cotallo GD, Fernandez Colomer B, et al. Neonatal invasive candidiasis: a prospective multicenter study of 118 cases. *Am J Perinatol.* 2003;20:153–163.

33. Hall JE, Cox F, Karlson K, et al. Amphotericin B dosage for disseminated candidiasis in premature infants. *J Perinatol.* 1987;7:194–198.

34. Koren G, Lau A, Klein J, et al. Pharmacokinetics and adverse effects of amphotericin B in infants and children. *J Pediatr.* 1988;113:559–563.

35. Starke JR, Mason EO Jr, Kramer WG, et al. Pharmacokinetics of amphotericin B in infants and children. *J Infect Dis.* 1987;155:766–774.

36. Wurthwein G, Groll AH, Hempel G, et al. Population pharmacokinetics of amphotericin B lipid complex in neonates. *Antimicrob Agents Chemother.* 2005;49:5092–5098.

37. Groll AH, Giri N, Petraitis V, et al. Comparative efficacy and distribution of lipid formulations of amphotericin B in experimental *Candida albicans* infection of the central nervous system. *J Infect Dis.* 2000;182:274–282.

38. Pappas PG, Kauffman CA, Andes D, et al. Clinical practice guidelines for the management of candidiasis: 2009 update by the Infectious Diseases Society of America. *Clin Infect Dis.* 2009;48:503–535.

39. Manzoni P, Rizzollo S, Franco C, et al. Role of echinocandins in the management of fungal infections in neonates. *J Matern Fetal Neonatal Med.* 2010;23(suppl 3):49–52.

40. Reboli AC, Rotstein C, Pappas PG, et al. Anidulafungin versus fluconazole for invasive candidiasis. *N Engl J Med.* 2007;356:2472–2482.

41. Yalaz M, Akisu M, Hilmioglu S, et al. Successful caspofungin treatment of multidrug resistant *Candida parapsilosis* septicaemia in an extremely low birth weight neonate. *Mycoses*. 2006;49:242–245.
42. Yamada N, Kumada K, Kishino S, et al. Distribution of micafungin in the tissue fluids of patients with invasive fungal infections. *J Infect Chemother*. 2011;17:731–734.
43. Stone JA, Xu X, Winchell GA, et al. Disposition of caspofungin: role of distribution in determining pharmacokinetics in plasma. *Antimicrob Agents Chemother*. 2004;48:815–823.
44. Hope WW, Mickiene D, Petraitis V, et al. The pharmacokinetics and pharmacodynamics of micafungin in experimental hematogenous *Candida* meningoencephalitis: implications for echinocandin therapy in neonates. *J Infect Dis*. 2008;197:163–171.
45. Groll AH, Mickiene D, Petraitiene R, et al. Pharmacokinetic and pharmacodynamic modeling of anidulafungin (LY303366): reappraisal of its efficacy in neutropenic animal models of opportunistic mycoses using optimal plasma sampling. *Antimicrob Agents Chemother*. 2001;45:2845–2855.
46. Odio CM, Araya R, Pinto LE, et al. Caspofungin therapy of neonates with invasive candidiasis. *Pediatr Infect Dis J*. 2004;23:1093–1097.
47. Saez-Llorens X, Macias M, Maiya P, et al. Pharmacokinetics and safety of caspofungin in neonates and infants less than 3 months of age. *Antimicrob Agents Chemother*. 2009;53:869–875.
48. Heresi GP, Gerstmann DR, Reed MD, et al. The pharmacokinetics and safety of micafungin, a novel echinocandin, in premature infants. *Pediatr Infect Dis J*. 2006;25:1110–1115.
49. Hope WW, Smith PB, Arrieta A, et al. Population pharmacokinetics of micafungin in neonates and young infants. *Antimicrob Agents Chemother*. 2010;54:2633–2637.
50. Auriti C, Falcone M, Ronchetti MP, et al. High-dose micafungin for preterm neonates and infants with invasive and central nervous system Candidiasis. *Antimicrob Agents Chemother*. 2016;60:7333–7339.
51. Wynn JL, Tan S, Gantz MG, et al. Outcomes following candiduria in extremely low birth weight infants. *Clin Infect Dis*. 2012;54:331–339.
52. European Medicines Agency: Mycamine—Summary of Product Characteristics. 2012.
53. Cohen-Wolkowiez M, Benjamin DK Jr, Piper L, et al. Safety and pharmacokinetics of multiple-dose anidulafungin in infants and neonates. *Clin Pharmacol Ther*. 2011;89:702–707.
54. Benjamin DK Jr, Driscoll T, Seibel NL, et al. Safety and pharmacokinetics of intravenous anidulafungin in children with neutropenia at high risk for invasive fungal infections. *Antimicrob Agents Chemother*. 2006;50:632–638.
55. Dowell JA, Knebel W, Ludden T, et al. Population pharmacokinetic analysis of anidulafungin, an echinocandin antifungal. *J Clin Pharmacol*. 2004;44:590–598.
56. Warn PA, Livermore J, Howard S, et al. Anidulafungin for neonatal hematogenous *Candida* meningoencephalitis: identification of candidate regimens for humans using a translational pharmacological approach. *Antimicrob Agents Chemother*. 2012;56:708–714.

15

CHAPTER 16

Antiviral Dosing Considerations for Term and Preterm Infants

Kelly C. Wade, MD, PhD, MSCE

- Antiviral agents typically require dose adjustment for prematurity and renal insufficiency.
- Myelosuppression is the most common toxicity associated with antiviral therapy.
- Acyclovir is recommended for treatment of neonatal HSV infections.
- Suppressive therapy with acyclovir for neonatal HSV or valganciclovir for symptomatic congenital CMV is associated with improved outcomes.
- Oral oseltamivir is approved for treatment of serious influenza infections in young infants >2 weeks of age.
- The antiretroviral drugs zidovudine and nevirapine are recommended for term and preterm newborns to reduce the risk of perinatal transmission of HIV.

Introduction

Neonatal viral infections are associated with significant morbidity and mortality. Antiviral medications have been shown to improve outcomes. Advances in availability of neonatal pharmacokinetics (PK) data and our understanding of pharmacodynamics (PD) have led to improved drug dosing.[1,2] The PK of a given drug describes the mathematical relationship between a given dose of a medication and the serum concentration achieved over time for a given dose regimen. The PD of a drug explains the relationship between the concentration of the drug over dosing interval time and the desired effect of killing the organism or the undesired effects of toxicity or resistance. PD exposure targets are mostly extrapolated from adult exposures in clinical trials, as well as animal and in vitro studies. With an adequate understanding of the PK of drug in preterm and term infants, we can define the dose that will achieve safe and effective drug concentrations.

Infants often exhibit highly variable drug concentrations over a dosing interval. This high variability reminds us that the PK of a drug can be affected by the patient's weight, postnatal age (PNA), gestational age (GA), postmenstrual age (PMA), hepatic and renal function, and fluid status. Population PK (popPK) approaches model interpatient variability in exposures by analyzing the impact of weight, PMA, serum creatinine, or other potential covariates. The method is commonly used in infants because it can accommodate preterm and term subjects who receive different dosing regimens and have PK samples obtained at different time points. Final models are used to predict drug exposures among different groups of neonates and to explore dose–exposure relationships.

This review will focus on the most common antiviral medications used for treatment of infections caused by herpes simplex virus (HSV), cytomegalovirus (CMV), influenza, and human immunodeficiency virus (HIV). For each antiviral drug in this review, we will explore what's known about three fundamental properties that guide dosing: (1) the clinical pharmacology and PK of the drug, (2) the PD drug exposures that have been associated with improved outcomes or toxicities, and (3) drug safety. Final dosing recommendations will be discussed.

Acyclovir and Valacyclovir for HSV Infections

Acyclovir is a synthetic nucleoside analogue that is active against HSV types 1 (HSV-1), 2 (HSV-2), and varicella zoster virus (VZV).[3,4] Acyclovir selectively targets HSV- and VZV-infected cells. The initial phosphorylation of acyclovir requires a specific viral thymidine kinase produced by HSV and VZV. After this first phosphorylation, cellular enzymes produce the final active compound: acyclovir triphosphate. Acyclovir triphosphate stops viral replication by inhibiting viral DNA polymerase and terminating the growing viral DNA chain. Acyclovir triphosphate attains up to 100-fold higher concentrations in HSV- and VZV-infected cells where the preferential inhibition of viral DNA polymerase leads to greater efficacy and lower toxicity. However, when acyclovir concentrations decrease, viral replication may resume.

Clinical Pharmacology and PK

Acyclovir is water soluble, exhibits low protein binding, and is widely distributed throughout the body.[3-5] It achieves high tissue concentrations in the kidneys, lung, liver, heart, and skin. In adults, acyclovir cerebrospinal fluid (CSF) concentrations are about 50% of plasma concentrations.[4] Acyclovir is eliminated primarily as active drug in the urine, through both glomerular filtration and tubular secretion. In infants, 60% to 70% of acyclovir is recovered in urine.[6] Hepatic metabolism accounts for the remaining drug elimination. Patients with significant renal insufficiency have higher acyclovir exposure due to reduced drug clearance, and therefore dose reduction is recommended.

Acyclovir is available in intravenous (IV) and oral (PO) suspensions. PO acyclovir has limited bioavailability, and higher doses are necessary to achieve adequate serum concentrations compared with IV.[4] Valacyclovir has not been adequately studied in infants and is not currently recommended.[7]

IV acyclovir demonstrates linear kinetics in term infants administered 5, 10, and 15 mg/kg dosing.[6] In 19 term infants <3 months of age who were receiving acyclovir at 15 mg/kg/dose every 8 hours, the mean ± SD maximal concentration (C_{max}) was 19 ± 5 µg/mL (range 11–33 µg/mL), trough (C_{min}) was 3 ± 2 µg/mL (range 0.7–8 µg/mL), and the half-life ($T_{1/2}$) was 3.8 ± 1.2 hours. In the dose escalation trial of 45 and 60 mg/kg/day, acyclovir levels from 13 infants showed similar exposures when normalized to 45 mg/kg/day; mean C_{max} 18.8 µg/mL, C_{min} 3.18 µg/mL, and $T_{1/2}$ 3 hours.[8] Although acyclovir concentrations are similar in these studies, there was significant interpatient variability. Neonatal exposures at this dose are similar to those in adults receiving 30 mg/kg/day.[4]

Acyclovir is eliminated through the kidney and has delayed clearance in infants with renal insufficiency or prematurity. In a PK study of acyclovir in 16 critically ill term and preterm infants with a mean GA 38 weeks (range 27–40), PNA of 9 days, and PMA of 38 weeks, the $T_{1/2}$ was 5 hours.[9] In this study, the $T_{1/2}$ of acyclovir in infants with renal insufficiency (defined as serum creatinine >1 mg/dL) was three times longer ($T_{1/2}$ 15 hours). Longer dosing intervals of 12 to 24 hours are recommended in infants with renal insufficiency.[4]

A popPK study recently explored acyclovir exposures in preterm and term infants.[10] In this study, 28 infants (23–40 weeks GA) less than 30 days old received acyclovir dosing that ranged from 10 to 20 mg/kg/dose every 12 hours, 20 mg/kg/dose every 8 hours, or 500 mg/m² every 8 hours. Infants who received body surface area–based dosing received higher doses; 15 infants received >80 mg/kg/day. Weight and PMA were the most important covariates affecting drug clearance. The impact of serum creatinine may have been minimized by the exclusion of infants with significant renal insufficiency. In the final model, acyclovir clearance increased 4.5-fold with advancing PMA from 25 to 41 weeks. Preterm infants with the longer half-life

($T_{1/2}$ = 13 hours) would accumulate high concentrations of acyclovir unless they received less frequent dosing.

PD Targets for Efficacy and Safety

The PD describing acyclovir exposures for optimal antiviral effect remains incompletely understood. Many propose that acyclovir exhibits time-dependent effects, meaning that viral replication can resume at low exposures. Acyclovir concentrations would be ideally maintained above a concentration that inhibits viral replication. Typically, drug exposures are described relative to the concentration that inhibits viral plaque formation in vitro by >50%, the inhibitory concentration (IC_{50}).[11] The typical IC_{50} for acyclovir is 1 µg/mL for HSV, and the breakpoint for acyclovir resistance is an IC_{50} >2 µg/mL.[11] For treatment of encephalitis, higher plasma exposures (>3 µg/mL) have been proposed to ensure adequate central nervous system (CNS) exposure. Most recommend that acyclovir concentrations are maintained >1 µg/mL (the typical HSV IC_{50}) or 3 µg/mL (accounting for CNS exposure) for >50% of the dosing interval. In term infants, average trough concentrations at both 45 mg/kg/day (C_{min} 3 µg/mL) and 60 mg/kg/day (C_{min} 4 µg/mL) are both well above this theoretical PD target. The higher dose, 60 mg/kg/day, showed significantly lower mortality in a clinical trial.[12] The higher dose may be necessary to ensure adequate exposure in most infants given interpatient variability and/or differences in CNS penetration.

The PD relationship between high acyclovir exposures and toxicity has also been described. Higher exposures in adults and children have been associated with neurotoxicity and renal toxicity. Given the time-dependent nature of antiviral activity, it is likely more important to focus on maintaining acyclovir concentrations over dosing interval rather than achieving high acyclovir concentration. In a few situations, continuous infusions have been effective in patients who failed traditional therapy.[13–16] Continuous infusions maintain consistent exposures while avoiding high peak concentrations. Some investigators recommend maintaining acyclovir concentrations <50 µg/mL as a PD safety exposure endpoint; neonatal exposures are typically below this theoretical metric.[10]

Safety Considerations

Overall, acyclovir is usually well tolerated at typical dosages in adults (30 mg/kg/day), children (45 mg/kg/day), and infants (60 mg/kg/day) (Table 16.1).[4] The most common adverse effects include phlebitis or inflammation at the injection site; gastrointestinal side effects (nausea, vomiting, diarrhea); rash; and laboratory abnormalities, including neutropenia and elevated levels of blood urea nitrogen, creatinine,

Table 16.1 DOSING OF ANTIVIRAL MEDICATIONS FOR TREATMENT OF HSV, CMV, AND INFLUENZA

Drug and Indication	Dosing in Term Infants	Dosing in Preterm Infants	Safety Concerns
Acyclovir for HSV treatment	20 mg/kg/dose q8h	<30 weeks PMA 20 mg/kg/dose q12h (based on PK)	Neutropenia Renal toxicity Neurotoxicity (older patients)
Acyclovir suppression after completing HSV treatment	300 mg/m²/dose q8h	Undefined	Neutropenia Less likely renal insufficiency or neurotoxicity
Valganciclovir for symptomatic congenital CMV	16 mg/kg/dose q12h IV ganciclovir (6 mg/kg/ dose q12h) if critically ill	Undefined	Neutropenia Anemia, thrombocytopenia
Oseltamivir for treatment of influenza in infants >14 days of age	3 mg/kg/dose q12h	1 mg/kg/dose q12h (based on PK)	Vomiting, diarrhea Rash

CMV, Cytomegalovirus; *HSV*, herpes simplex virus; *PK*, pharmacokinetics; *PMA*, postmenstrual age; *Q*, frequency of dosing interval.

and liver transaminases. Acyclovir injection solution should not be administered via intramuscular, subcutaneous, or PO routes. IV infusions should be administered over 1 hour to reduce the risk of renal tubular damage associated with precipitation of acyclovir crystals in the renal tubules.[4] Clinical monitoring of renal function and complete blood counts are recommended.

In neonatal studies, IV acyclovir at the typical dosage, 60 mg/kg/day divided every 8 hours, was well tolerated.[3] The most common adverse effect was neutropenia, defined as absolute neutrophil count (ANC) <1000 cells/mm^3. There was no significant difference in laboratory abnormalities between infants exposed to 45 or 60 mg/kg/day.[8] Neutropenia is expected in 10% to 20% of infants receiving 60 mg/kg/day IV acyclovir. Most neutropenia occurred early in the course of therapy and resolved without dose modification. Thrombocytopenia, as well as elevated creatinine, bilirubin, and aspartate aminotransferase, occurs primarily in patients with disseminated HSV and is likely related to HSV disease. The incidence of neutropenia was somewhat higher at 20% to 25% during oral suppressive therapy.[12] Neutropenia resolved with or without dose modification, and there were no reported complications. Transient high acyclovir exposures of 100 μg/mL were tolerated in two infants who received an inadvertent overdose.[17] Drug-related adverse effects typically resolve at the end of therapy or with dose reduction.

Nephrotoxicity is an important acyclovir-associated adverse effect primarily seen in children and adults.[4] Concerns of nephrotoxicity led to the recommendation for a lower daily dose of 45 mg/kg/day in children.[7] Nephrotoxicity typically occurs shortly after initiation of acyclovir, but can occur later in therapy. The most commonly described mechanism is an obstructive tubulopathy caused by precipitation of acyclovir crystals. Avoiding bolus administration and maintaining adequate patient hydration may minimize this risk.[4] More recently, reports of non-obstructive, nonoliguric nephrotoxicity have been described that likely reflect tubular injury.[18] One proposed mechanism involves the production of acyclovir metabolites, specifically acyclovir aldehydes, in renal tubule cells.[18] Risk factors for nephrotoxicity include impaired renal function at drug initiation, age >8 years, higher dose, concomitant ceftriaxone, or exposure to other nephrotoxic medications.[19,20] Renal function typically improves after discontinuation of acyclovir or dose reduction. Nephrotoxicity is less common in neonates, possibly due to the higher urine flow rates and decreased concentrating ability.

Acyclovir-associated neurotoxicity is a rare but serious adverse effect reported in <1% of patients.[4,21] Neurotoxicity has not been reported in young infants with current dosing; however, it may be possible at higher exposures. Neurotoxicity often is manifested as tremors, myoclonus, confusion, lethargy, agitation, hallucination, ataxia, and, less often, seizure.[21] Symptoms typically appear within the first 72 hours but have occurred later. Risk factors for neurotoxicity include the elderly, severe renal insufficiency, or concomitant neurotoxic medications, typically in transplant patients.[21,22] Neurotoxicity most often occurs in patients with high acyclovir concentrations and renal insufficiency; however, toxicity has been reported in patients without excessive exposure. Neurotoxicity may be due to accumulation of metabolites in the setting of renal insufficiency.[23,24] Symptoms of neurotoxicity typically resolve upon discontinuation of acyclovir.

Dosing Considerations for Neonatal HSV

Most infectious disease experts recommend infants with HSV receive an IV acyclovir dose of 60 mg/kg/day divided every 8 hours, based on improved survival in clinical trials conducted primarily in term infants (see Table 16.1).[12] With this dose, mean trough acyclovir concentrations at the end of the dosing intervals are more than three times the typical IC$_{50}$ of 1 μg/mL. This dose leads to acyclovir exposures that are safe and effective in adults and children. This acyclovir dose (60 mg/kg/day) is higher than what is recommended in the acyclovir label because it takes into consideration safety and efficacy from the dose escalation trial.[7,8] For disseminated or CNS disease, IV acyclovir is administered for 21 days. It is important to ensure that CSF is negative for HSV at the end of therapy because persistence of the virus in

CSF is associated with worse outcomes. Neutropenia is expected to occur in 10% to 20%. Monitoring blood counts and renal function is recommended.

One study recommends higher dosing (80 mg/kg/day divided every 6 hours) for infants whose PMA is 36 to 41 weeks with good renal function. However, the safety of this higher daily dose has not been explored. In simulated exposure, 87% of infants receiving 80 mg/kg/day divided every 6 hours maintained acyclovir concentrations >3 μg/mL for >50% of the dosing interval compared with 70% who received standard dosing (60 mg/kg/day divided every 8 hours). This PD target is designed to achieve adequate CNS exposure but has not been confirmed in clinical trials. Because renal function improves with postnatal age, every-6-hour dosing seems reasonable in infants >14 days old with good renal function. Ideally, the safety and efficacy of alternative dosing would be evaluated in a randomized controlled trial.

There is no definitive dosing guidance for IV acyclovir in extremely preterm infants. Extremely preterm infants have reduced acyclovir clearance and a longer half-life; therefore longer dosing intervals are recommended to prevent acyclovir accumulation. Proposed dosing guidance for preterm infants is based on simulated exposures derived from a popPK model that accounts for the effect of PMA on clearance. In infants <30 weeks PMA, a dose of 20 mg/kg/dose every 12 hours maintains acyclovir exposure >3 μg/mL for at least 50% of the dosing interval. In infants PMA 30 to <36 weeks, traditional dosing (20 mg/kg/dose every 8 hours) maintains similar acyclovir exposures. A prospective study of exposure and safety would strengthen these recommendations.

Oral Suppressive Therapy

After completion of IV treatment, ongoing viral suppression with oral acyclovir is recommended for 6 months.[7,12] The recommended suppressive dose is 900 mg/m²/day divided every 8 hours, based on a placebo-controlled randomized clinical trial that showed reduction in recurrence of skin vesicles and improved neurologic outcomes.[12] Neutropenia occurred in 20% to 25% of infants; therefore serial monitoring of blood counts is recommended. Given low bioavailability, exposures during suppressive therapy are less than that achieved during IV therapy. Some authors recommend a higher suppressive dose for a longer duration. In one small observational study, infants receiving 1200 to 1600 mg/m²/dose every 12 hours for 2 years had improved neurodevelopmental outcomes.[25] The safety and efficacy of this higher dose and longer duration have not been studied in randomized clinical trials.

Ganciclovir and Its Oral Prodrug Valganciclovir

CMV is another member of the Herpes virus family. Infants with symptomatic congenital CMV infections can exhibit a variety of signs and symptoms, including neurologic injury, sensorineural hearing loss, hepatitis, retinitis, bowel injury, and myelosuppression.[7,26] Sensorineural hearing loss due to congenital CMV is not necessarily present at birth and can progress in infancy and early childhood.

Ganciclovir, administered IV or using its oral prodrug valganciclovir, is recommended by many infectious disease experts for infants with symptomatic congenital CMV based on modest improvement in hearing and neurodevelopmental outcomes in a randomized clinical trial.[7,26–29] It is important to note that the US Food and Drug Administration (FDA)–approved ganciclovir label contains the following black box warning: "The clinical toxicity of ganciclovir includes granulocytopenia, anemia, and thrombocytopenia. In animal studies, ganciclovir was carcinogenic, teratogenic, and caused aspermatogenesis. Ganciclovir for injection is indicated for use only in the treatment of CMV retinitis in immunocompromised patients and for the prevention of CMV disease in transplant patients at risk for CMV disease."[30]

Clinical Pharmacology and PK

Ganciclovir is a synthetic guanine derivative that is active against CMV and available for IV injection.[30] Selective activity against CMV is conferred by initial phosphorylation to ganciclovir monophosphate by CMV-derived thymidine kinase. Cellular kinases provide the additional phosphorylation steps to generate the active ganciclovir triphosphate. Ganciclovir triphosphate inhibits CMV replication by inhibiting viral DNA polymerase and termination of viral DNA elongation. The requirement for initial phosphorylation by CMV-derived thymidine kinase confers selective accumulation of ganciclovir triphosphate in CMV-infected cells.

Ganciclovir is widely distributed throughout the body and achieves CSF concentrations that are 24% to 70% of plasma concentrations.[3,30] Plasma protein binding is minimal. Ganciclovir is eliminated primarily through the kidneys and excreted as active drug in the urine. Dose adjustment is recommended for patients with renal insufficiency.

Ganciclovir has limited oral bioavailability and therefore is only available for IV administration. Valganciclovir is the monovalyl ester prodrug of ganciclovir that offers improved bioavailability.[31] Once absorbed into the bloodstream, valganciclovir is rapidly converted to ganciclovir and maintains the same activity as IV ganciclovir. Valganciclovir can provide similar plasma concentrations of ganciclovir as achieved with IV therapy.[31] Bioavailability is improved when valganciclovir is coadministered with food.

The PK of IV ganciclovir has been evaluated in 27 term infants <2 months of age with symptomatic CMV.[32] Ganciclovir clearance varied with weight and creatinine clearance. Ganciclovir had a median half-life of 2.4 hours, but longer half-lives of 4.6 hours were seen in infants with decreased creatinine clearance. An IV ganciclovir dose of 6 mg/kg/dose every 12 hours achieved a mean area under the concentration curve (AUC) of 25 mg•h/L. These neonatal exposures were similar to the target exposures demonstrated in older patients.

The PK of valganciclovir has been evaluated in 24 infants at 34 to 41 weeks GA.[33,34] Valganciclovir bioavailability ranged from 41% to 54%. Infants receiving valganciclovir 16 mg/kg/dose every 12 hours or IV ganciclovir 6 mg/kg/dose every 12 hours have similar exposures, both providing a mean AUC_{12} 25 to 27 mg•h/L during a 12-hour dosing interval.

Ganciclovir is eliminated in urine. Not surprisingly, ganciclovir clearance increases and drug exposures decrease in the first month of life as kidney function improves. In neonates receiving IV ganciclovir, clearance increased 73% and the median AUC_{12} decreased 41% between day 4 and 34.[33] Infants receiving valganciclovir had a less dramatic decline in ganciclovir exposure with a 16% decrease in AUC_{12} between day 6 and 36.[33] Valganciclovir more consistently maintains ganciclovir exposure because at the same time clearance becomes faster, bioavailability also increases, allowing for higher serum ganciclovir exposure for a given oral dose of valganciclovir. Maintaining ganciclovir exposure is thought to confer greater efficacy.

PD Targets for Efficacy and Safety

The PD relationships between ganciclovir exposure, in vitro sensitivity of CMV strains, and clinical response or toxicity have not been clearly established. In infants with symptomatic congenital CMV, ganciclovir exposure has been associated with significant reduction in viral load.[33] Like other nucleoside analogues, ganciclovir likely exhibits time-dependent effects, because ongoing exposure is necessary to inhibit viral replication. Plasma concentrations of ganciclovir underestimate the concentrations achieved in viral infected cells. In vitro, ganciclovir concentrations of 0.02 to 2.45 µg/mL inhibit CMV replication by at least 50% (IC_{50}), and the breakpoint for ganciclovir resistance is reported to be IC_{50} >3 µg/mL.[30] Bone marrow–derived colony-forming units are sensitive to similar ganciclovir concentrations of 0.028 to 0.7 µg/mL.[30] Most agree that maintaining adequate ganciclovir exposure as measured by AUC_{12} is important for efficacy.

In infants receiving valganciclovir, CMV viral load decreases during 42 days of treatment; however, viral load rebounds after discontinuation of therapy unless suppressive therapy is continued.[33] Ganciclovir PK parameters such as C_{max}, C_{min}, or AUC did not correlate with changes in CMV viral load over the course of treatment.[33] Higher ganciclovir plasma C_{max} and AUC were significantly correlated with neutropenia.[33]

Safety Considerations

Ganciclovir and valganciclovir drug labels both contain black box warnings regarding the risk of neutropenia, anemia, and thrombocytopenia (see Table 16.1).[30,31] In animal studies, high exposures to ganciclovir have demonstrated potential carcinogenic effects, teratogenic effects, and inhibition of spermatogenesis. It is unclear if this animal information is relevant to humans. Ganciclovir is typically administered over 1 hour by infusion, and bolus administration is not recommended.[30] Phlebitis and serious infusion site reactions have occurred with ganciclovir administration.

Neutropenia and thrombocytopenia are the most common adverse events reported in young infants receiving ganciclovir or valganciclovir.[3,27,29] CMV infection without treatment is also associated with myelosuppression. In the 6-week IV ganciclovir trial, 63% of infants developed neutropenia (ANC <1000 cells/m^3).[28,29] Among infants with neutropenia, half required dose reduction and 13% had the drug discontinued. In comparison, fewer infants in the 6-month valganciclovir trial had neutropenia.[27] Neutropenia occurred in 19% of participants during the first 6 weeks of valganciclovir and in 21% over the subsequent 4.5 months. Ganciclovir should not be administered to patients if the ANC is <500 cells/mm^3 or the platelet count is <25,000 cells/mm^3.[30,31] Neutropenia typically resolves with dose reduction or discontinuation. Monitoring of blood counts is recommended during ganciclovir therapy.

Dosing Considerations for Symptomatic Congenital CMV

Many pediatric infectious disease experts recommend that infants with symptomatic congenital CMV receive a 6-month course of valganciclovir, 16 mg/kg/dose every 12 hours (see Table 16.1).[7] IV ganciclovir (6 mg/kg/dose every 12 hours) is reserved for those who cannot tolerate enteral medication and exhibit severe illness. Dosing of ganciclovir and valganciclovir is designed to achieve plasma ganciclovir exposures that are effective in adults and children (AUC$_{12}$ = 27 mg•h/L). At these doses, ganciclovir and valganciclovir significantly reduce CMV viral load and are associated with modest improvement in hearing and neurodevelopment in randomized clinical trials.[7,27]

In infants tolerating enteral nutrition, valganciclovir is preferred over IV ganciclovir because valgancyclovir maintains more consistent exposures over the 6 months of therapy when renal clearance of ganciclovir improves.[33] Valgancyclovir also confers a somewhat lower risk of neutropenia. Blood count monitoring is advised in infants receiving ganciclovir or valganciclovir.[7] Dose adjustment is warranted in patients with sustained renal insufficiency.

Ganciclovir and valganciclovir have not been adequately studied in preterm infants. There are no dose recommendations for very preterm infants. Preterm infants have delayed renal clearance of medications that are eliminated through the kidneys. Therefore, preterm infants would be expected to be at risk of higher ganciclovir exposures if they receive the traditional term-infant dosing.

Oseltamivir for Treatment of Influenza Infections

Influenza infections cause serious morbidity and mortality in children, and particularly in young infants <6 months old.[35] The best way to protect young infants is through passive immunity with maternal vaccination during pregnancy.[35,36]

Oseltamivir is the only antiviral medicine recommended by the Centers for Disease Control and Prevention (CDC) and the FDA for treatment of young children.[35,37–39] Oseltamivir is indicated for the treatment of acute illness due to influenza A and B in patients >2 weeks old who have been symptomatic for <48 hours.[39] Prophylaxis is not routinely recommended in infants <1 year of age unless the risk of illness after exposure is considered extreme. The oseltamivir drug label contains the essential clinical pharmacology, PK, PD, safety, and dosing considerations that support dosing in young infants >2 weeks of age.[39]

16

Brief Synopsis: Clinical Pharmacology, PK, and PD

Oseltamivir is an oral prodrug that is rapidly converted by hepatic carboxylesterase to the active neuraminidase inhibitor oseltamivir carboxylate.[39,40] Oseltamivir carboxylate inhibits influenza virus neuraminidase and blocks the release of viral particles from infected cells. Early initiation of oseltamivir after viral infection is necessary to limit release of progeny virus and prevent infection of new host cells.

Although the PK–PD relationship is variable, most agree that oseltamivir exhibits a primarily time-dependent relationship between drug exposure and effect.[2] In vitro and clinical models both suggest that AUC of the active metabolite, oseltamivir carboxylate, is the most important determinant of efficacy, relative to the effective concentration that reduces the viral plaque in vitro by 50% (EC_{50}). The EC_{50} of oseltamivir against clinical isolates has wide variability and ranges from 0.0008 to >35 μM.[39] Decreased susceptibility to oseltamivir in different influenza strains has been demonstrated during treatment and community surveillance. The CDC provides up-to-date information regarding circulating strains of influenza and their sensitivity patterns.[38]

The active drug, oseltamivir carboxylate, is widely distributed throughout the body and concentrated to levels higher than blood in fluid in the lung, middle ear, nasal mucosa, and saliva, where the viral burden is typically high.[39] Drug levels reflect oral absorption, conversion to active metabolite by hepatic carboxylesterase, release of oseltamivir carboxylate from hepatic cells to plasma, and renal elimination of active metabolite. Oseltamivir carboxylate accumulates to higher levels in patients with renal insufficiency; therefore dose adjustment is indicated. Metabolism of oseltamivir to active oseltamivir carboxylate seems to be maintained in adults with mild to moderate hepatic impairment; therefore dose adjustment is typically not necessary.

In adults, the half-life of oral oseltamivir is 6 hours, much of this time due to activation of oseltamivir carboxylate and release from hepatic cells into the circulation.[39] The rate-limiting step in the presence of oseltamivir carboxylate in plasma appears to be release of the active metabolite from hepatic cells. Formation of the active compound oseltamivir carboxylate is slower than elimination of the active metabolite. This means that plasma drug levels of oseltamivir carboxylate will continue to accumulate for the first few days of therapy as more is released from hepatic cells than is eliminated in urine.

The complexity of oseltamivir drug disposition makes careful PK analysis of oseltamivir in young infants essential.[2,40,41] Expression of the predominant activating enzyme, hepatic carboxylesterase-1, increases rapidly during the first year of life such that increasing production of active metabolite is expected as infants get older. Carboxylation is a highly efficient process compared with rate-limiting release of active compound from hepatic cells. Therefore, changes in carboxylase expression may have little impact on the amount of metabolite in the plasma. Renal clearance of active metabolite is delayed in young infants and also expected to increase as glomerular filtration and tubular secretion improved during the first year. In general, PK studies in infants have demonstrated a slower rate of oseltamivir carboxylate appearance in plasma and slower drug clearance compared with older infants and children. In young infants, delays in appearance of active oseltamivir carboxylate means that the first dose may need to be higher to acheive the target concentration on day 1 of therapy. However, in infants as in adults, the active metabolite, oseltamivir carboxylate, appears more quickly than it can be eliminated such that accumulation of active oseltamivir carboxylate is expected over the first few days of therapy.

PK studies have demonstrated wide interindividual variability between measured drug concentration (reported as AUC) after standard dosing. Variation is particularly high in young children. Children <2 years of age had twofold to fivefold variation in AUC exposure, and the youngest infants (0–2 months) had greater than 10-fold variation.[42]

Oseltamivir dosing in infants 2 weeks to 12 months of age is primarily based on PK analysis of 136 infants enrolled in two prospective open-label studies.[39,42,43] The disposition of oseltamivir and oseltamivir carboxylate was described using the popPK approach on pooled data of the 604 oseltamivir and 648 oseltamivir carboxylate plasma samples from these prior studies.[43] On average, infants were 23.5 weeks old (range 1.9–49), had a PMA of 62 weeks (range 38–90), and weighed 6.5 kg (range 2.9–12.4). A popPK model was used to assess individual estimates of AUC, C_{max}, and C_{min} at steady state. There was no clear association between drug exposures and PD efficacy outcomes (temperature, fever, viral load, viral shedding, or viral resistance) or gastrointestinal side effects. Simulation was used to determine the neonatal dose that would best accomplish exposure targets in adults and children that correlate with safety and efficacy.

Safety Considerations

Overall, oseltamivir is well tolerated. The most common reported side effects include vomiting, diarrhea, or rash (see Table 16.1).[39] Gastrointestinal side effects are usually self-limited. In a retrospective study of infants, diarrhea was the most frequent adverse event.[44] In children <2 years old, a dose of 3 to 3.5 mg/kg every 12 hours was well tolerated without drug discontinuation.[42] The most common adverse events were vomiting (6%) or skin rash (2%). One serious adverse event was reported for an infant with a skin hypersensitivity reaction. Mild transient elevation in liver transaminases has been reported.

In teens and adults, postmarketing surveillance identified a possible association with oseltamivir and transient neuropsychiatric events of self-injury or delirium.[39] It is unclear if neuropsychiatric changes were related to oseltamivir or influenza. Individuals receiving oseltamivir should be monitored for abnormal behavior.

Dosing Considerations for Influenza Infections

The recommended dose of oseltamivir in infants >2 weeks of age with symptomatic influenza infection is 3 mg/kg/dose twice daily for 5 days (see Table 16.1).[39,43] Simulated exposures in infants receiving this dose were at or above the upper interquartile bounds of adults receiving 75 mg/dose twice daily but still below the median exposure for adults receiving 150 mg/dose twice daily, a dose that is well tolerated. Higher exposures were particularly noted among the youngest infants (0–2 months), yet this is also the group with the highest interpatient variability. The higher exposure in the youngest infants is reasonable, given the desire to achieve adequate exposure in nearly all infants, the safety profile at these exposures in older patients, and the desire to prevent subtherapeutic exposures. This analysis excluded premature infants with PMA <36 weeks. In patients with significant, sustained renal insufficiency, dose adjustment is recommended.[39]

Dosing of oseltamivir for very preterm infants is less well defined. PK was studied using sparse plasma samples collected from infants receiving off-label oseltamivir after inadvertent influenza exposure in the newborn intensive care unit. One study evaluated oseltamivir exposure in 20 infants (mean GA 29 weeks and PNA 4.6 weeks) who received 1.5 mg/kg/dose every 12 hours.[45] Despite this lower dose, exposures in preterm infants were almost twofold higher than expected among older infants receiving the 3 mg/kg/dose every 12 hours dosing. In another study, 22 infants received oseltamivir 1 to 3 mg/kg/dose every 12 to 24 hours and 9 infants (PMA 28–52 weeks) submitted multiple blood samples for PK analysis.[46] Simulated drug exposure using the derived popPK model was used to explore dose–exposure relationships. Both PK studies concluded that an oseltamivir dose of 1 mg/kg/dose every 12 hours was reasonable for infants ≤37 weeks PMA.

Resistance to neuraminidase inhibitors has been described, and resistance patterns are being monitored given increased use of oseltamivir. Resistance rates appear to be higher in children compared with adults.[2,42] It is unclear if differences in resistant patterns in children reflect differences in immune response to infection or variations in drug exposure in children.

16

Medications Used to Prevent Perinatal Transmission of HIV

Recent recommendations for the use of antiretroviral drugs in pregnant HIV-1–infected women for maternal health and interventions to reduce perinatal HIV transmission in the United States are publicly available on the AIDSinfo website (http://aidsinfo.nih.gov/guidelines).[47] The US National Perinatal HIV hotline (1-888-448-8765) also provides free clinical consultation on all aspects of perinatal HIV. It is important to follow the most recent guidance provided by national organizations. The following review is abbreviated.

All HIV-exposed infants should receive postpartum antiretroviral drug therapy as soon after birth as possible to reduce the risk of prenatal transmission of HIV.[47] Choice of medication and duration of prophylaxis are dependent on GA of neonate, maternal treatment regimen, and maternal viral load. The most common drugs used for neonatal prophylaxis include zidovudine, nevirapine, and lamivudine. However, for premature infants, only zidovudine and nevirapine are recommended due to limited dosing and safety information on other drugs.

Single-Drug Prevention With Zidovudine

Zidovudine is a nucleoside reverse transcriptase inhibitor that effectively reduces perinatal HIV transmission and is recommended for all term and preterm infants born to mothers with HIV infection.[47,48] Zidovudine is a nucleoside analogue that, once activated by phosphorylation, is incorporated into the elongating DNA strand by HIV reverse transcriptase, whereby it prevents further transcription. Infants born to mothers who received antiretroviral therapy during pregnancy and who achieved viral suppression are typically treated with zidovudine as single-drug therapy. Zidovudine is available as an IV preparation or an oral suspension. It demonstrates good bioavailability and is widely distributed. Unlike other nucleoside analogues, zidovudine is eliminated through hepatic metabolism to an inactive metabolite. However, 14% of active zidovudine is recovered in the urine; therefore renal insufficiency can lead to drug accumulation. Zidovudine can be administered with or without food.

Zidovudine is approved for the prevention of perinatal transmission of HIV in newborns based on PK, safety, and efficacy data.[47–49] Infants in the first 14 days of life and those born prematurely have reduced clearance and longer half-life. Bioavailability remains adequate (>60%) in young infants. Zidovudine is associated with increased risk of anemia and neutropenia as specified in the black box warning on the drug label.[48]

The recommended dose of zidovudine for prevention of perinatal transmission of HIV varies with prematurity (Table 16.2).[47,48] IV zidovudine is reserved for infants unable to tolerate enteral medications. The dose of IV zidovudine is 75% of the oral dose. Premature infants require dose adjustment with advancing PNA to account for changes in drug elimination with maturation. Blood count monitoring is recommended.

Combination Antiretroviral Prophylaxis Therapy

Combination antiretroviral prophylaxis therapy is recommended for infants at higher risk of HIV acquisition, including infants born to HIV-infected women who did not receive antepartum and intrapartum therapy or if antepartum therapy did not achieve viral suppression near delivery.[47] Nevirapine is a nonnucleoside reverse transcriptase inhibitor that is available in an oral solution appropriate for pediatric use and approved for treatment of HIV in infants >2 weeks old.[47,49–51] The nevirapine drug label contains an important black box warning regarding hepatotoxicity and severe skin reactions at treatment doses.[51] Lamivudine is another nucleoside reverse transcriptase inhibitor that is available in an oral solution approved for HIV treatment in infants >3 months of age, and sometimes used in combination therapy for neonatal prophylaxis.[50,52] Protease inhibitors are being evaluated in young infants but are not recommended in the first few weeks of life due to lack of dosing and safety information.[47]

Combination prophylaxis has been evaluated in one large randomized trial of infants at high risk of perinatal transmission. This trial compared the following drug

Table 16.2 DRUG DOSING REGIMENS FOR THE PREVENTION OF PERINATAL TRANSMISSION OF HIV

Drug	Safety	Duration and Dosing
Single-drug therapy Zidovudine *75% dose reduction if administered IV	Anemia Neutropenia	Start soon after birth Duration 4–6 wk Dosing based on GA at birth GA >35 wk 4 mg/kg/dose q12h (PNA 0–42) GA 30–34 wk 2 mg/kg/dose q12h (PNA 0–14 days) 3 mg/kg/dose q12h (PNA 15–42 days) GA <30 wk 2 mg/kg/dose q12h (PNA 0–28 days) 3 mg/kg/dose q12h (PNA 29–42 days)
Combination therapy Nevirapine (+ zidovudine)	Anemia Neutropenia Hepatotoxicity Rash	Three doses in first week* First dose shortly after birth Second dose 48 hr after first dose Third dose 96 hr after second dose Dose based on BW BW 1.5–2 kg 8 mg/dose BW >2 kg 12 mg/dose

BW, Body weight; *GA*, gestational age; *PNA*, postnatal age; *q*, frequency of dosing interval.
*Optimal dose duration of nevirapine is being evaluated. Some recommend a higher dose and longer course.
Table modified from AIDSinfo Panel Recommendations available at http://aidsinfo.nih.gov/contentfiles/lvguidelines/PerinatalGL.pdf.[47]

16

regimens: one-drug regimen (zidovudine 6 weeks), two-drug regimen (zidovudine + nevirapine three doses), and three-drug regimen (zidovudine, + 2 weeks lamivudine/nelfinavir).[50] The risk of intrapartum transmission was significantly lower in combination therapy groups (2.2%–2.5%) compared with zidovudine alone (4.9%). Neutropenia was the most common side effect of antiretroviral therapy. Neutropenia occurred more often with the three-drug regimen compared with the two-drug or single-drug regimen: 27.5%, 15%, and 16%, respectively.[50] Combination therapy has been associated with higher incidences of vomiting, diarrhea, rash, jitteriness, and irritability that potentially could be nonspecific signs of medication-related adverse effects not otherwise reported in infants on single therapy with zidovudine. For combination therapy, the two-drug regimen (6 weeks zidovudine plus three doses nevirapine) is most often recommended.[47] Some experts recommend the three-drug regimen and higher treatment doses of antiretroviral drugs in infants at the highest risk of HIV acquisition. Ongoing clinical trials investigating PK, safety, and efficacy of three-drug regimens will inform future decisions.

Conclusion

Guidance for dosing of antiviral medications in term and preterm infants has improved over the last decade. PK studies in term and preterm infants have demonstrated important exposure differences associated with maturity and renal functions. Studies are ongoing to better define dosing in preterm populations. Beyond dosing, a high index of suspicion and prompt initiation of antiviral therapies are needed to reduce mortality and morbidity associated with viral infections.

REFERENCES

1. Roberts JK, Stockmann C, Constance JE, et al. Pharmacokinetics and pharmacodynamics of antibacterials, antifungals, and antivirals used most frequently in neonates and infants. *Clin Pharmacokinet.* 2014;53(7): 581–610.
2. Standing JF, Tsolia M, Lutsar I. Pharmacokinetics and pharmacodynamics of oseltamivir in neonates, infants and children. *Infect Disord Drug Targets.* 2013;13(1):6–14.

3. Whitley RJ. The use of antiviral drugs during the neonatal period. *Clin Perinatol.* 2012;39(1):69–81.
4. Food and Drug Administration. Acyclovir Drug Label, available at DailyMed website maintained by National Library of Medicine. https://dailymed.nlm.nih.gov/dailymed/drugInfo.cfm?setid=cb64dfab -52ee-4312-bc9c-c3d04efe9109. Accessed November 28, 2016.
5. Wagstaff AJ, Faulds D, Goa KL. Aciclovir. A reappraisal of its antiviral activity, pharmacokinetic properties and therapeutic efficacy. *Drugs.* 1994;47(1):153–205.
6. Hintz M, Connor JD, Spector SA, et al. Neonatal acyclovir pharmacokinetics in patients with herpes virus infections. *Am J Med.* 1982;73(1A):210–214.
7. Committee on Infectious Disease of the American Academy of Pediatrics, Kimberlin DW, Brady MT, et al. The Red Book Online. https://redbook.solutions.aap.org/book.aspx?bookid=1484. American Academy of Pediatrics; 2015. Accessed November 10, 2016.
8. Kimberlin DW, Lin CY, Jacobs RF, et al. Safety and efficacy of high-dose intravenous acyclovir in the management of neonatal herpes simplex virus infections. *Pediatrics.* 2001;108(2):230–238.
9. Englund JA, Fletcher CV, Balfour HH. Acyclovir therapy in neonates. *J Pediatr.* 1991;119(1 Pt 1): 129–135.
10. Sampson MR, Bloom BT, Lenfestey RW, et al. Population pharmacokinetics of intravenous acyclovir in preterm and term infants. *Pediatr Infect Dis J.* 2014;33(1):42–49.
11. Piret J, Boivin G. Resistance of herpes simplex viruses to nucleoside analogues: mechanisms, prevalence, and management. *Antimicrob Agents Chemother.* 2011;55(2):459–472.
12. Kimberlin DW, Whitley RJ, Wan W, et al. Oral acyclovir suppression and neurodevelopment after neonatal herpes. *N Engl J Med.* 2011;365(14):1284–1292.
13. Cies JJ, Moore WS, Miller K, et al. Therapeutic drug monitoring of continuous-infusion acylovir for disseminated herpes simplex virus infection in a neonate receiving concurrent extracorporeal life support and continuous renal replacement therapy. *Pharmacotherapy.* 2015;35(2):229–233.
14. Kim JH, Schaenman JM, Ho DY, et al. Treatment of acyclovir-resistant herpes simplex virus with continuous infusion of high-dose acyclovir in hematopoietic cell transplant patients. *Biol Blood Marrow Transplant.* 2011;17(2):259–264.
15. Kakisaka Y, Ishitobi M, Wakusawa K, et al. Efficacy of continuous acyclovir infusion in neonatal herpes virus encephalitis. *Neuropediatrics.* 2009;40(4):199–200.
16. Funaki T, Miyata I, Shoji K, et al. Therapeutic drug monitoring in neonatal hsv infection on continuous renal replacement therapy. *Pediatrics.* 2015;136(1):e270–e274.
17. McDonald LK, Tartaglione TA, Mendelman PM, et al. Lack of toxicity in two cases of neonatal acyclovir overdose. *Pediatr Infect Dis J.* 1989;8(8):529–532.
18. Gunness P, Aleksa K, Bend J, et al. Acyclovir-induced nephrotoxicity: the role of the acyclovir aldehyde metabolite. *Transl Res.* 2011;158(5):290–301.
19. Rao S, Abzug MJ, Carosone-Link P, et al. Intravenous acyclovir and renal dysfunction in children: a matched case control study. *J Pediatr.* 2015;166(6):1462–1468, e1461–e1464.
20. Schreiber R, Wolpin J, Koren G. Determinants of aciclovir-induced nephrotoxicity in children. *Paediatr Drugs.* 2008;10(2):135–139.
21. Ernst ME, Franey RJ. Acyclovir- and ganciclovir-induced neurotoxicity. *Ann Pharmacother.* 1998; 32(1):111–113.
22. Haefeli WE, Schoenenberger RA, Weiss P, et al. Acyclovir-induced neurotoxicity: concentration-side effect relationship in acyclovir overdose. *Am J Med.* 1993;94(2):212–215.
23. Bean B, Aeppli D. Adverse effects of high-dose intravenous acyclovir in ambulatory patients with acute herpes zoster. *J Infect Dis.* 1985;151(2):362–365.
24. Helldén A, Odar-Cederlöf I, Diener P, et al. High serum concentrations of the acyclovir main metabolite 9-carboxymethoxymethylguanine in renal failure patients with acyclovir-related neuropsychiatric side effects: an observational study. *Nephrol Dial Transplant.* 2003;18(6):1135–1141.
25. Tiffany KF, Benjamin DK, Palasanthiran P, et al. Improved neurodevelopmental outcomes following long-term high-dose oral acyclovir therapy in infants with central nervous system and disseminated herpes simplex disease. *J Perinatol.* 2005;25(3):156–161.
26. James SH, Kimberlin DW. Advances in the prevention and treatment of congenital cytomegalovirus infection. *Curr Opin Pediatr.* 2016;28(1):81–85.
27. Kimberlin DW, Jester PM, Sánchez PJ, et al. Valganciclovir for symptomatic congenital cytomegalovirus disease. *N Engl J Med.* 2015;372(10):933–943.
28. Oliver SE, Cloud GA, Sánchez PJ, et al. Neurodevelopmental outcomes following ganciclovir therapy in symptomatic congenital cytomegalovirus infections involving the central nervous system. *J Clin Virol.* 2009;46(suppl 4):S22–S26.
29. Kimberlin DW, Lin CY, Sánchez PJ, et al. Effect of ganciclovir therapy on hearing in symptomatic congenital cytomegalovirus disease involving the central nervous system: a randomized, controlled trial. *J Pediatr.* 2003;143(1):16–25.
30. Food and Drug Administration. Ganciclovir Drug Label. Available at DailyMed website maintained by National Library of Medicine. http://dailymed.nlm.nih.gov/dailymed/drugInfo.cfm?setid=b47f5d1c -36b8-49b6-a410-3b3f4661dde7. Accessed November 28, 2016.
31. Food and Drug Administration. Valganciclovir Drug Label. Available at DailyMed website maintained by National Library of Medicine. https://dailymed.nlm.nih.gov/dailymed/drugInfo.cfm?setid=9228130 1-5fb5-4eea-8766-4863e241c234. Accessed November 28, 2016.
32. Zhou XJ, Gruber W, Demmler G, et al. Population pharmacokinetics of ganciclovir in newborns with congenital cytomegalovirus infections. NIAID Collaborative Antiviral Study Group. *Antimicrob Agents Chemother.* 1996;40(9):2202–2205.

33. Kimberlin DW, Acosta EP, Sánchez PJ, et al. Pharmacokinetic and pharmacodynamic assessment of oral valganciclovir in the treatment of symptomatic congenital cytomegalovirus disease. *J Infect Dis*. 2008;197(6):836–845.

34. Acosta EP, Brundage RC, King JR, et al. Ganciclovir population pharmacokinetics in neonates following intravenous administration of ganciclovir and oral administration of a liquid valganciclovir formulation. *Clin Pharmacol Ther*. 2007;81(6):867–872.

35. Centers for Disease Control and Prevention, National Center for Immunization and Respiratory Diseases (NCIRD). Protecting against influenza (Flu): Advice for Caregivers of Young Children. 2016. http://www.cdc.gov/flu/protect/infantcare.htm. Accessed December 1, 2016.

36. Eick AA, Uyeki TM, Klimov A, et al. Maternal influenza vaccination and effect on influenza virus infection in young infants. *Arch Pediatr Adolesc Med*. 2011;165(2):104–111.

37. Food and Drug Administration. Influenza antiviral drugs and related information. 2016. http://www.fda.gov/Drugs/DrugSafety/InformationbyDrugClass/ucm100228.htm. Accessed December 1, 2016.

38. Centers for Disease Control and Prevention, National Center for Immunization and Respiratory Diseases (NCIRD). Antiviral drugs for seasonal influenza. 2016. http://www.cdc.gov/flu/professionals/antivirals/links.htm. Accessed December 1, 2016.

39. Food and Drug Administration. Oseltamivir Drug Label. Available at DailyMed website maintained by National Library of Medicine. https://dailymed.nlm.nih.gov/dailymed/drugInfo.cfm?setid=ee3c9555-60f2-4f82-a760-11983c86e97b. Accessed November 28, 2016.

40. Karadag-Oncel E, Ceyhan M. Oseltamivir in neonates, infants and young children: a focus on clinical pharmacology. *Infect Disord Drug Targets*. 2013;13(1):15–24.

41. Muñoz FM, Anderson EJ, Deville JG, et al. Pharmacokinetics and safety of intravenous oseltamivir in infants and children in open-label studies. *Int J Clin Pharmacol Ther*. 2015;53(7):531–540.

42. Kimberlin DW, Acosta EP, Prichard MN, et al. Oseltamivir pharmacokinetics, dosing, and resistance among children aged <2 years with influenza. *J Infect Dis*. 2013;207(5):709–720.

43. Kamal MA, Acosta EP, Kimberlin DW, et al. The posology of oseltamivir in infants with influenza infection using a population pharmacokinetic approach. *Clin Pharmacol Ther*. 2014;96(3):380–389.

44. Jefferson T, Jones M, Doshi P, et al. Oseltamivir for influenza in adults and children: systematic review of clinical study reports and summary of regulatory comments. *BMJ*. 2014;348:g2545.

45. Acosta EP, Jester P, Gal P, et al. Oseltamivir dosing for influenza infection in premature neonates. *J Infect Dis*. 2010;202(4):563–566.

46. Standing JF, Nika A, Tsagris V, et al. Oseltamivir pharmacokinetics and clinical experience in neonates and infants during an outbreak of H1N1 influenza A virus infection in a neonatal intensive care unit. *Antimicrob Agents Chemother*. 2012;56(7):3833–3840.

47. Panel on Treatment of HIV-Infected Pregnant Women and Prevention of Perinatal Transmission. Recommendations for Use of Antiretroviral Drugs in Pregnant HIV-1-Infected Women for Maternal Health and Interventions to Reduce Perinatal HIV transmission in the United States. 2016 AIDSinfo website. http://aidsinfo.nih.gov/contentfiles/lvguidelines/PerinatalGL.pdf. Accessed November 9, 2016.

48. Food and Drug Administration. Zidovudine syrup Drug Label. Available at DailyMed website maintained by National Library of Medicine. https://dailymed.nlm.nih.gov/dailymed/drugInfo.cfm?setid=51abd2ce-6be1-412d-b806-5f24935ac5e3. Accessed December 1, 2016.

49. King JR, Kimberlin DW, Aldrovandi GM, et al. Antiretroviral pharmacokinetics in the paediatric population: a review. *Clin Pharmacokinet*. 2002;41(14):1115–1133.

50. Nielsen-Saines K, Watts DH, Veloso VG, et al. Three postpartum antiretroviral regimens to prevent intrapartum HIV infection. *N Engl J Med*. 2012;366(25):2368–2379.

51. Food and Drug Administration. Nevirapine Drug Label. Available at DailyMed website maintained by National Library of Medicine. https://dailymed.nlm.nih.gov/dailymed/drugInfo.cfm?setid=8dfe86aa-ea5d-48d2-94a8-1a5506055d70. Accessed December 1, 2016.

52. Mirochnick M, Nielsen-Saines K, Pilotto JH, et al. Nelfinavir and Lamivudine pharmacokinetics during the first two weeks of life. *Pediatr Infect Dis J*. 2011;30(9):769–772.

16

CHAPTER 17

Antiepileptic Drug Therapy in Neonates

Amanda G. Sandoval Karamian, MD, Courtney J. Wusthoff, MD, MS

- Initial/emergent management of neonatal seizures includes stabilization of the neonate, assessment and correction of reversible causes of seizures, and evaluation for sepsis/meningitis at the same time as AEDs are initiated.

- Despite limited efficacy data and concern for adverse effects, phenobarbital remains the first-line treatment for most neonatal seizures.

- Limited evidence supports phenytoin, benzodiazepines, lidocaine, and levetiracetam as second- or third-line agents.

- Other third-line agents may also be used for refractory seizures, but there is limited evidence regarding their safety and efficacy.

- Empiric pyridoxine, pyridoxal 5'-phosphate (PLP), and folinic acid trials should be considered in neonates with seizures refractory to therapy with multiple AEDs while diagnostic biochemical and genetic testing is performed.

Introduction

Goals of Therapy

Untreated neonatal seizures have been shown to cause neuronal apoptosis and are associated with poor neurodevelopmental outcomes in both animal and human studies.[1-5] Although controversy remains regarding the degree to which seizure treatment might affect outcomes, most providers attempt to control neonatal seizures with the use of antiepileptic drugs (AEDs). As such, the overarching goal of treatment is usually to minimize acute seizure burden for the neonate. At the same time, different providers and specific clinical scenarios may warrant a distinct consideration of the potential benefits of seizure treatment against the potential risks. When selecting AEDs, it is helpful to be explicit about the goals of therapy for each individual case.

The majority of neonatal seizures are acute, symptomatic seizures.[1] That is, they are symptomatic of acute brain injury such as hypoxic-ischemic encephalopathy (HIE) or stroke. Animal models and observational studies suggest that increased seizure burden in the setting of acute neonatal brain injury is associated with worsened outcomes.[2-4] For this reason, when treating acute symptomatic seizures, the initial goal of treatment is typically resolution of all seizures. Of note, this includes both clinical seizures and subclinical (electrographic-only) seizures. Over 85% of neonatal seizures are subclinical, with no outward clinical signs visible.[6] Subclinical seizures can only be identified through use of electroencephalography (EEG). As such, continuous electroencephalography (cEEG) is required for accurate diagnosis of neonatal seizures.[6–8] If cEEG is not available, amplitude integrated EEG (aEEG) may be used, though aEEG is known to have lower sensitivity and specificity compared with cEEG. With treatment for neonatal seizures, about half of neonates will have electroclinical dissociation, meaning outward signs might resolve even as EEG seizures continue.[9] cEEG monitoring is therefore particularly important after initiating treatment to accurately evaluate response as treatment is continued and to target complete resolution of seizures.

In contrast, approximately 20% of neonatal seizures are symptomatic of underlying brain malformation or neonatal-onset epilepsy, meaning ongoing seizures are expected. In these cases, the goal of treatment is more likely to reduce seizure burden as much as possible using oral agents, but with the knowledge that some breakthrough seizures may continue. cEEG may be useful in these cases to clarify which clinical events are true seizures with an electrographic correlate.

In rare cases, such as when palliative care has been selected, the goal of treatment might be only suppression of clinical seizures to maximize patient and parental comfort. In these cases, EEG is not necessary. The main consideration is efficacy of the AED for outward control of symptoms.

Regardless, it is essential to establish and communicate the goals of treatment for each neonate with seizures when initiating therapy. Treatment choices are heavily influenced by a shared understanding of the goal of treatment (e.g., complete resolution of seizures, seizure control as best as possible with oral agents, suppression of clinical seizures). These goals may be revisited throughout the course of treatment; good communication as goals are revised is essential in treating neonatal seizures.

Overview of Therapy

In any case of suspected neonatal seizures, the first steps in management are securing and maintaining the infant's airway, confirming adequate ventilation, and ensuring adequate circulation and perfusion. cEEG should be placed as soon as possible after the infant is stabilized, and can be placed concurrently with subsequent steps in evaluation and treatment. Interventions should not be delayed for EEG placement. The next step in acute management is to assess for reversible causes of seizure, including hypocalcemia, hypoglycemia, and hypomagnesemia. Electrolytes and glucose should be rapidly obtained and any electrolyte abnormalities or hypoglycemia corrected. Infants should also be evaluated for infectious causes of seizures, such as meningitis and sepsis, with appropriate antimicrobial therapy initiated. If seizures are highly suspected clinically or confirmed on EEG, a loading dose of an AED should be given as soon as possible. See Table 17.1 for dosing guidelines and Fig. 17.1 for a suggested treatment algorithm.

Current International League Against Epilepsy (ILAE) and World Health Organization (WHO) recommendations and expert consensus support phenobarbital as the first-line agent for the treatment of neonatal seizures.[8] Seizures unresponsive or only partially responsive to phenobarbital should be treated with an additional second-line agent: either phenytoin, benzodiazepines, or lidocaine.[8] Although not yet included in official guidelines, levetiracetam is increasingly popular as a second-line agent as well. No clear guidelines exist for third-line treatment, other than use of second-line agents already noted. Choice of third-line agent is largely dependent on clinician and institutional preference. In neonates with seizures refractory to adequate doses of multiple AEDs and when there is no clear etiology for seizures identified, vitamin-responsive epileptic encephalopathies should be considered. Trials of pyridoxine, pyridoxal 5′-phosphate (PLP), and folinic acid should be performed. Evaluation for specific genetic and metabolic causes of neonatal seizures should also be performed, with consideration of the ketogenic diet in select cases. Neuroimaging should be obtained to evaluate for acute causes of seizure and structural abnormalities as soon as possible; magnetic resonance imaging is the preferred imaging modality.[10,11] Identification of the underlying cause of seizures can be helpful in guiding choice of treatment and informing duration of anticipated treatment.

Table 17.1 ANTIEPILEPTIC DRUG DOSING AND SERUM LEVELS

AED	Loading Dose	Maintenance Dosing	Target Serum Level
Phenobarbital	20 mg/kg IV, may give additional doses of 10 mg/kg up to 40 mg/kg total	5 mg/kg/day divided in one to two doses	Obtain level 1–2 hr after loading dose, target range 20–40 µg/mL
Phenytoin/ fosphenytoin	15–20 mg PE/kg IV, may give additional 10 mg PE/kg once	3–5 mg/kg/day divided in two to four doses	Obtain level 1 hr after loading dose, target level 10–20 µg/mL total or 1–2 µg/mL free phenytoin
Midazolam	0.05 mg/kg IV over 10 min	Continuous infusion of 0.15 mg/kg/hr, may increase stepwise by 0.05 mg/kg/hr up to maximum of 0.5 mg/kg/hr	No established drug-level monitoring
Lorazepam	0.05–0.1 mg/kg IV given over 2–5 min, may repeat up to total dose of 0.15 mg/kg		
Clonazepam	0.01 mg/kg IV	0.01 mg/kg/dose for 3–5 doses	
Levetiracetam	20–50 mg/kg IV	30–50 mg/kg/day divided in two doses	No established drug-level monitoring
Topiramate	5–10 mg/kg enteral	1–5 mg/kg/day	5–20 µg/mL in adults, not established in neonates

Please see separate table (Table 17.2) for lidocaine dosing.
AED, antiepileptic drug; PE, phenytoin equivalents.

Antiepileptic Drugs

Phenobarbital

Phenobarbital, although an older AED, remains the mainstay of treatment for neonatal seizures. The 2011 WHO guidelines on neonatal seizures designate phenobarbital as a first-line treatment.[8] Similarly, surveys of child neurologists and neonatologists confirm that phenobarbital remains the first-choice medication for most physicians treating neonatal seizures.[12–15] This is largely because phenobarbital has the largest evidence base, with the most animal model data and the greatest clinical experience.[16–21]

Mechanism of Action

Phenobarbital is a barbiturate, which acts as an agonist at the gamma-aminobutyric acid-(GABA) A receptor to enhance inhibitory neurotransmission. Phenobarbital binding to the GABA-A receptor triggers opening of the postsynaptic chloride ion channel, which in mature neurons results in chloride entering the cell, hyperpolarizing the cell, and thus reducing excitability (see Fig. 17.2A). In immature neurons, however, a different mechanism exists that may explain why phenobarbital is only incompletely effective for neonatal seizures. In immature neurons, there is age-specific increased expression of a specific sodium-potassium-chloride cotransporter, NKCC1, that causes immature neurons to have much higher intracellular chloride levels than exist in mature neurons. Due to this high intracellular concentration of chloride in an immature neuron, when the GABA-A receptor is activated to open the chloride ion channel, there is not an influx of chloride. There may be little change, or even an outflow of chloride, with resulting depolarization (excitation). This correlates with the clinical finding that phenobarbital is incompletely effective for controlling neonatal seizures.[22] Ongoing research investigates whether adjunctive agents might enhance the efficacy of phenobarbital by manipulating chloride concentrations (see later discussion of bumetanide). It has also been proposed that phenobarbital reduces excitatory neurotransmission across the glutamatergic synapse through action on the alpha-amino-3-hydroxy-5-methyl-4-isoxazolepropionic acid (AMPA)/kainite glutamate receptor (see Fig. 17.2B).[19] It is possible that phenobarbital's partial efficacy is through an alternative mechanism to its GABAergic effects, such as this.

Neonate with suspected seizures:
- ABCs: secure and maintain airway, breathing/ ventilation, adequate circulation
- Assess for reversible causes: check electrolytes, glucose and correct if needed
- Evaluate for infection and consider antimicrobial therapy
- Obtain EEG when infant stabilized

concurrently with

Initial AED treatment for confirmed seizures:
Phenobarbital load 20 mg/kg IV

Continued seizures:
Phenobarbital 10 mg/kg IV, may repeat up to a total of 40 mg/kg IV

Persistent seizures: Use a second-line agent

Phenytoin/fosphenytoin 15-20 mg PE/kg IV

Or

Benzodiazepine, midazolam 0.05 mg/kg IV over 10 minutes

Or

Lidocaine 2 mg/kg IV infusion over 10 minutes

Persistent seizures after second-line agent: Use other second-line agent or levetiracetam

Levetiracetam 20-50 mg/kg IV

Or

Use second-line agent listed above not already given
*Note: do not give phenytoin and lidocaine together, as there is increased risk for cardiac toxicity

Seizures refractory to therapy:
- Pyridoxine IV 100 mg, repeat 100 mg every 5-10 minutes up to 500 mg
- PLP 10 mg/kg x2-3 doses 2 hours apart
- Folinic acid 5 mg x2 6 hours apart
- Obtain plasma (amino acids), CSF (pyridoxal phosphate, biogenic amines), and urine studies (AASA, pipecolic acid)

Concurrently with

Further evaluation/treatment:
- Consider other third-line agents: topiramate, others (see text for further details)
- Evaluate for genetic/metabolic causes
- Consider ketogenic diet or surgical interventions

Figure 17.1   General treatment algorithm, guided by WHO and ILAE recommendations.

Efficacy

Despite extensive clinical use, there is a paucity of high-grade clinical evidence supporting phenobarbital's efficacy. The only published randomized trial of phenobarbital for treatment of neonatal seizures was conducted by Painter and colleagues in 1999.[23] This study included 59 neonates with acute seizures confirmed on EEG. The majority had identified acute causes of seizure, such as HIE or stroke. Subjects were randomized to receive either phenobarbital first or phenytoin first. If seizures continued, the other drug was added. Among subjects receiving phenobarbital first, only 43% had control of seizures (versus 45% response rate with phenytoin). With the addition of phenytoin, this increased to 57%. Subsequent retrospective and small prospective studies have similarly reported phenobarbital monotherapy to provide seizure control rates of 43% to 63%.[24-26] Consistent across these studies has been lower efficacy in neonates with significantly abnormal background EEG[24,27] or with worse initial seizure burden.[23]

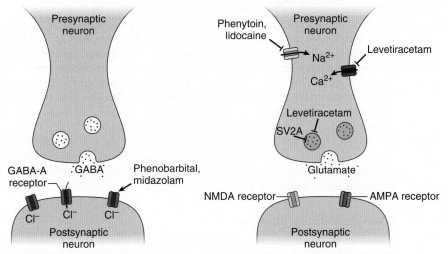

Figure 17.2 (A) Mechanism of action of AEDs at the GABAergic synapse. Phenobarbital and midazolam both act via the GABA-A receptor to open postsynaptic chloride channels. (B) Mechanism of action of AEDs at the glutamatergic synapse. Phenytoin/fosphenytoin and lidocaine both inhibit presynaptic voltage-gated sodium channels. Levetiracetam blocks presynaptic glutamate release via synaptic vesicle protein 2A and inhibits presynaptic calcium channels to prevent calcium influx into the neuron.

Of note, evidence suggests that phenobarbital should only be used for treatment of existing seizures and not for prophylaxis before seizures in neonates with encephalopathy.[28] A Cochrane review found that although prophylactic phenobarbital did reduce the risk of seizures for neonates with perinatal asphyxia, there was no reduction in mortality and no data to suggest improved long-term outcomes.[29] Similarly, prophylactic phenobarbital does not enhance the efficacy of hypothermia in limiting brain injury from HIE.[30]

Dosing

Initial phenobarbital treatment for confirmed seizures is a loading dose of 20 mg/kg intravenous (IV). After the initial load, neonates are typically started on short-term maintenance therapy of 5 mg/kg/day, divided into either twice-daily doses or as one daily dose.[16,17,19,31] The recommended loading dose is the same in the setting of therapeutic hypothermia.[31] If seizures do not subside on EEG after the initial 20 mg/kg loading dose, additional doses of 10 mg/kg can be given up to a total load of 40 mg/kg.[16,26] A phenobarbital level should be checked 1 to 2 hours after the loading dose is given, with a target level of 20 to 40 µg/mL.[16,17,23] Some patients may require levels up to 60 µg/mL to achieve seizure control,[32] although increased sedation is noted with levels >50 µg/mL.[17]

The half-life of phenobarbital varies widely with postnatal age, especially if given orally. In the first 10 days of life, there is delayed and incomplete absorption of phenobarbital from the gastrointestinal tract and the half-life is typically long, with increasing clearance in days 11 to 30 and 31 to 70.[32,33] Therefore, neonates may require increasing doses to achieve the same therapeutic effect after the first few weeks of life.

Metabolism of phenobarbital is inhibited by several drugs, including phenytoin. These medications may increase serum phenobarbital concentrations.[33] There are conflicting reports in the current literature regarding the effect of hypothermia on phenobarbital clearance. Shellhaas et al.[34] found that therapeutic hypothermia did not influence clearance of phenobarbital in a study of 39 infants with seizures undergoing cooling for hypoxic ischemic encephalopathy. In a small single-center study of 19 neonates, however, Filippi et al.[31] found that hypothermic infants had higher plasma concentrations and longer half-lives of phenobarbital compared with their normothermic counterparts.

Adverse Effects, Contraindications, and Monitoring

The most commonly encountered side effects with phenobarbital use are sedation and respiratory depression.[17,32,33] Other potential adverse effects include hypotension, skin rash, hepatotoxicity, and blood dyscrasia.[32] A large retrospective study showed an association between increased neonatal exposure to phenobarbital and worse neurodevelopmental outcomes. This included cognitive and motor scores on the Bayley Scales of Infant Development (8- and 9-point decrease per 100 mg/kg cumulative dose) and increased rates of cerebral palsy (2.3-fold increase per 100 mg/kg phenobarbital).[4] This is in keeping with the body of animal evidence demonstrating increased neuronal apoptosis, altered synaptic development, and long-term behavioral changes with early phenobarbital use.[2,35,36] Thus, although phenobarbital remains commonly used, there are concerns regarding overuse and adverse neurodevelopmental effects and an urgent need for alternative drugs.

Phenytoin/Fosphenytoin

Phenytoin/fosphenytoin is a common second-line agent for the treatment of neonatal seizures.[13,37] A recent systematic review demonstrated that there is no strong evidence that phenytoin is superior or inferior to alternative second-line AEDs levetiracetam or lidocaine.[16] WHO guidelines on the treatment of neonatal seizures also recommend phenytoin as a second-line treatment after phenobarbital, along with consideration of a benzodiazepine or lidocaine.[8] A 2009 survey of European neonatologists found phenytoin was most commonly used as a third-line treatment after benzodiazepines.[14]

Mechanism of Action

Phenytoin primarily acts at the glutamatergic synapse by inhibiting voltage-gated sodium channels (see Fig. 17.2B). In doing so, phenytoin prevents depolarization of the presynaptic neuron, which in turn inhibits excitatory neurotransmission at the glutamatergic synapse.[19] Fosphenytoin is a phosphate ester prodrug of phenytoin that can be given parenterally and is associated with fewer infusion-related adverse effects, but it is more expensive.[14]

Efficacy

In the only randomized controlled trial of phenytoin versus phenobarbital for first-line treatment of neonatal seizures, phenytoin had a response rate of 45% with complete seizure cessation, similar to phenobarbital.[23] In a later study, among neonates with seizures refractory to phenobarbital, phenytoin achieved seizure control in 16%.[38] There have been specific reports of phenytoin's efficacy in treating neonatal-onset encephalopathies, including SCN2A and KCNQ2 encephalopathy.[39,40] Further work is needed to clarify whether phenytoin has superior efficacy to other agents for these diseases.

Dosing

The typical loading dose of phenytoin is 15 to 20 mg/kg IV.[16,21] Of note, fosphenytoin is typically dosed in "PE," or "phenytoin equivalents," and thus a dose of 20 mg/kg phenytoin is equivalent to fosphenytoin 20 mg PE/kg. Neonates receiving phenytoin must have cardiac monitoring during infusion therapy per current WHO guidelines, given the risk for arrhythmia and/or bradycardia.[8] An additional 10 mg/kg load may be considered if seizures persist.[21] Further repeat boluses are to be avoided due to the risks of toxicity with higher serum levels. Phenytoin levels should be obtained 1 hour after the loading dose is given[16] with the goal range being 10 to 20 μg/mL.[33] Increasing adverse effects are seen at concentrations >30 μg/mL.[33] Because phenytoin is albumin bound, in patients with abnormal albumin levels, a free phenytoin level may be more reliable. A therapeutic range for free phenytoin is typically 1 to 2 μg/mL.

Maintenance dosing is typically 3 to 5 mg/kg/day divided two to four times daily.[16,21] However, because of rapid hepatic metabolism in the neonate, it can be challenging to maintain therapeutic phenytoin levels even with four-times-daily dosing. Thus dosing is frequently adjusted to target a blood level in the goal range and is rarely continued beyond the acute period.

Adverse Effects, Contraindications, and Monitoring

There are several drug–drug interactions to consider when using phenytoin. Acutely, the most important is avoidance of phenytoin when lidocaine has recently been given, as these drugs have a similar mechanism of action and combined have a much increased risk for cardiovascular effects. When considering chronic use, aluminum-, magnesium-, or calcium-containing antacids reduce the absorption of phenytoin, and valproic acid displaces phenytoin from albumin-binding sites and inhibits its metabolism.[33] Phenobarbital and carbamazepine may also have variable effects on the serum concentration of phenytoin.[33]

Several adverse effects have been seen with phenytoin use in neonates and older children. In the trial by Painter and colleagues, there were no significant adverse effects, with no changes in heart rate, heart rhythm, or respiratory status observed.[23] However, phenytoin has been described to cause arrhythmias, hypotension, and hepatotoxicity.[32,41,42] Soft tissue injury from extravasation of phenytoin has also been described, with the development of blue discoloration and blistering noted.[32,43,44] All of these effects are less severe with fosphenytoin versus phenytoin.[21,32,44] One case report in a 1-month-old infant described ileus at toxic phenytoin levels (serum concentration 91.8 μg/mL).[45]

The long-term risks of phenytoin administration are less clear. Similar to effects seen with phenobarbital, phenytoin has been demonstrated to cause neuronal apoptosis in the developing white matter of rat pups.[2] Widespread dose-dependent neurodegeneration has been demonstrated in rat pups, with a threshold dose of 20 mg/kg.[46] Specific effects on the cerebellum have also been studied, with cerebellar cells and motor coordination deficits seen in rat pups exposed to phenytoin.[47] Further study is needed to determine whether these animal studies translate to clinical deficits in humans.

Lidocaine

Lidocaine is widely used as a second- or third-line agent for neonatal seizures in Europe, though less often used in North America. In a survey of European neonatologists, providers from all hospitals except one reported using lidocaine as the third-line treatment for refractory neonatal seizures, after phenobarbital and benzodiazepines.[14] The 2011 WHO guidelines include lidocaine as a second-line agent, along with phenytoin or benzodiazepines, for neonatal seizures that do not respond to initial treatment with phenobarbital.[8] There is no high-quality evidence to clearly support efficacy of any one of the second-line therapies over the others.[16]

Mechanism of Action

An amine derivative of cocaine, lidocaine has many applications, including use as an anesthetic, sedative, antiarrhythmic, and anticonvulsant.[48] As an AED, lidocaine reduces excitatory neurotransmission at the glutamatergic synapse (see Fig. 17.2B). It does so by inhibiting voltage-gated sodium channels, in turn preventing depolarization of the presynaptic neuron.[19]

Efficacy

There have been no randomized, controlled trials to demonstrate the efficacy of lidocaine, though other evidence supports its use. Variable response rates have been reported with lidocaine, ranging from 53% to 76%,[25,49–51] with a particularly high seizure control rate of 91% reported in one small series of hypothermic infants receiving lidocaine as add-on therapy.[52] In a large retrospective study of 413 term and preterm infants, 71% had "good" (no seizures for >4 hours, no need for rescue medication) or "intermediate" (no seizures for 0–2 hours, but rescue medication needed after 2–4 hours) response to lidocaine.[53] Lidocaine response rates may vary based on gestational age, with one study finding seizure control in 76% of full-term infants versus only 55% of preterm neonates.[54] Limited evidence suggests lidocaine may be more efficacious than midazolam, but larger prospective studies are needed to confirm these findings.[50,54]

Dosing

Lidocaine is primarily metabolized by hepatic cytochrome P450 into two bioactive anticonvulsant metabolites that are renally excreted. Thus lidocaine elimination involves both hepatic and renal clearance.[48,55] It has a short half-life of 90 to 100 minutes and therefore is typically given as a continuous infusion.[55] Acceptable dosing regimens vary. Most begin with a loading dose of 2 mg/kg IV over 10 minutes, followed by a maintenance infusion of 2 to 6 mg/kg/hr titrated to seizure control; it is then typically continued for 12 to 24 hours and then rapidly weaned off for a total infusion duration of <48 hours.[14] A loading dose of 2 mg/kg IV over 10 minutes is used for neonates regardless of gestational age, birth weight, or cooling status.[18] The most commonly used maintenance regimen consists of an infusion over a total of 30 hours, with the infusion rate initially 6 mg/kg/hr for 6 hours, followed by a reduction to 4 mg/kg/hr for 12 hours, and then another reduction to 2 mg/kg/hr for 12 hours, for a total dosage of 110 mg/kg.[51,54] Care must be used when setting or adjusting lidocaine infusion rates, as some protocols list rates as mg/min, whereas others list as mg/kg/hr or mg/hr.

Preterm neonates have a lower clearance of lidocaine.[48,56] A proposed weight-adjusted regimen for low birth weight and very low birth weight neonates was developed to avoid supratherapeutic lidocaine levels in these patients; several variations of this regimen have been described.[18] In one pharmacokinetic study, therapeutic hypothermia reduced clearance of lidocaine in neonates by 24% compared with historic normothermic controls; therefore, a decreased dosing regimen was proposed for this population as well.[52] See Table 17.2 for further details.

Adverse Effects, Contraindications, and Monitoring

Lidocaine levels can be checked after completion of the initial infusion dose, with a goal concentration of 6 to 7 µg/mL.[48] A practical limitation of this is that lidocaine is typically used for <48 hours, and so results of level checks may not return in sufficient time to be relevant for treatment decisions. When levels are rapidly available, plasma concentrations of >9 µg/mL should be avoided given the increased risk for adverse effects. Because of the risk for arrhythmias, neonates treated with lidocaine require continuous cardiac monitoring throughout infusion.[8,57]

The adverse effect of most concern with lidocaine is cardiac toxicity, including bradycardia, ventricular tachycardia, prolonged QRS complex, and irregular heart rate.[19,51,57] There is increased risk of cardiac effects with plasma concentrations >9 µg/mL and after use of other cardiotoxic agents, including phenytoin.[19] For this reason, lidocaine should be avoided in neonates with congenital heart disease and infants who

Table 17.2   LIDOCAINE DOSING

	Loading Dose	First Infusion	Second Infusion	Third Infusion
General dosing[54]	2 mg/kg IV, given over 10 min	6 mg/kg/hr for 6 hr	4 mg/kg/hr for 12 hr	2 mg/kg/hr for 12 hr
Birth weights 0.8–1.5 kg[48]		5 mg/kg/hr for 4 hr	2.5 mg/kg/hr for 6 hr	1.25 mg/kg/hr for 12 hr
Birth weights 1.6–2.5 kg[48]		6 mg/kg/hr for 4 hr	3 mg/kg/hr for 6 hr	1.5 mg/kg/hr for 12 hr
Birth weights 2.6–4.5 kg[48]		7 mg/kg/hr for 4 hr	3.5 mg/kg/hr for 6 hr	1.75 mg/kg/hr for 12 hr
Hypothermia, birth weights 2.0–2.5 kg[52]		6 mg/kg/hr for 3.5 hr	3 mg/kg/hr for 12 hr	1.5 mg/kg/hr for 12 hr
Hypothermia, birth weights 2.5–4.5 kg[52]		7 mg/kg/hr for 3.5 hr	3.5 mg/kg/hr for 12 hr	1.75 mg/kg/hr for 12 hr

have received phenytoin in the preceding 24 hours.[18,32] Rates of cardiotoxicity range from 0% to 5% across multiple studies.[49,52,57] A large retrospective study reported a cardiac event rate of 1.3% to 1.9% in term and preterm neonates due to lidocaine. However, this rate was only 0.4% with appropriately dosed regimens.[54] The common practice of limiting lidocaine use to 48 hours or less is based on hopes of limiting the accumulation of lidocaine and its metabolites to limit the risk for cardiotoxicity.[51]

Paradoxically, lidocaine has proconvulsant activity at higher concentrations, though this mechanism is not well understood.[51,55] Several case reports describe seizure after lidocaine administration for circumcision in otherwise healthy neonates.[58,59] It has been speculated that these cases may reflect inadvertent intravenous administration instead of local administration of lidocaine at anesthetic does. At the doses used for neonatal seizure treatment, however, there is no evidence of a proconvulsant effect. When appropriately dosed and monitored, lidocaine can provide good efficacy for treatment of seizures in cases where phenobarbital has failed to provide complete seizure control.

Benzodiazepines

Benzodiazepines, including midazolam, lorazepam, and clonazepam, are a second- or third-line treatment option for neonatal seizures. In a survey of European neonatologists, 85% reported use of midazolam as their second-line treatment for neonatal seizures after phenobarbital.[14] In an international survey of primarily American neurologists and neonatologists, lorazepam was the first treatment choice of 22% for preterm neonates and 23% for term neonates.[15] When asked about using lorazepam as a second- or third-line treatment, 27% endorsed use in preterm infants and 26% endorsed use in term infants.[15] Midazolam was used as a first-line therapy by 3% of providers in term or preterm infants and was used as a second- or third-line treatment by 24% for preterm and 25% for term infants.[15] The 2011 WHO guidelines include benzodiazepines as second-line agents, along with phenytoin or lidocaine, for neonatal seizures that do not respond to initial treatment with phenobarbital.[8] Given the potential effects of sedation and respiratory depression, some authors recommend this class of medications as second- or third-line therapy and use it primarily in already-intubated neonates.[16]

Mechanism of Action

Benzodiazepines act on the postsynaptic side of the GABAergic synapse, modulating the chloride channel in the GABA-A receptor to increase inhibitory neurotransmission (see Fig. 17.2A).[19] It has been proposed that because midazolam is more lipophilic than lorazepam, midazolam crosses the blood–brain barrier more easily and has a more rapid onset of action.[17]

Efficacy

As with many other AEDs discussed here, a variable response to treatment has been observed with benzodiazepines, and high-quality evidence for efficacy is lacking. A very small study randomized neonates to benzodiazepines or lidocaine as second-line treatment after phenobarbital failure; this study found no effect on seizure burden with midazolam (three neonates) or clonazepam (three neonates).[25] In contrast, in a study with eight neonates receiving midazolam, 50% had a partial response,[50] with higher rates of seizure control reported in other series, ranging from 67% to 100%.[26,60–62] In two small studies of lorazepam, there was good to immediate response in 86% to 100% after treatment; however, both studies suffered from small sample size, with only seven patients each, and inconsistent use of EEG to confirm electrographic seizure activity.[63,64]

Dosing

Midazolam is primarily metabolized by cytochrome P450 enzymes in the liver, relying on hepatic clearance.[60] Typical midazolam dosing is a load of 0.05 mg/kg given intravenously over 10 minutes, followed by a continuous infusion of 0.15 mg/kg/hr to a maximum of 0.5 mg/kg/hr, increasing stepwise by 0.05 mg/kg/hr as needed

17

for seizure control.[17,18,60,65] Clonazepam may be given as a 0.01 mg/kg intravenous loading dose followed by 0.01 mg/kg/dose for an additional three to five doses if needed.[17] Lorazepam is typically given only as a loading dose of 0.05 to 0.1 mg/kg IV over 2 to 5 minutes, with no maintenance regimen.[17,18,21,63,64] The loading dose may be repeated up to a total dose 0.15 mg/kg if needed.[17,18,64] There have been no reported effects of hypothermia on the pharmacokinetics of midazolam; however, concomitant use of inotropes was shown to decrease midazolam clearance by 33%.[65]

Adverse Effects, Contraindications, and Monitoring

Potential adverse effects with benzodiazepines include hypotension, sedation, and respiratory depression, though some studies report no significant adverse effects within their cohorts.[26,63,64] Reported rates of hypotension vary widely, with as many as 33% to 38% of neonates treated with midazolam requiring inotropic support for hypotension in two small studies.[62,66] An inverse relationship between midazolam plasma concentration and mean arterial blood pressure was described in a prospective pharmacokinetic study of midazolam.[65] Lower rates were reported in a review of midazolam and lorazepam for both sedation and seizure control in neonates, with hypotension in only 8% and respiratory depression in 5%.[67] Midazolam may cause less respiratory depression and sedation than lorazepam because it is relatively faster acting.[21] The potential for adverse effects is greater when benzodiazepines are used in combination or when benzodiazepines are used in combination with barbiturates.

Of note, a retrospective study reported better neurodevelopmental outcomes at 1 year of life in infants treated with midazolam compared with infants who did not respond to treatment with phenobarbital/phenytoin.[26] This, however, may be more reflective of the damage caused by untreated seizures in neonates with improved neurodevelopmental outcomes in infants with better seizure control, rather than a specific benefit of midazolam. Of the benzodiazepines used for neonatal seizures, the largest body of evidence exists for midazolam; however, more studies are needed to evaluate its safety and efficacy in this population.

Levetiracetam

Levetiracetam is an increasingly common second- or third-line treatment for neonatal seizures. It has been approved by the US Food and Drug Administration (FDA) for children as young as 1 month,[16] and use has been described in neonates as young as 23 weeks' gestational age with no adverse effects reported.[68] It has also been described as treating seizures of various etiologies in term and preterm infants without significant adverse effects.[69,70] Because of this lack of significant adverse effects, levetiracetam is increasingly popular. In a 2007 survey of child neurologists, 47% reported using levetiracetam as second- or third-line treatment for neonatal seizures.[71] Though there is no evidence-based recommendation by the ILAE regarding use of any current agent used to treat neonatal seizures, they acknowledge that there is evidence to support levetiracetam as a therapy for seizures in older infants.[72] Levetiracetam is not, however, currently included in the WHO guidelines for treatment of neonatal seizures.[8,73]

Mechanism of Action

Levetiracetam inhibits excitatory neurotransmission at the glutamatergic synapse through inhibition of N-type calcium channels on the presynaptic neuron (see Fig. 17.2B). This prevents the influx of calcium into the cell, which in turn blocks exocytosis of intracellular vesicles containing glutamate.[19] Levetiracetam additionally prevents the release of glutamate from intracellular vesicles through modulation of synaptic vesicle protein 2A.[19,55,73,74]

Efficacy

There is no published randomized controlled trial data as of yet to demonstrate the efficacy of levetiracetam in neonatal seizures; limited evidence is available from other types of studies. In one retrospective cohort of 23 neonates treated with levetiracetam, 35% had reduction in seizures by >50% within 24 hours, with an additional 17% of neonates showing improvement within 24 to 72 hours.[75] In another retrospective study of 22 neonates, 32% had complete cessation of seizures on EEG after a loading dose of levetiracetam, 64% had seizure cessation within 24 hours, and up to 86% were seizure free by 48 hours.[76] In a separate retrospective study of 12 preterm neonates by the same author, 82% had complete cessation of seizures on EEG within 24 hours.[68] A prospective study of levetiracetam pharmacokinetics in 18 neonates showed similar results, with cessation of seizures in 33% of neonates treated with lower doses (20 mg/kg load) versus 42% at higher doses (40 mg/kg load).[77] In a prospective feasibility study of levetiracetam administered as the first-line antiepileptic agent to 38 neonates, 79% were seizure free by the end of the first week of treatment. However, >50% of the study population required 20 to 40 mg/kg phenobarbital loading doses as adjunctive therapy.[70] It is difficult to draw conclusions about the efficacy of levetiracetam as monotherapy for neonatal seizures, given the limitations of studies to date.

At the writing of this chapter, a phase II randomized blinded controlled trial is underway comparing levetiracetam and phenobarbital as first-line agents for treatment of neonatal seizures, with results eagerly awaited.[78]

Dosing

Most authors recommend a loading dose of 40 to 50 mg/kg IV levetiracetam,[16,76,77] though some extend this range to 20 to 50 mg/kg.[17,76] Maintenance dosing ranges from 20 to 25 mg/kg every 12 hours[76] or 30 mg/kg/day divided into twice- or three-times-daily dosing.[55] A small prospective pharmacokinetic study of levetiracetam concluded that the best levels were achieved using a loading dose of 40 mg/kg IV, followed by maintenance dosing of 10 mg/kg every 8 hours to keep trough levels >20 μg/mL in the first 3 days, then to keep trough levels >10 μg/mL in the rest of the first week, although goal levels are unclear in neonates.[77] A different prospective pharmacokinetic modeling study suggested higher loading doses are needed for neonates compared with older children and adults, due to the higher volume of distribution in neonates. These authors also recommended only twice-daily dosing in the first few weeks of life, even with a levetiracetam half-life of 8.9 hours, due to immature renal function in neonates.[79] Other authors have similarly advised higher loading doses for this reason.[55] Similarly, because preterm neonates have less mature renal function, longer half-lives may be seen in preterm compared with term newborns.[55]

Adverse Effects, Contraindications, and Monitoring

Levetiracetam does not require routine drug-level monitoring,[16,73] as there is a limited side effect profile and no well-established reference ranges for neonates.[73] Metabolism does not involve the cytochrome P450 system, and it is primarily renally excreted. There are no known clinically relevant drug–drug interactions with levetiracetam.[17]

Unlike many other AEDs, levetiracetam is not thought to cause neuronal apoptosis or disrupt synaptic development.[80–82] Some animal data suggest that levetiracetam may exert neuroprotective effects after hypoxic injury, with reduced neuronal apoptosis noted in rat pups treated with levetiracetam.[83]

Levetiracetam has been well tolerated in several study populations, with no acute adverse effects reported in term and preterm neonates,[68,75–77] though some infants were noted to be somnolent in the first 24 hours after the loading dose was given.[79] Temporary irritability reported in one patient improved with pyridoxine supplementation.[76] There is one case report of a neonate developing anaphylactic shock after 10 mg/kg of IV levetiracetam.[84]

In one follow-up study, levetiracetam use correlated with decreased cognitive and motor scores on the Bayley Scales of Infant Development at 24-month follow-up; however, this was to a much lesser degree than was associated with phenobarbital use (2- versus 8-point cognitive score and 3- versus 9-point motor score decreases with levetiracetam versus phenobarbital, respectively). Similarly, no association was found between levetiracetam exposure and development of cerebral palsy.[4] Although further research is needed to fully understand long-term outcomes after levetiracetam use, the adverse effect profile demonstrated to date makes this an attractive treatment option for neonatal seizures.

Emerging Therapies

Topiramate

Topiramate is a second-generation AED sometimes used to treat refractory neonatal seizures, despite a lack of data in neonates.[16,17] In a 2007 survey of pediatric neurologists, 54% recommended treatment of neonatal seizures with topiramate in at least some circumstances, either alone or with other agents.[71] This drug is not included in the current WHO guidelines for treatment of neonatal seizures.

Topiramate is thought to have multiple mechanisms of action, the most well characterized being inhibition of voltage-gated sodium channels on the presynaptic glutamatergic neuron to prevent depolarization.[19] It is also thought to act as a GABA-A receptor agonist, as well as an AMPA/kainite glutamate receptor antagonist.[85,86]

Small case series have reported efficacy in neonatal seizures. One retrospective cohort of six term newborns reported seizure reduction in 67%,[87] and 100% seizure control was achieved in a case series of three neonates with refractory seizures.[88] There is one reported ongoing trial of topiramate therapy in the setting of therapeutic hypothermia for HIE. This study is investigating the primary outcome of clinical or EEG seizures before hospital discharge.[89]

No intravenous formulation of topiramate is currently available commercially, limiting its use for acute seizures.[71] Topiramate is given to neonates as crushed tablets or extemporaneous liquid suspension, either orally or via nasogastric tube. Different doses have been reported, with loading doses typically 5 to 10 mg/kg and a maintenance dose of 1 to 5 mg/kg/day.[87,90] The therapeutic range for blood levels in adults is 5 to 20 μg/mL, but no therapeutic range of levels has been established for neonates.[17,90] Clearance may be prolonged in hypothermia, meaning that doses may need to be administered less often.[91]

No adverse effects have been noted in the published case series of topiramate in neonates.[87,90,91] Due to its inhibition of carbonic anhydrase in the renal tubules, topiramate can cause metabolic acidosis. However, no clinically significant decreases in bicarbonate were noted in a study of neonates receiving topiramate and undergoing hypothermia, a population already at risk for metabolic acidosis due to asphyxia and renal impairment.[91] Anecdotal reports of metabolic acidosis, transient hyperammonemia, and irritability or feeding problems were reported in a survey of pediatric neurologists.[71]

There has been concern for neurodevelopmental consequences of chronic administration, given the well-described cognitive effects in older children and adults.[92–95] However, animal studies suggest that topiramate may have neuroprotective effects and does not increase apoptosis.[96,97] Some animal studies even demonstrate improved cognitive function after treatment with topiramate, though this may be reflective of the detrimental effects of uncontrolled seizures on the developing brain rather than a specific benefit of topiramate.[98,99]

Carbamazepine

Carbamazepine is rarely used for neonatal seizures, though it may have a role in specific neonatal-onset epilepsies. Mutations in the KCNQ2 gene affect voltage-gated potassium channels and cause 10% of early infantile epileptic encephalopathies associated with intractable seizures and developmental delay.[40] Carbamazepine blocks sodium channels that colocalize with KCNQ potassium channels, which is hypothesized to affect the function of the potassium channel complex. As such, carbamazepine, along with other sodium channel blockers including phenytoin, may be a preferred therapy for seizures in neonates with KCNQ2 encephalopathy.[40,100]

A small study of preterm infants with refractory seizures reported that 90% achieved good clinical seizure control with carbamazepine. The true efficacy is unknown, however, as this study did not use EEG monitoring to assess response.[101] Carbamazepine has been given as an initial dose of 10 mg/kg, followed by maintenance therapy of 5 to 7 mg/kg every 8 hours starting 24 hours after the loading dose.[102] A drop in serum concentrations between days 8 and 15 of life has been observed due to increased capacity of liver cytochrome CYP3A4 to metabolize the drug.[55] Of note, enzyme induction by phenobarbital and phenytoin may cause increased elimination of carbamazepine.[55] In the few studies of carbamazepine in neonates, no significant adverse effects were reported.[101,102] Generally, this agent is used only when other treatments have failed or when a specific neonatal-onset epilepsy diagnosis suggests potential efficacy.

Valproic Acid

Little literature exists to support the use of valproic acid in neonates. There is generally reluctance to use valproic acid due to the known risk of (and black box warning for) hepatic failure with this drug in young children. In particular, valproate should not be used when there is the possibility of a metabolic or mitochondrial disorder. At the same time, some providers do still use valproic acid for refractory seizures with a clearly identified cause that is not metabolic or mitochondrial. In a survey of Israeli neurologists and neonatologists, neurologists were more likely to recommend valproic acid and topiramate for the treatment of intractable neonatal seizures versus lidocaine and benzodiazepines recommended by neonatologists.[103] The mechanism of action of valproic acid is not completely understood, with multiple targets including inhibition of sodium channels and increased GABA function.[55] A loading dose of 20 to 30 mg/kg of rectal valproic acid in two neonates followed by maintenance therapy in one patient of 30 mg/kg/day rectally divided twice daily achieved good seizure control in a case report of two neonates who failed phenobarbital and phenytoin.[104] If valproic acid is used in a neonate, it should be in close consultation with a child neurologist.

Bumetanide

Though phenobarbital is currently used as a monotherapy for first-line treatment of neonatal seizures, there is some evidence for a potential role for chloride cotransporters as adjunctive therapies with phenobarbital to reduce phenobarbital resistance. However, recent safety concerns have tempered early enthusiasm for these agents.

Bumetanide is a loop diuretic that inhibits sodium–potassium–chloride cotransporters NKCC1 and NKCC2, which both move chloride into cells. NKCC2 is expressed in renal tubular cells, whereas neurons express NKCC1 with increased expression in immature neurons, making this a potential target for AEDs in neonates. As mentioned previously (see the earlier discussion of phenobarbital), GABA may be excitatory in immature neurons with higher intracellular levels of chloride, due to high NKCC1 expression with low KCC2 potassium chloride cotransporter expression. By blocking NKCC1, bumetanide may prevent intracellular chloride accumulation, which may then allow GABA agonists to have greater effect.[17,19,32,86]

In two recent studies of neonatal rat pups, one demonstrated increased efficacy of phenobarbital with bumetanide versus phenobarbital alone.[105] However, the other demonstrated no difference between phenobarbital plus adjunctive therapy with bumetanide versus phenobarbital alone.[106] Unfortunately, a large phase I/II trial assessing use of bumetanide was stopped early due to hearing loss and poor efficacy. A review of this study emphasized that there was a reduced seizure burden seen with bumetanide use and argued that hearing loss may not be entirely attributable to the study drug.[107,108] An additional randomized trial of bumetanide remains underway.[109] With the evidence currently available, the use of bumetanide for the treatment of neonatal seizures cannot be recommended at this time.

Other Therapies

Ketogenic Diet

The ketogenic diet is a dietary therapy in which the majority of caloric intake is fat to put the body in a state of chronic ketosis, in turn altering energy supply to the brain. The ketogenic diet is used in children with intractable epilepsy with good evidence, though it is used less commonly in neonates and there is less published evidence for use in this population.[110,111] There may be a role for the ketogenic diet in certain cases of inborn errors of metabolism, and it is the treatment of choice in patients with pyruvate dehydrogenase complex deficiency and glucose transporter 1 (GLUT-1) deficiency.[72,112] A case series of three neonates with early myoclonic epilepsy and nonketotic hyperglycinemia demonstrated good seizure response to the ketogenic diet after failure of multiple AEDs.[113] More high-quality evidence is needed to determine the safety and efficacy of the ketogenic diet in neonates.

Surgery

With technologic advances enhancing the precision of epilepsy surgery, more options are now available for neonates with intractable seizures. Current ILAE recommendations state that standard care for infants with seizures should include identifying patients who are potential candidates for epilepsy surgery.[72] Although not common among neonates, surgery may be considered as an option in select cases of refractory seizures.

Vitamin Supplementation

A minority of neonates with seizures have underlying disorders of metabolism that respond to specific vitamin supplementation. These conditions are sometimes described as *vitamin-responsive epilepsies*. In addition, there are reports of vitamin supplementation reducing neonatal seizures due to other causes, though these are less consistent. For neonates with seizures of unknown etiology that remain refractory to conventional AEDs, an empiric trial of vitamin supplementation is warranted. After an empiric vitamin treatment has been started, it should be continued until confirmatory testing returns, unless another clear etiology for seizures is found. This may be up to several weeks, depending on laboratory capabilities.

Pyridoxine

Pyridoxine-dependent epilepsy (PDE) is a rare cause of intractable seizures in neonates due to a deficiency of alpha-aminoadipic semialdehyde dehydrogenase (antiquitin).[114] Neonates with intractable seizures not responsive to therapy with AEDs should receive an empiric trial of pyridoxine (vitamin B_6) therapy.[17,18,32]

Patients should be monitored with cEEG and given 100 mg of pyridoxine intravenously, watching for response on EEG. In some regimens, it is proposed that doses of 100 mg may be repeated every 5 to 10 minutes up to a cumulative dose of 500 mg, at which point no further pyridoxine should be loaded.[114] This should be done only in an intensive care unit setting with respiratory support resources readily available, as first administration of pyridoxine may result in respiratory arrest in neonates responsive to treatment.[115,116] Patients with a positive response to intravenous pyridoxine should be maintained on enteral pyridoxine 15 to 18 mg/kg/day divided into twice-daily doses,[114] though ranges up to 15 to 30 mg/kg/day divided into two or three doses up to a maximum of 200 mg/day have been reported in neonates.[117] Lifelong therapy with pyridoxine is required in patients with PDE.[114] Adjuvant therapy with folinic acid 3 to 5 mg/kg/day has been suggested for infants with PDE.[117]

The diagnosis of pyridoxine-dependent seizures is typically made by clinical and electrographic response to intravenous pyridoxine, though biochemical tests (elevated serum pipecolic acid levels and elevated serum, cerebrospinal fluid [CSF], or urine levels of alpha-aminoadipic semialdehyde [AASA]) and testing of the *ALDH7A1* gene are becoming available.[114,118–120] It is important to note that pipecolic acid and AASA levels cannot be followed as a measure of treatment response, as these will remain elevated with treatment.[118,119] Conversely, these markers may remain abnormal and be useful to identify affected patients even if drawn after a trial of pyridoxine has been initiated.

Pyridoxine therapy is known to cause dorsal root ganglionopathy and sensory neuropathy at high doses; therefore, the maximum dose of 30 mg/kg/day should be observed.[114,116,117]

Pyridoxal 5′-phosphate (PLP)

PLP-dependent seizures are caused by a deficiency of pyridox(am)ine 5′-phosphate oxidase (PNPO) encoded by the *PNPO* gene.[114,121] Similar to PDE, PNPO deficiency should be suspected in neonates with intractable seizures unresponsive to AED treatment, and empiric PLP therapy should be trialed.[17,18,32] Because PLP is less readily available than pyridoxine, in practice many neonates have completed a pyridoxine trial before initiating a PLP trial. However, if PLP is available, this can be given as empiric therapy for both PDE and PLP-dependent seizures.

PLP is given enterally, with a recommended dose of 30 mg/kg/day divided into three or four doses, given for at least three to five days to observe for clinical and EEG response.[114,116] Acutely, a trial of 10 mg/kg/dose for 2 doses given 2 hours apart can be considered.[121] If the diagnosis is confirmed, maintenance therapy of 30 to 50 mg/kg/day divided in four to six doses should be continued.[114,121] As with PDE, lifelong therapy is required, and hepatic function should be monitored given reports of cirrhosis with treatment.[117,122]

A diagnosis of PLP can be confirmed by serum, urine, and CSF metabolic studies. Increased CSF L-DOPA, 3-methoxytyrosine, threonine, and glycine, with decreased CSF homovanillic acid and 5-hydroxyindoleacetic acid, increased urine vanillactic acid, and increased plasma levels of threonine and glycine are characteristic of PNPO deficiency.[123,124] This may be more directly tested with demonstration of decreased levels of PLP in the CSF or *PNPO* gene sequencing.[125]

Folinic Acid

First described in 1995, folinic acid–responsive seizures are another cause of vitamin-responsive epileptic encephalopathy.[126] Treatment with folinic acid should be considered in neonates with intractable seizures not responsive to pyridoxine or with a transient response to pyridoxine.[127] There is some crossover between patients who respond to pyridoxine and those who respond to folinic acid, as patients with a yet-to-be-identified folinic acid–responsive CSF marker (termed *peak X*)[116] also have antiquin mutations, and patients with PDE also often have the same elevated peak in their CSF.[114,128] Patients should be treated with enteral folinic acid (5-formyltetrahydrofolate) 3 to 5 mg/kg/day for 3 to 5 days to evaluate for response to treatment, followed by maintenance therapy of 3 to 5 mg/kg/day divided into three doses.[114] A trial of 5 mg for 2 doses given 6 hours apart in the acute period can be considered.[121] Care must be used to avoid confusion with folic acid, a common mistake when folinic acid is prescribed.

Biotin

Biotinidase deficiency is another rare cause of intractable epilepsy in neonates caused by mutations of the biotinidase *BTD* gene.[129] It is associated with optic atrophy with visual loss, sensorineural hearing loss, conjunctivitis, cheilosis, and alopecia.[117] Testing for this disorder is included in most newborn screening programs. Profound or severe deficiency is characterized by <10% enzymatic activity, whereas 10% to 30% of activity is retained in cases of partial deficiency. Patients with both partial and severe deficiency should be treated with 5 to 20 mg of biotin daily, and patients must continue lifelong therapy.[117,129,130]

Discontinuation of Therapy

After acute seizures resolve, there is controversy regarding how long AED treatment must be continued. In cases of neonatal-onset epilepsy, AEDs will likely be required in the long term and thus should be continued at the time of hospital discharge. For neonates with acute symptomatic seizures or seizures of unknown cause, however, the appropriate duration of treatment is unclear. The 2015 ILAE Task Force Report does not include recommendations for how long neonates with seizures should be treated, given there is no clear evidence to advise this.[72] The 2011 WHO guidelines on this topic, based on expert opinion in the absence of supporting data, state that medication may be discontinued abruptly before hospital discharge without tapering

17

in neonates who achieve seizure control on a single AED. However, if more than one AED is required for seizure control, that expert consensus recommends discontinuing medications one by one, with phenobarbital being the final medication to discontinue.[8]

Historically, providers had recommended continuation of AED therapy for several months before tapering medications.[131] More recent practice is trending toward discontinuation of AED therapy during the neonatal period to avoid the potential neurodevelopmental problems linked to chronic AED administration. In a large multicenter prospective cohort study, practices varied widely, with timing of medication discontinuation largely dependent on the institution, etiology of seizures, and EEG and examination findings.[132] There was large variability in practice between hospitals; some sites sent the vast majority of neonates home on AEDs (>85%), whereas others discontinued medication in almost all patients before discharge. Patients with EEG-confirmed seizures, seizures refractory to initial AED loading doses, an abnormal neurologic exam, and status epilepticus were more likely to be discharged home on medication.[132]

An older retrospective study demonstrated no significant correlation between seizure etiology or initial examination with recurrence of seizures during the tapering of AEDs. The presence of normal background on EEG and normal computed tomography findings were correlated with successful tapering of AEDs.[133]

As there are no clear recommendations on this topic with little available evidence, providers must evaluate each case of neonatal seizures individually when deciding when to discontinue therapy. Given the concerns for long-term adverse effects with chronic AED administration, we recommend early discontinuation of AEDs for neonates with acute symptomatic seizures. Our own practice is to continue maintenance AED dosing until seizures are totally controlled for at least 48 hours. Subsequently, for neonates with seizures due to ischemic injury or with no cause identified, AEDs are stopped before hospital discharge. If multiple AEDs were required in the acute period, it may be that one or more AEDs are stopped before discharge, with the last AED continued until follow-up with a neurologist a few weeks after discharge. In acute symptomatic seizures with a higher risk for recurrence (e.g., hemorrhage), we do consider a longer initial treatment period.

Ideally, medication tapering and discontinuation are performed in the neonatal intensive care unit, where the infant can be closely monitored for seizure recurrence. In neonates with neonatal-onset epilepsy, AEDs most often should be continued at hospital discharge. Discontinuation of therapy, however, is ultimately provider and institution dependent.

Conclusion

Current recommendations for the treatment of neonatal seizures are largely based on historical experience, with a dearth of high-quality evidence to support the use of the aforementioned therapies. Currently available AEDs have been demonstrated to achieve only a partial response, and further research into optimal treatment regimens for this population is needed. The suggested treatments in this chapter are based on the recommendations of ILAE and WHO guidelines, experts in the field, and the evidence available in the literature, but should be tailored and adjusted for each individual patient.

REFERENCES

1. Glass HC, Shellhaas RA, Wusthoff CJ, et al. Contemporary profile of seizures in neonates: a prospective cohort study. *J Pediatr*. 2016;174:98–103.
2. Kaushal S, Tamer Z, Opoku F, et al. Anticonvulsant drug-induced cell death in the developing white matter of the rodent brain. *Epilepsia*. 2016;57(5):727–734.
3. Kang SK, Kadam SD. Neonatal seizures: impact on neurodevelopmental outcomes. *Front Pediatr*. 2015;3:101.
4. Maitre NL, Smolinsky C, Slaughter JC, et al. Adverse neurodevelopmental outcomes after exposure to phenobarbital and levetiracetam for the treatment of neonatal seizures. *J Perinatol*. 2013;33(11): 841–846.
5. van Rooij LG, Toet MC, van Huffelen AC, et al. Effect of treatment of subclinical neonatal seizures detected with aEEG: randomized, controlled trial. *Pediatrics*. 2010;125(2):e358–e366.

6. Shellhaas RA, Chang T, Tsuchida T, et al. The American Clinical Neurophysiology Society's Guideline on Continuous Electroencephalography Monitoring in Neonates. *J Clin Neurophysiol.* 2011;28(6): 611–617.
7. Boylan GB, Stevenson NJ, Vanhatalo S. Monitoring neonatal seizures. *Semin Fetal Neonatal Med.* 2013;18(4):202–208.
8. WHO Guidelines Approved by the Guidelines Review Committee. Guidelines on Neonatal Seizures. Geneva: World Health Organization. Copyright (c) World Health Organization; 2011.
9. Scher MS, Alvin J, Gaus L, et al. Uncoupling of EEG-clinical neonatal seizures after antiepileptic drug use. *Pediatr Neurol.* 2003;28(4):277–280.
10. Weeke LC, Groenendaal F, Toet MC, et al. The aetiology of neonatal seizures and the diagnostic contribution of neonatal cerebral magnetic resonance imaging. *Dev Med Child Neurol.* 2015;57(3): 248–256.
11. Osmond E, Billetop A, Jary S, et al. Neonatal seizures: magnetic resonance imaging adds value in the diagnosis and prediction of neurodisability. *Acta Paediatr.* 2014;103(8):820–826.
12. Wickstrom R, Hallberg B, Bartocci M. Differing attitudes toward phenobarbital use in the neonatal period among neonatologists and child neurologists in Sweden. *Eur J Paediatr Neurol.* 2013;17(1):55–63.
13. Hellstrom-Westas L, Boylan G, Agren J. Systematic review of neonatal seizure management strategies provides guidance on anti-epileptic treatment. *Acta Paediatr.* 2015;104(2):123–129.
14. Vento M, de Vries LS, Alberola A, et al. Approach to seizures in the neonatal period: a European perspective. *Acta Paediatr.* 2010;99(4):497–501.
15. Glass HC, Kan J, Bonifacio SL, et al. Neonatal seizures: treatment practices among term and preterm infants. *Pediatr Neurol.* 2012;46(2):111–115.
16. Slaughter LA, Patel AD, Slaughter JL. Pharmacological treatment of neonatal seizures: a systematic review. *J Child Neurol.* 2013;28(3):351–364.
17. van Rooij LG, van den Broek MP, Rademaker CM, et al. Clinical management of seizures in newborns : diagnosis and treatment. *Paediatr Drugs.* 2013;15(1):9–18.
18. van Rooij LG, Hellstrom-Westas L, de Vries LS. Treatment of neonatal seizures. *Semin Fetal Neonatal Med.* 2013;18(4):209–215.
19. Donovan MD, Griffin BT, Kharoshankaya L, et al. Pharmacotherapy for neonatal seizures: current knowledge and future perspectives. *Drugs.* 2016;76(6):647–661.
20. Brodie MJ, Kwan P. Current position of phenobarbital in epilepsy and its future. *Epilepsia.* 2012;53(suppl 8):40–46.
21. Sankar JM, Agarwal R, Deorari A, et al. Management of neonatal seizures. *Indian J Pediatr.* 2010; 77(10):1129–1135.
22. Booth D, Evans DJ. Anticonvulsants for neonates with seizures. *Cochrane Database Syst Rev.* 2004;(4):CD004218.
23. Painter MJ, Scher MS, Stein AD, et al. Phenobarbital compared with phenytoin for the treatment of neonatal seizures. *N Engl J Med.* 1999;341(7):485–489.
24. Spagnoli C, Seri S, Pavlidis E, et al. Phenobarbital for Neonatal Seizures: Response Rate and Predictors of Refractoriness. *Neuropediatrics.* 2016;47(5):318–326.
25. Boylan GB, Rennie JM, Chorley G, et al. Second-line anticonvulsant treatment of neonatal seizures: a video-EEG monitoring study. *Neurology.* 2004;62(3):486–488.
26. Castro Conde JR, Hernandez Borges AA, Domenech Martinez E, et al. Midazolam in neonatal seizures with no response to phenobarbital. *Neurology.* 2005;64(5):876–879.
27. Boylan GB, Rennie JM, Pressler RM, et al. Phenobarbitone, neonatal seizures, and video-EEG. *Arch Dis Child Fetal Neonatal Ed.* 2002;86(3):F165–F170.
28. Evans DJ, Levene MI, Tsakmakis M. Anticonvulsants for preventing mortality and morbidity in full term newborns with perinatal asphyxia. *Cochrane Database Syst Rev.* 2007;(3):CD001240.
29. Young L, Berg M, Soll R. Prophylactic barbiturate use for the prevention of morbidity and mortality following perinatal asphyxia. *Cochrane Database Syst Rev.* 2016;(5):CD001240.
30. Sarkar S, Barks JD, Bapuraj JR, et al. Does phenobarbital improve the effectiveness of therapeutic hypothermia in infants with hypoxic-ischemic encephalopathy? *J Perinatol.* 2012;32(1):15–20.
31. Filippi L, la Marca G, Cavallaro G, et al. Phenobarbital for neonatal seizures in hypoxic ischemic encephalopathy: a pharmacokinetic study during whole body hypothermia. *Epilepsia.* 2011;52(4): 794–801.
32. Glass HC. Neonatal seizures: advances in mechanisms and management. *Clin Perinatol.* 2014; 41(1):177–190.
33. Patsalos PN, Berry DJ, Bourgeois BF, et al. Antiepileptic drugs–best practice guidelines for therapeutic drug monitoring: a position paper by the subcommission on therapeutic drug monitoring, ILAE Commission on Therapeutic Strategies. *Epilepsia.* 2008;49(7):1239–1276.
34. Shellhaas RA, Ng CM, Dillon CH, et al. Population pharmacokinetics of phenobarbital in infants with neonatal encephalopathy treated with therapeutic hypothermia. *Pediatr Crit Care Med.* 2013; 14(2):194–202.
35. Gutherz SB, Kulick CV, Soper C, et al. Brief postnatal exposure to phenobarbital impairs passive avoidance learning and sensorimotor gating in rats. *Epilepsy Behav.* 2014;37:265–269.
36. Bittigau P, Sifringer M, Ikonomidou C. Antiepileptic drugs and apoptosis in the developing brain. *Ann N Y Acad Sci.* 2003;993:103–114.
37. Shetty J. Neonatal seizures in hypoxic-ischaemic encephalopathy–risks and benefits of anticonvulsant therapy. *Dev Med Child Neurol.* 2015;57(suppl 3):40–43.
38. Bye A, Flanagan D. Electroencephalograms, clinical observations and the monitoring of neonatal seizures. *J Paediatr Child Health.* 1995;31(6):503–507.

39. Howell KB, McMahon JM, Carvill GL, et al. SCN2A encephalopathy: A major cause of epilepsy of infancy with migrating focal seizures. *Neurology*. 2015;85(11):958–966.

40. Pisano T, Numis AL, Heavin SB, et al. Early and effective treatment of KCNQ2 encephalopathy. *Epilepsia*. 2015;56(5):685–691.

41. Pathak G, Upadhyay A, Pathak U, et al. Phenobarbitone versus phenytoin for treatment of neonatal seizures: an open-label randomized controlled trial. *Indian Pediatr*. 2013;50(8):753–757.

42. Appleton RE, Gill A. Adverse events associated with intravenous phenytoin in children: a prospective study. *Seizure*. 2003;12(6):369–372.

43. Sharief N, Goonasekera C. Soft tissue injury associated with intravenous phenytoin in a neonate. *Acta Paediatr*. 1994;83(11):1218–1219.

44. Mueller EW, Boucher BA. Fosphenytoin: current place in therapy. *J Pediatr Pharmacol Ther*. 2004;9(4):265–273.

45. Lowry JA, Vandover JC, DeGreeff J, et al. Unusual presentation of iatrogenic phenytoin toxicity in a newborn. *J Med Toxicol*. 2005;1(1):26–29.

46. Bittigau P, Sifringer M, Genz K, et al. Antiepileptic drugs and apoptotic neurodegeneration in the developing brain. *Proc Natl Acad Sci USA*. 2002;99(23):15089–15094.

47. Ohmori H, Ogura H, Yasuda M, et al. Developmental neurotoxicity of phenytoin on granule cells and Purkinje cells in mouse cerebellum. *J Neurochem*. 1999;72(4):1497–1506.

48. van den Broek MP, Huitema AD, van Hasselt JG, et al. Lidocaine (lignocaine) dosing regimen based upon a population pharmacokinetic model for preterm and term neonates with seizures. *Clin Pharmacokinet*. 2011;50(7):461–469.

49. Lundqvist M, Agren J, Hellstrom-Westas L, et al. Efficacy and safety of lidocaine for treatment of neonatal seizures. *Acta Paediatr*. 2013;102(9):863–867.

50. Shany E, Benzaqen O, Watemberg N. Comparison of continuous drip of midazolam or lidocaine in the treatment of intractable neonatal seizures. *J Child Neurol*. 2007;22(3):255–259.

51. Malingre MM, Van Rooij LG, Rademaker CM, et al. Development of an optimal lidocaine infusion strategy for neonatal seizures. *Eur J Pediatr*. 2006;165(9):598–604.

52. van den Broek MP, Rademaker CM, van Straaten HL, et al. Anticonvulsant treatment of asphyxiated newborns under hypothermia with lidocaine: efficacy, safety and dosing. *Arch Dis Child Fetal Neonatal Ed*. 2013;98(4):F341–F345.

53. Weeke LC, Toet MC, van Rooij LG, et al. Lidocaine response rate in aEEG-confirmed neonatal seizures: retrospective study of 413 full-term and preterm infants. *Epilepsia*. 2016;57(2):233–242.

54. Weeke LC, Schalkwijk S, Toet MC, et al. Lidocaine-associated cardiac events in newborns with seizures: incidence, symptoms and contributing factors. *Neonatology*. 2015;108(2):130–136.

55. Tulloch JK, Carr RR, Ensom MH. A systematic review of the pharmacokinetics of antiepileptic drugs in neonates with refractory seizures. *J Pediatr Pharmacol Ther*. 2012;17(1):31–44.

56. Rey E, Radvanyi-Bouvet MF, Bodiou C, et al. Intravenous lidocaine in the treatment of convulsions in the neonatal period: monitoring plasma levels. *Ther Drug Monit*. 1990;12(4):316–320.

57. van Rooij LG, Toet MC, Rademaker KM, et al. Cardiac arrhythmias in neonates receiving lidocaine as anticonvulsive treatment. *Eur J Pediatr*. 2004;163(11):637–641.

58. Rezvani M, Finkelstein Y, Verjee Z, et al. Generalized seizures following topical lidocaine administration during circumcision: establishing causation. *Paediatr Drugs*. 2007;9(2):125–127.

59. Moran LR, Hossain T, Insoft RM. Neonatal seizures following lidocaine administration for elective circumcision. *J Perinatol*. 2004;24(6):395–396.

60. van Leuven K, Groenendaal F, Toet MC, et al. Midazolam and amplitude-integrated EEG in asphyxiated full-term neonates. *Acta Paediatr*. 2004;93(9):1221–1227.

61. Sheth RD, Buckley DJ, Gutierrez AR, et al. Midazolam in the treatment of refractory neonatal seizures. *Clin Neuropharmacol*. 1996;19(2):165–170.

62. Sirsi D, Nangia S, LaMothe J, et al. Successful management of refractory neonatal seizures with midazolam. *J Child Neurol*. 2008;23(6):706–709.

63. Deshmukh A, Wittert W, Schnitzler E, et al. Lorazepam in the treatment of refractory neonatal seizures. A pilot study. *Am J Dis Child*. 1986;140(10):1042–1044.

64. Maytal J, Novak GP, King KC. Lorazepam in the treatment of refractory neonatal seizures. *J Child Neurol*. 1991;6(4):319–323.

65. van den Broek MP, van Straaten HL, Huitema AD, et al. Anticonvulsant effectiveness and hemodynamic safety of midazolam in full-term infants treated with hypothermia. *Neonatology*. 2015;107(2):150–156.

66. Hu KC, Chiu NC, Ho CS, et al. Continuous midazolam infusion in the treatment of uncontrollable neonatal seizures. *Acta Paediatr Taiwan*. 2003;44(5):279–281.

67. Ng E, Klinger G, Shah V, et al. Safety of benzodiazepines in newborns. *Ann Pharmacother*. 2002; 36(7–8):1150–1155.

68. Khan O, Cipriani C, Wright C, et al. Role of intravenous levetiracetam for acute seizure management in preterm neonates. *Pediatr Neurol*. 2013;49(5):340–343.

69. Shoemaker MT, Rotenberg JS. Levetiracetam for the treatment of neonatal seizures. *J Child Neurol*. 2007;22(1):95–98.

70. Ramantani G, Ikonomidou C, Walter B, et al. Levetiracetam: safety and efficacy in neonatal seizures. *Eur J Paediatr Neurol*. 2011;15(1):1–7.

71. Silverstein FS, Ferriero DM. Off-label use of antiepileptic drugs for the treatment of neonatal seizures. *Pediatr Neurol*. 2008;39(2):77–79.

72. Wilmshurst JM, Gaillard WD, Vinayan KP, et al. Summary of recommendations for the management of infantile seizures: Task Force Report for the ILAE Commission of Pediatrics. *Epilepsia*. 2015; 56(8):1185–1197.

73. Mruk AL, Garlitz KL, Leung NR. Levetiracetam in neonatal seizures: a review. *J Pediatr Pharmacol Ther*. 2015;20(2):76–89.
74. Lynch BA, Lambeng N, Nocka K, et al. The synaptic vesicle protein SV2A is the binding site for the antiepileptic drug levetiracetam. *Proc Natl Acad Sci USA*. 2004;101(26):9861–9866.
75. Abend NS, Gutierrez-Colina AM, Monk HM, et al. Levetiracetam for treatment of neonatal seizures. *J Child Neurol*. 2011;26(4):465–470.
76. Khan O, Chang E, Cipriani C, et al. Use of intravenous levetiracetam for management of acute seizures in neonates. *Pediatr Neurol*. 2011;44(4):265–269.
77. Sharpe CM, Capparelli EV, Mower A, et al. A seven-day study of the pharmacokinetics of intravenous levetiracetam in neonates: marked changes in pharmacokinetics occur during the first week of life. *Pediatr Res*. 2012;72(1):43–49.
78. Haas RH. Efficacy of Intravenous Levetiracetam in Neonatal Seizures (NEOLEV2). In: ClinicalTrials. gov [Internet]. Bethesda (MD): National Library of Medicine (US); 2000. Available from: http:// clinicaltrials.gov/show/NCT01720667. Cited November 10, 2016. NLM Identifier: NCT01720667.
79. Merhar SL, Schibler KR, Sherwin CM, et al. Pharmacokinetics of levetiracetam in neonates with seizures. *J Pediatr*. 2011;159(1):152–154.e153.
80. Forcelli PA, Janssen MJ, Vicini S, et al. Neonatal exposure to antiepileptic drugs disrupts striatal synaptic development. *Ann Neurol*. 2012;72(3):363–372.
81. Kim JS, Kondratyev A, Tomita Y, et al. Neurodevelopmental impact of antiepileptic drugs and seizures in the immature brain. *Epilepsia*. 2007;48(suppl 5):19–26.
82. Manthey D, Asimiadou S, Stefovska V, et al. Sulthiame but not levetiracetam exerts neurotoxic effect in the developing rat brain. *Exp Neurol*. 2005;193(2):497–503.
83. Kilicdag H, Daglioglu K, Erdogan S, et al. The effect of levetiracetam on neuronal apoptosis in neonatal rat model of hypoxic ischemic brain injury. *Early Hum Dev*. 2013;89(5):355–360.
84. Koklu E, Ariguloglu EA, Koklu S. Levetiracetam-induced anaphylaxis in a neonate. *Pediatr Neurol*. 2014;50(2):192–194.
85. Vesoulis ZA, Mathur AM. Advances in management of neonatal seizures. *Indian J Pediatr*. 2014; 81(6):592–598.
86. Pressler RM, Mangum B. Newly emerging therapies for neonatal seizures. *Semin Fetal Neonatal Med*. 2013;18(4):216–223.
87. Glass HC, Poulin C, Shevell MI. Topiramate for the treatment of neonatal seizures. *Pediatr Neurol*. 2011;44(6):439–442.
88. Riesgo R, Winckler MI, Ohlweiler L, et al. Treatment of refractory neonatal seizures with topiramate. *Neuropediatrics*. 2012;43(6):353–356.
89. University of California D. Topiramate in Neonates Receiving Whole Body Cooling for Hypoxic Ischemic Encephalopathy. In: ClinicalTrials.gov [Internet]. Bethesda (MD): National Library of Medicine (US); 2000. Available from: http://clinicaltrials.gov/show/NCT01765218. Cited November 15, 2016. NLM Identifier: NCT01765128.
90. Filippi L, la Marca G, Fiorini P, et al. Topiramate concentrations in neonates treated with pro- longed whole body hypothermia for hypoxic ischemic encephalopathy. *Epilepsia*. 2009;50(11): 2355–2361.
91. Filippi L, Poggi C, la Marca G, et al. Oral topiramate in neonates with hypoxic ischemic encephalopathy treated with hypothermia: a safety study. *J Pediatr*. 2010;157(3):361–366.
92. Ortinski P, Meador KJ. Cognitive side effects of antiepileptic drugs. *Epilepsy Behav*. 2004;5(suppl 1):S60–S65.
93. Thompson PJ, Baxendale SA, Duncan JS, et al. Effects of topiramate on cognitive function. *J Neurol Neurosurg Psychiatr*. 2000;69(5):636–641.
94. Lee S, Sziklas V, Andermann F, et al. The effects of adjunctive topiramate on cognitive function in patients with epilepsy. *Epilepsia*. 2003;44(3):339–347.
95. Meador KJ, Loring DW, Hulihan JF, et al. Differential cognitive and behavioral effects of topiramate and valproate. *Neurology*. 2003;60(9):1483–1488.
96. Schubert S, Brandl U, Brodhun M, et al. Neuroprotective effects of topiramate after hypoxia-ischemia in newborn piglets. *Brain Res*. 2005;1058(1–2):129–136.
97. Glier C, Dzietko M, Bittigau P, et al. Therapeutic doses of topiramate are not toxic to the developing rat brain. *Exp Neurol*. 2004;187(2):403–409.
98. Zhao Q, Hu Y, Holmes GL. Effect of topiramate on cognitive function and activity level following neonatal seizures. *Epilepsy Behav*. 2005;6(4):529–536.
99. Cha BH, Silveira DC, Liu X, et al. Effect of topiramate following recurrent and prolonged seizures during early development. *Epilepsy Res*. 2002;51(3):217–232.
100. Kato M, Yamagata T, Kubota M, et al. Clinical spectrum of early onset epileptic encephalopathies caused by KCNQ2 mutation. *Epilepsia*. 2013;54(7):1282–1287.
101. Hoppen T, Elger CE, Bartmann P. Carbamazepine in phenobarbital-nonresponders: experience with ten preterm infants. *Eur J Pediatr*. 2001;160(7):444–447.
102. Singh B, Singh P, al Hifzi I, et al. Treatment of neonatal seizures with carbamazepine. *J Child Neurol*. 1996;11(5):378–382.
103. Bassan H, Bental Y, Shany E, et al. Neonatal seizures: dilemmas in workup and management. *Pediatr Neurol*. 2008;38(6):415–421.
104. Steinberg A, Shalev RS, Amir N. Valproic acid in neonatal status convulsivus. *Brain Dev*. 1986; 8(3):278–279.
105. Cleary RT, Sun H, Huynh T, et al. Bumetanide enhances phenobarbital efficacy in a rat model of hypoxic neonatal seizures. *PLoS ONE*. 2013;8(3):e57148.

17

106. Kang SK, Markowitz GJ, Kim ST, et al. Age- and sex-dependent susceptibility to phenobarbital-resistant neonatal seizures: role of chloride co-transporters. *Front Cell Neurosci.* 2015;9:173.

107. Pressler RM, Boylan GB, Marlow N, et al. Bumetanide for the treatment of seizures in newborn babies with hypoxic ischaemic encephalopathy (NEMO): an open-label, dose finding, and feasibility phase 1/2 trial. *Lancet Neurol.* 2015;14(5):469–477.

108. Thoresen M, Sabir H. Epilepsy: Neonatal seizures still lack safe and effective treatment. *Nat Rev Neurol.* 2015;11(6):311–312.

109. Soul J. Pilot Study of Bumetanide for Newborn Seizures. In: ClinicalTrials.gov [Internet]. Bethesda (MD): National Library of Medicine (US). 2000. Available from: http://clinicaltrials.gov/show/ NCT00830531. Cited November 15, 2016. NLM Identifier: NCT00830531.

110. Freeman JM, Kossoff EH. Ketosis and the ketogenic diet, 2010: advances in treating epilepsy and other disorders. *Adv Pediatr.* 2010;57(1):315–329.

111. Martin K, Jackson CF, Levy RG, et al. Ketogenic diet and other dietary treatments for epilepsy. *Cochrane Database Syst Rev.* 2016;(2):CD001903.

112. Rubenstein JE. Use of the ketogenic diet in neonates and infants. *Epilepsia.* 2008;49(suppl 8):30–32.

113. Cusmai R, Martinelli D, Moavero R, et al. Ketogenic diet in early myoclonic encephalopathy due to non ketotic hyperglycinemia. *Eur J Paediatr Neurol.* 2012;16(5):509–513.

114. Gospe SM Jr. Neonatal vitamin-responsive epileptic encephalopathies. *Chang Gung Med J.* 2010; 33(1):1–12.

115. Bass NE, Wyllie E, Cohen B, et al. Pyridoxine-dependent epilepsy: the need for repeated pyridoxine trials and the risk of severe electrocerebral suppression with intravenous pyridoxine infusion. *J Child Neurol.* 1996;11(5):422–424.

116. Stockler S, Plecko B, Gospe SM Jr, et al. Pyridoxine dependent epilepsy and antiquitin deficiency: clinical and molecular characteristics and recommendations for diagnosis, treatment and follow-up. *Mol Genet Metab.* 2011;104(1–2):48–60.

117. Pearl PL. Amenable treatable severe pediatric epilepsies. *Semin Pediatr Neurol.* 2016;23(2):158–166.

118. Plecko B, Paul K, Paschke E, et al. Biochemical and molecular characterization of 18 patients with pyridoxine-dependent epilepsy and mutations of the antiquitin (ALDH7A1) gene. *Hum Mutat.* 2007;28(1):19–26.

119. Bok LA, Struys E, Willemsen MA, et al. Pyridoxine-dependent seizures in Dutch patients: diagnosis by elevated urinary alpha-aminoadipic semialdehyde levels. *Arch Dis Child.* 2007;92(8):687–689.

120. Baxter P. Pyridoxine-dependent seizures: a clinical and biochemical conundrum. *Biochim Biophys Acta.* 2003;1647(1–2):36–41.

121. Pearl PL. New treatment paradigms in neonatal metabolic epilepsies. *J Inherit Metab Dis.* 2009; 32(2):204–213.

122. Sudarsanam A, Singh H, Wilcken B, et al. Cirrhosis associated with pyridoxal 5'-phosphate treatment of pyridoxamine 5'-phosphate oxidase deficiency. *JIMD Rep.* 2014;17:67–70.

123. Brautigam C, Hyland K, Wevers R, et al. Clinical and laboratory findings in twins with neonatal epileptic encephalopathy mimicking aromatic L-amino acid decarboxylase deficiency. *Neuropediatrics.* 2002;33(3):113–117.

124. Clayton PT, Surtees RA, DeVile C, et al. Neonatal epileptic encephalopathy. *Lancet.* 2003;361(9369):1614.

125. Van Hove JL, Lohr NJ. Metabolic and monogenic causes of seizures in neonates and young infants. *Mol Genet Metab.* 2011;104(3):214–230.

126. Hyland K, Buist NR, Powell BR, et al. Folinic acid responsive seizures: a new syndrome? *J Inherit Metab Dis.* 1995;18(2):177–181.

127. Nicolai J, van Kranen-Mastenbroek VH, Wevers RA, et al. Folinic acid-responsive seizures initially responsive to pyridoxine. *Pediatr Neurol.* 2006;34(2):164–167.

128. Gallagher RC, Van Hove JL, Scharer G, et al. Folinic acid-responsive seizures are identical to pyridoxine-dependent epilepsy. *Ann Neurol.* 2009;65(5):550–556.

129. Zempleni J, Hassan YI, Wijeratne SS. Biotin and biotinidase deficiency. *Expert Rev Endocrinol Metab.* 2008;3(6):715–724.

130. Wolf B. Clinical issues and frequent questions about biotinidase deficiency. *Mol Genet Metab.* 2010;100(1):6–13.

131. Volpe JJ. Neonatal seizures: current concepts and revised classification. *Pediatrics.* 1989;84(3):422–428.

132. Shellhaas R, Chang T, Wusthoff C, et al. Treatment duration after acute symptomatic seizures in neonates: a multicenter cohort study. *J Pediatr.* 2016;published online ahead of press at: http://www .jpeds.com/article/S0022-3476(16)31172-6/pdf. November 8, 2016.

133. Brod SA, Ment LR, Ehrenkranz RA, et al. Predictors of success for drug discontinuation following neonatal seizures. *Pediatr Neurol.* 1988;4(1):13–17.

CHAPTER 18

Neuroprotective Therapies in Infants

Sonia L. Bonifacio, MD, Krisa VanMeurs, MD

- Preterm and term infants are at risk of acquiring brain injury with lasting neurodevelopmental sequelae.
- Mechanisms of brain injury in the developing brain are related to unique vulnerabilities due to the maturational stage of the various types of cells in the brain.
- The pathogenesis of brain injury in both preterm and term infants provides multiple opportunities for therapeutic intervention, such as addressing excitotoxicity, inflammation, oxidative stress, cytokines, and mechanisms of repair and regeneration.
- In the future, it is plausible that a cocktail of medications may be prescribed to address the mechanisms of brain injury at different time points during the injury and repair process.
- Antenatal steroids and magnesium sulfate should be administered to women at risk of delivering a premature infant, as they have been proven to reduce the risk of developing intraventricular hemorrhage (IVH).
- Therapeutic hypothermia is standard of care for term infants with hypoxic-ischemic encephalopathy (HIE). Additional drugs such as erythropoiesis-stimulating agents (ESAs), xenon, melatonin, and allopurinol are being studied as adjunctive treatments to further reduce the risk of death or disability in these patients.

Introduction

Sick infants are at significant risk for acquisition of perinatal brain injury. Concerns about long-term neurologic sequelae have increased along with improved survival rates of extremely premature infants, movement of the limits of viability toward earlier gestational ages, and increased survival among infants with complex medical and surgical conditions. According to the Centers for Disease Control and Prevention, 1 in 10 infants born in the United States in 2015 was premature. Mortality is highest among the smallest and youngest premature infants, and 40% of survivors have cognitive or physical disabilities. The lifetime cost associated with cognitive and physical disabilities is >$1,000,000 per family, without accounting for parental loss of work to care for a disabled child or family emotional burdens.

Despite advances in respiratory and cardiovascular care, fewer advances have been made in prevention and treatment of brain injury in premature infants. The best protective strategy remains prevention of preterm birth. Neuroprotective strategies for premature infants focus on providing thermoregulation and maintenance of hemodynamic and respiratory stability, particularly in the first 3 to 7 days after birth. Current regimens thought to further improve neurologic outcomes in preterm infants include administration of antenatal betamethasone and magnesium sulfate and postnatal treatment with indomethacin, caffeine citrate, or erythropoiesis-stimulating agents (ESAs; erythropoietin [EPO] and darbepoetin).

For term infants, there has been significant progress over the last 15 years for those with neonatal encephalopathy due to presumed perinatal asphyxia, also known as *hypoxic-ischemic encephalopathy (HIE)*. Eleven randomized controlled trials (RCTs) that enrolled >1500 infants demonstrated efficacy of therapeutic hypothermia in reducing the risk of death and neurodevelopmental impairment in infants with HIE.[1] Therapeutic hypothermia is the only clinically available treatment for moderate to severe HIE and is considered the standard of care for this patient population.[2] Several medications, including EPO and darbepoetin, xenon, topiramate, melatonin, magnesium sulfate, and stem cells, are under evaluation to determine if they provide neuroprotection in addition to that of hypothermia. Other agents have been evaluated in animals but are not yet ready for clinical trials. In this chapter, we will review neuroprotective strategies and therapies currently in use or being evaluated for use in preterm or term infants.

Neuroprotective Therapies and Strategies for Premature Infants

The pathophysiology of brain injury in premature infants is complex, reflecting developmental susceptibility of the immature and rapidly changing preterm brain,[3,4] fragility of the vascular germinal matrix (where intraventricular hemorrhages [IVHs] originate),[5] and the impacts of various measures needed to sustain life outside of the womb.[6,7] The chronic inflammatory state often associated with life-sustaining intensive care is postulated to interfere with normal brain development and may account for the focal injuries to and abnormal maturation of white matter detected using advanced magnetic resonance and diffusion tensor imaging techniques.[8-14] Chronic mechanical ventilation, oxygen exposure, sepsis, necrotizing enterocolitis, surgery (e.g., ligation of a patent ductus arteriosus [PDA]), and suboptimal nutrition all likely contribute to the brain pathology observed in this population. At 24 weeks gestation, the white matter is predominated by immature oligodendrocytes and lacks myelination, and the cortex is undergoing development and reorganization via neuronal migration and synaptogenesis. Over the next 12 to 16 weeks, while the extremely premature infant is cared for in the neonatal intensive care unit (NICU), the brain undergoes tremendous growth and development (Fig. 18.1). Abnormal development of the brain may be

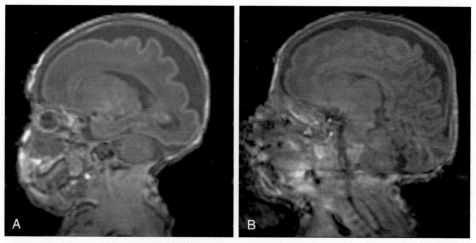

Figure 18.1 MRI images of a preterm infant born at 26 weeks gestation. (A) Shows a midline sagittal image acquired between 26 and 27 weeks. (B) Is the same infant imaged 7 weeks later. Note the growth and development of complexity during the interval while the infant was cared for in the intensive care nursery.

caused by direct damage to the brain tissue (as occurs in periventricular hemorrhagic infarction or PVHI, previously known as grade 4 IVH) or by interruption of normal development without tissue disruption.[15] Between 24 and 32 weeks postmenstrual age, preoligodendrocytes and the subplate neurons are highly vulnerable to oxidative injury, hypoxia, and excitotoxicity.[15] Impaired maturation of preoligodendrocytes leads to abnormalities of the white matter on ultrasound and magnetic resonance imaging (MRI), and later poor head growth, motor abnormalities such as cerebral palsy, and other neurodevelopmental disabilities.

Care Bundles to Reduce IVH and Improve Neurodevelopmental Outcome

Care practices during the antenatal and perinatal period may affect the pathogenesis of brain injury. Due to the complex pathophysiology that leads to the development of IVH, care bundles based on avoidance of abnormal physiologic or coagulopathic states have been used in quality improvement studies to attempt to reduce rates of IVH and ultimately improve neurodevelopmental outcome.[16] Antenatal steroids and magnesium sulfate are both associated with lower rates of IVH. Management at the time of delivery, including delayed cord clamping,[17] resuscitation practices such as early continuous positive airway pressure,[18] volume administration (both volume and rate of infusion), and gentle or noninvasive ventilation strategies, may also reduce brain injury.[18] Midline head positioning, minimal handling, reduction of stress and painful procedures, and addressing nutritional deficiencies have been identified as potentially helpful.[16,19] Given the premature infant's limited ability to autoregulate cerebral blood flow, measures should be taken to avoid hypotension, hypertension, and hypocarbia or hypercarbia. Hyperoxia is also toxic to the developing brain by promoting production of oxygen free radicals.[20] Targeted oxygen saturation goals may help prevent exposure to high oxygen levels. Early introduction of breast milk may improve immune status and early gut function and thus reduce the risk of developing necrotizing enterocolitis.[21] Developmental care practices such as containment devices, protection from noise and light, and kangaroo or skin-to-skin care are also frequently included in care bundles.[22] However, evidence that demonstrates efficacy of these methods to prevent high-grade IVH, PVHI, periventricular leukomalacia, or long-term motor or cognitive impairment remains limited.

Antenatal Betamethasone

Among very low birth weight (VLBW) infants (<1500 g) the current incidence of IVH is about 20%.[23] In extremely low birth weight infants (<1000 g), the incidence of IVH remains high at about 45%.[23] Increasing use of antenatal betamethasone since the 1980s has been associated with a commensurate reduction in the rate of IVH.[24] The initial studies of antenatal steroids in the 1970s and 1980s, including the landmark study of Liggins and Howie in 1972,[25] had the primary goal of improving respiratory outcomes. The most recent Cochrane review, which includes data on >8000 infants, shows that antenatal steroid treatment is also associated with decreased risk of perinatal death (RR 0.72, 95% confidence interval [CI] 0.58–0.89), neonatal death (RR 0.69, 95% CI 0.59–0.81), any grade of IVH (RR 0.55, 95% CI 0.40–0.76), and severe (grade 3 or 4) IVH (RR 0.26, 95% CI 0.11–0.60).[26] Despite these and other benefits, meta-analyses have not shown an improvement in long-term developmental outcomes.

The mechanisms by which antenatal steroid treatment reduces IVH is thought to be similar to those of indomethacin, including structural stabilization and reduced permeability of the basement membrane of the germinal matrix vasculature. In theory, these changes should make the fragile germinal matrix more tolerant to changes in cerebral blood flow caused by episodes of hypoxia, hypercarbia or hypocarbia, or unstable blood pressure.

Recent work has focused on the relationships between the risk of IVH and the proximity of antenatal betamethasone exposure to delivery or repeated courses of antenatal steroids. A recent study by Liebowitz and Clyman of 429 infants <28 weeks at birth evaluated the impact of proximity of steroid exposure and severe IVH (grade

3, 4).[27] In premature infants born ≥10 days after a course of maternal betamethasone, the rate of severe IVH was 17% compared with 7% for those born <10 days after steroid exposure (adjusted odds ratio [OR] 4.16, 95% CI 1.59–10.87, $P = 0.004$). This higher risk of IVH potentially could be reversed by a repeat course of steroids, because infants who received a second course had a rate of IVH of 8%, similar to that for infants born <10 days after the first course. Given the beneficial impact of antenatal steroids on both respiratory and neurologic outcomes, it should be the goal to administer betamethasone to all women at risk of preterm delivery at <34 weeks gestation.

Magnesium Sulfate

Magnesium sulfate was introduced to prevent maternal eclampsia, then used as a tocolytic agent, and later recognized in the late 1980s and early 1990s to have neuroprotective effects, with a reduction in the rate of IVH after treatment of mothers with preeclampsia. Concurrently, animal evidence of neuroprotection in age-appropriate models suggested benefit for human fetuses in the 26- to 34-week gestation time period.[28] Several subsequent controlled trials, including four in which the primary outcome was neuroprotection of the fetus, have confirmed this effect. Meta-analyses demonstrate a clear reduction in the risk of cerebral palsy at 18 to 24 months corrected age, but data on whether this benefit is sustained at early childhood are conflicting.[29] Antenatal administration to mothers at risk of preterm delivery reduces the risk of cerebral palsy (RR 0.68, 95% CI 0.54–0.97) and the rate of substantial gross motor dysfunction (unable to walk without assistance at age 2 years; RR 0.61, 95% CI 0.44–0.85).[29] Antenatal magnesium sulfate administration is considered standard of care by the American College of Obstetricians and Gynecologists for women presenting with preterm labor at <32 weeks gestation and expected to deliver within 7 days. Dosing regimens vary, in the range of a 4- to 6-g loading dose followed by 1 to 2 g/hour by continuous infusion for 12 to 24 hours.

The mechanism of neuroprotective action of magnesium sulfate is not well understood. Magnesium is important for key cellular processes such as glycolysis, oxidative phosphorylation, protein synthesis, DNA and RNA aggregation, and maintenance of cell membrane integrity. Magnesium is also involved in mechanisms of cell death and dysfunction. modulating inflammatory cytokines and free radicals, as well as preventing excitotoxic calcium injury by reducing calcium entry into cells. Finally, magnesium may have important hemodynamic effects that stabilize cerebral blood flow and thus reduce the risk of IVH.[28]

Caffeine

Apnea, defined as cessation of breathing for more than 15 seconds, occurs in at least 85% of infants born at <34 weeks gestation and is frequently accompanied by bradycardia and desaturation. Caffeine, a methylxanthine respiratory stimulant, is one of the most commonly used medications in premature infants.[30] Methylxanthines reduce both apnea and the need for mechanical ventilation. However, methylxanthines inhibit adenosine receptors, and adenosine preserves brain adenosine triphosphate (ATP) levels during experimental hypoxia and ischemia.[31] They also increase oxygen consumption and may diminish growth.[32] Accordingly, there was uncertainty about short- and long-term benefits or risks of methylxanthine treatment.[33]

This uncertainty was addressed by the Caffeine for Apnea of Prematurity (CAP) trial, an RCT in infants with birth weights of 500 to 1250 g (n = 2006).[34] The primary outcome was a composite outcome of death, cerebral palsy or cognitive delay, deafness, or blindness assessed at 18 to 21 months of age.[35] Caffeine decreased death or survival with neurodevelopmental disability (40.2% versus 46.2%; adjusted OR 0.77, 95% CI 0.64–0.93; $P = 0.008$). Significant reductions in cerebral palsy and cognitive delay were observed without any difference in the rates of death, deafness, or blindness. The number of infants needed to prevent one adverse outcome was 16 (95% CI 9–56).

When CAP Trial participants were seen at 5 years of age, caffeine therapy was no longer associated with a significantly lower risk of death or disability (21.1%

versus 24.8%; adjusted OR 0.82; 95% CI 0.65–1.03; P = 0.09).[36] Interestingly, the incidence of cognitive impairment at 5 years was similar in the placebo- and caffeine-treated groups and was lower than at 18 months, but gross motor impairment was less severe in the caffeine-treated infants, who had better motor coordination and visual perception. The rate of developmental coordination disorder (DCD; a form of motor dysfunction not associated with cerebral palsy or cognitive dysfunction defined as motor performance less than the fifth percentile on the Movement Assessment Battery for Children) was lower in the caffeine-treated group (11.3% versus 15.2%; OR 0.71; 95% CI 0.52–0.97; P = .032).[37] This was felt to be an important finding, because DCD is associated with learning disabilities, poor school performance, behavioral problems, poor social skills, and low self-esteem. The CAP Trial has now followed 76% of the original cohort to 11 years of age, when the primary outcome was functional impairment defined as a composite of poor academic performance, motor impairment, and behavior problems. Rates of functional impairment were not significantly different between the groups, but caffeine therapy was associated with a reduced risk of motor impairment (19.7% versus 27.5%; OR 0.66; 95% CI 0.48–0.90; P = .009).[38]

Caffeine has been called a silver bullet in neonatology because of its wide therapeutic index, tolerability, and efficacy in reducing bronchopulmonary dysplasia, PDA, severe retinopathy of prematurity, and neurodevelopmental disability. Few drugs used in the neonatal period have been tested in RCTs with follow-up out to 11 years with continued evidence of benefit. The exact mechanisms responsible for neuroprotection remain incompletely elucidated. Brain microstructural changes consisting of improved myelination have been seen in the caffeine-treated group, and larger MRI studies are underway to better understand this finding.[39]

Indomethacin

Indomethacin, a nonsteroidal antiinflammatory drug, diminishes prostaglandin production by inhibiting the activity of cyclooxygenase. Indomethacin was initially used in neonatology to promote closure of the ductus arteriosus, but administration within hours after birth also has independent effects that reduce the rate of early IVH. Meta-analyses show that indomethacin administered prophylactically (within 24 hours of birth) can reduce the risk of grade III or IV IVH (RR 0.66, 95% CI 0.53–0.82; number needed to treat 20). Despite a reduction in severe IVH, prophylactic indomethacin has not been shown to improve longer-term neurodevelopment in VLBW infants.[40] The mechanisms of IVH prevention are thought to include promotion of vascular stability during episodes of hypoxia or hypercapnia, preventing ischemia-related hyperperfusion. Indomethacin is also thought to promote maturation of the germinal matrix.[41,42]

Erythropoiesis-Stimulating Agents (ESAs): Erythropoietin/Darbepoetin

Preclinical studies have found neuronal repair, regeneration, antioxidant, antiinflammatory, and antiapoptotic effects of ESAs.[43] EPO is an endogenous cytokine produced by the liver in the fetus and in the kidney postnatally. Although primarily known for its effects on erythropoiesis, EPO is also produced in the brain, where it acts as a growth factor and neuroprotectant for the developing brain.[44] Several cell types in the brain, including neurons, oligodendrocytes, astrocytes, and microglia, produce EPO. Neuroprotective properties include promoting transcription of antiapoptotic genes, reduction of inflammation and oxidation, and long-term effects that promote healing, such as angiogenesis, neurogenesis, and olidendrogenesis. EPO production is stimulated by hypoxia, although prolonged periods of hypoxia are thought to be required to upregulate production. In rodent and nonhuman primate models of hypoxia-ischemia, EPO has demonstrated both histologic and functional benefit. A surprising and clinically appealing property identified in rodent model of hypoxia-ischemia is that EPO could provide functional and histologic neuroprotection even if administered 7 days after the insult.[45] These characteristics make ESAs promising therapeutic agents for brain injury in preterm infants and for term infants with HIE.

18

ESAs appear to be ideal neuroprotectants to combat brain injury in premature infants. As reviewed earlier, inflammation and arrest of cellular development are characteristics of brain injury in preterm infants. EPO combats inflammation and promotes neurogenesis. It has been widely used to stimulate erythropoiesis in preterm infants, who often are exposed to EPO for several weeks during their hospital course, providing ample data on safety and tolerability. Neuroprotective doses are higher than those needed to stimulate red blood cell production. Animal and human studies have been performed to elucidate appropriate dosing strategies.[46] Darbepoetin alfa (Darbe) is a long-acting form of EPO. An RCT comparing Darbe (10 μg/kg/week), EPO (400 U/kg three times per week), and placebo with dosing starting at <48 hours after birth and continuing through 35 weeks was performed to evaluate if Darbe and EPO would reduce transfusion needs in premature infants born weighing 500 to 1250 g.[47] At follow-up of 80 of the 102 randomized infants at 18 to 22 months of age, infants in the Darbe and EPO groups had significantly higher cognitive scores than those in the placebo group.[48] In addition, none of the ESA-treated patients developed cerebral palsy, compared with five in the placebo group, and the odds of neurodevelopmental impairment were lower in the ESA-treated group (OR 0.18, 95% CI 0.05–0.63). This benefit of ESAs persisted at 3.5 to 4 years of age, with higher full-scale and performance IQ in treated infants compared with those who received placebo.[49] A large phase III trial of darbepoetin to improve red cell mass and provide neuroprotection is now open for enrollment. This trial will recruit 650 infants born at 23 to 28 weeks gestation for enrollment within 24 hours after birth. Darbe or placebo will be administered weekly at a dose of 10 μg/kg weekly. The primary outcome will be the composite cognitive score on the Bayley III examination at a corrected gestational age of 26 months (NCT03169881).

Neuroprotective effects of EPO have also been directly studied in premature infants. The Swiss EPO Neuroprotection Trial Group recently reported neurodevelopmental outcomes for preterm infants (26–32 weeks gestation at birth; mean 29 weeks) who were randomized to receive high-dose EPO (3000 U/kg) or placebo at 3, 12 to 18, and 36 to 42 hours after birth. There were no differences in the primary outcome between the study groups. The mean mental developmental index (MDI) of the Bayley II at 2 years of age was 93.5 (95% CI 91.2–95.8) in the EPO group and 94.5 (95% CI 90.8–98.5) in the placebo group.[50] Compared with other trials of ESAs, which showed benefit in this population, this trial enrolled slightly older infants, the control group had a higher-than-expected MDI score, and duration of the EPO dosing regimen was much shorter. The latter may not adequately address the mechanism of brain injury in premature infants. A US trial of EPO in preterm infants (PENUT, NCT01378273) is now closed to enrollment and awaiting final outcome assessment. This is a multicenter, placebo-controlled, randomized trial of 941 preterm infants (24–28 weeks) randomized to placebo or high-dose EPO (1000 U/kg IV every 48 hours for 6 doses for the first 2 weeks after birth) followed by low-dose EPO (400 U/kg subcutaneous three times per week until $32\frac{6}{7}$ weeks) with neurodevelopmental outcome to be determined at 24 to 26 months of age.

Management of Pain Versus Impact of Analgesics and Sedatives on the Developing Brain

The impact of pain on the developing brain and neurodevelopmental outcome is a recent area of focus in neonatal care. Measures to provide comfort and developmentally appropriate care are emphasized to support the developing brain. The NICU in no way resembles the relatively quiet, dark, and insulated environment in which the fetus develops in utero. Premature infants in the NICU are constantly stimulated and have interrupted sleep–wake cycles. The optimal balance between overstimulation and understimulation is uncertain, as leaving a developing infant in a dark incubator without interaction is also unlikely to promote healthy development. Recent studies have addressed the importance of the NICU environment and parental interaction on neurodevelopment.[51,52] Exposure to maternal voice improves infant physiologic stability and reduces pain.[53,54] In contrast, a growing body of literature describes ill effects of painful procedures on brain development, as measured by MRI or by neurodevelopment at school age. Routine procedures in the NICU, such as heel sticks for laboratory monitoring or placement of intravenous lines, are painful. Many patients experience more than 100 of these procedures while under our care. Recent investigations have identified that the number of painful procedures affects white matter development and is associated with lower IQ at age 7.[55] Some painful procedures cannot be avoided, so treatment with analgesics and sedatives may be warranted. However, there is also a growing body of evidence demonstrating adverse impacts of some of these medications on the developing brain. Fentanyl and morphine have been associated with both injury to and abnormal growth of the cerebellum,[56,57] and midazolam has been associated with abnormalities of the hippocampus.[58] Although not frequently used in the NICU environment, animal data suggest that inhaled anesthetics may trigger neuronal apoptosis (programed cell death).[59] Best practices to better balance the need for painful procedures and sedation or analgesia need to be developed to minimize the risk of iatrogenic neurodevelopmental harm.

Neuroprotective Strategies for Term Infants

Brain injury due to hypoxia-ischemia is an important cause of death or significant neurodevelopmental disability. HIE is a major cause of neonatal death across the globe, with an incidence of 1 to 3 per 1000 live births.

Hypoxic or ischemic insults may trigger multiple pathways that result in cell death. The initial event can result in immediate cell death (cellular necrosis) or trigger processes that evolve over a period of hours to days or weeks postinsult[60] (Fig. 18.2).

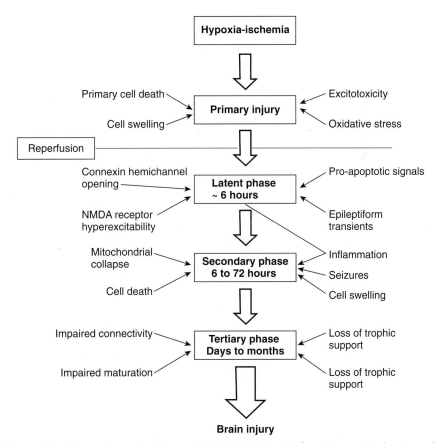

Figure 18.2 Mechanisms of evolving neuronal injury cascade after an hypoxic-ischemic insult during the primary, latent, secondary, and tertiary phases of injury that occur over hours, days, weeks, and months, highlighting potential therapeutic targets for prevention and repair. (Image taken from an open access publication: Davidson JO et al: Therapeutic hypothermia for neonatal hypoxic-ischemic encephalopathy: where to go from here? *Front Neurol* 2015;6:198.)

These pathways include oxidative stress, inflammation, and excitatory pathways, which lead to both early and late cellular dysfunction and may trigger programmed cell death (apoptosis). Immediately after an hypoxic-ischemic insult there is cellular depolarization, release of excitotoxins, calcium entry into cells, and cell lysis. After the insult there is a period of reperfusion, which may correlate with clinical resuscitation, during which aerobic metabolism recovers but the earlier mentioned deleterious pathways have been triggered. The insult itself is a trigger that causes downstream cascades that are thought to occur in a latent phase (6–15 hours postinsult) and a secondary phase (6 hours to 3 days postinsult) during which secondary energy failure may occur (see Fig. 18.2). Drugs that may ameliorate or block these pathways, reducing apoptosis and neuronal injury, thereby preventing neurodevelopmental impairments will be discussed later.

Clinically Available Treatments

Therapeutic Hypothermia

Therapeutic hypothermia was first identified in the mid-1900s to provide neuroprotection after hypoxic-ischemic insults in animal studies. As early as the 1950s, improved outcomes were reported in small studies of immersing infants who were not breathing at birth in water baths until the onset of spontaneous respiration.[61] Hypothermia was not tested again in large RCTs until the late 1990s. In 2013 a meta-analysis of 11 RCTs including >1500 infants found that therapeutic hypothermia significantly decreased the rate of death or moderate to severe neurodisability.[1] Treatment with hypothermia resulted in a significant reduction in the risk of death or disability (RR 0.75, 95% CI 0.68–0.83; NNT 7, 95% CI 5–10). Therapeutic hypothermia appears to be most beneficial when initiated within 6 hours after birth. Although not yet proven, some data suggest that initiating treatment within 4 hours after birth may optimize efficacy.[62,63] Infants are cooled to 33.5°C ± 0.5°C for 72 hours, then rewarmed slowly over 6 hours. Most centers use servo-regulated cooling devices that circulate cold water through a blanket that is either placed underneath or wrapped around the infant, although cooling caps with moderate body hypothermia have also been used. Overall, the treatment is safe, with few adverse effects. Some adverse effects, including persistent pulmonary hypertension (about 25% of patients), coagulopathy, and thrombocytopenia, may be related directly to perinatal asphyxia itself.

The mechanisms by which hypothermia provides neuroprotection are not completely understood. Hypothermia likely affects many of the pathways triggered by hypoxic-ischemic insults.[64] One primary effect is a reduction in the metabolic rate. The metabolic rate decreases by 5% with each reduction in body temperature by 1°C, resulting in decreased energy consumption and delay of anoxic cell depolarization. The neonatal brain is one of the most metabolically active organs, with the neurons in the cortex and the deep gray structures being much more metabolically active than the white matter. Reducing the metabolic rate in these areas of the brain may impede the injurious cellular cascades that are triggered after an hypoxic-ischemic insult.

Recent trials of longer and deeper hypothermia and late-onset hypothermia (onset between >6 and <24 hours after birth) have been completed. The longer and deeper cooling trial was terminated early due to safety concerns in the deeper and longer arms of the study, with increased mortality compared with the standard cooling arm, although death in all arms was lower than in the initial trials of hypothermia.[65] Using Bayesian statistics, the late hypothermia trial (as presented at Hot Topics 2016) demonstrated a 77% chance of some benefit but only a 58% chance that late hypothermia would result in a 10% or greater reduction in the risk of death or disability. Treatment of premature infants (33–35 weeks gestation) is currently being studied in an RCT (NCT01793129).

Therapies Under Study

Erythropoiesis-Stimulating Agents (ESAs)

An appealing aspect of ESAs is that they are thought to promote neurogenesis and repair postinjury and have efficacy even when administered 24 hours or more after an insult.[45,66] Several human studies have evaluated ESAs, either alone or in combination with hypothermia, as a treatment for infants with HIE. A phase I dose escalation safety and pharmacokinetics study identified the dose of 1000 U/kg intravenously every 48 hours as providing serum concentrations equivalent to the neuroprotective ranges identified in animal studies (NCT00719407).[67] The phase I/II NEATO trial aimed at determining safety and feasibility of enrolling infants with HIE treated with hypothermia into an RCT of EPO or placebo within 24 hours of delivery. The dosing regimen was 1000 U/kg at 1, 2, 3, 5, and 7 days of age. Secondary outcomes included brain injury on MRI within the first week after birth and motor and developmental testing at 1 year of age. EPO was associated with decreased brain injury and improved motor performance.[68] Larger studies with longer neurodevelopmental follow-up are needed to confirm the efficacy of ESAs in HIE patients. A large phase III trial is currently ongoing (HEAL Trial, NCT02811263).

ESAs are also being studied in infants with stroke, a focal hypoxic-ischemic injury. A double-blinded, placebo-controlled, randomized trial of darbepoetin for perinatal arterial ischemic stroke is being planned. Infants will be eligible if they are identified to have a middle cerebral artery stroke within 1 week of birth and will receive two doses of darbepoetin 10 µg/kg IV or placebo. The study will include 80 patients to be enrolled at two centers in Canada and one in Utrecht, the Netherlands (NCT03171818). Primary outcome is stroke tissue volume loss at 6 to 8 weeks after birth, and secondary outcomes include neurodevelopment at 18 months of age.

Topiramate

Topiramate, an anticonvulsant, is thought to act by inhibiting activation of glutamate receptors, thus preventing programmed cell death. Topiramate also blocks sodium and calcium channels, inhibits carbonic anhydrase, and affects mitochondrial permeability. In vitro and in vivo animal data suggest a beneficial effect of topiramate. A safety and feasibility study in 44 infants with HIE, comparing topiramate 10 mg/kg for 3 days with placebo, was recently completed (NCT01241019).[69] There were no differences in safety or other outcome measures, but epilepsy was less frequent in treated infants. Larger trials are needed to determine if adding topiramate to hypothermia further improves outcomes.

Xenon

Xenon is a rare and inert noble gas known for its anesthetic and neuroprotective properties. Neuroprotective effects of xenon are likely mediated by inhibition of the N-methyl-D aspartate glutamate receptor, dampening the excitotoxic phase of acute neurologic injury. Other neuroprotective actions of xenon may include activation of two-pore potassium channels, modulation of neuroapoptosis and inflammation, induction of hypoxia-inducible factor alpha, and activation of ATP-sensitive potassium channels. Xenon crosses the blood–brain barrier rapidly as a result of a low blood/gas partition coefficient. Xenon is used in Europe as an anesthetic but is not FDA approved in the United States. Its high cost makes use as an anesthetic difficult to justify; however, it may have a role in pediatric anesthesia where anesthetic-induced neurotoxicity is a concern. Xenon is attractive for use in sick newborns due to cardiovascular stability and myocardial protective properties.

In in vitro and in vivo animal models, xenon and hypothermia together provide greater neuroprotection after hypoxic-ischemic injury than either treatment alone.[70,71] In an animal model of hypoxia-ischemia, dramatic improvements in function and histology were observed after administration of xenon.[71] The combination of xenon with therapeutic hypothermia is effective even when xenon administration is delayed.[72,73] However, a recent study by Sabir et al. cautioned that animals subjected to severe hypoxia-ischemia and either hypothermia alone or hypothermia plus 50% xenon did not demonstrate a benefit as measured by hemispheric brain area or subventricular zone neuronal cell counts.[74]

Clinical data on xenon use in human newborns with HIE are limited. A feasibility study in 14 newborns with moderate to severe HIE who were receiving less than 35% oxygen increased xenon treatment time stepwise from 3 to 18 hours.[75] Xenon was delivered using a closed-circuit delivery system utilizing a modified standard anesthesia workstation with modified breathing hoses.[76] Xenon caused sedation and attenuated background amplitude integrated electroencephalogram. Seizures occurred with rapid xenon tapering but not with slow weaning. There were no adverse cardiovascular or respiratory effects. Mortality in this small study was 20%; 64% of survivors had Bayley II mental and motor scores >70.

A recently published trial randomized 92 newborns with HIE to either 30% xenon for 24 hours along with cooling or to cooling alone at a median age of 11 hours.[77] There were no significant differences in the primary MRI outcomes of reduced lactate–to–N-acetyl aspartate ratio in the thalamus and preserved fractional anisotropy (FA) in the posterior limb of the internal capsule. The authors concluded that treatment with 30% xenon for 24 hours started more than 6 hours after birth did not have additional neuroprotective benefits when compared with cooling alone. The study was adequately powered to detect changes in FA but not for the other MRI outcome measure. The timing, dose, or duration of xenon use may not have been optimal. Another trial currently enrolling is the CoolXenon3 trial (NCT02071394). Newborns are randomized to 50% xenon for 18 hours or hypothermia alone. The primary outcome is survival without moderate or severe disability, defined as Bayley III composite score <85. A transport device to deliver xenon in an ambulance to allow earlier initiation of treatment has been developed.[78]

Xenon has potent anticonvulsant effects that are likely due to glutamate receptor blockade. In five infants treated with 30% xenon, seizures stopped during xenon therapy but recurred within minutes after xenon was stopped.[79] Suppression of seizures may contribute to the neuroprotective effect of xenon. Further clinical trial results with long-term outcome measures in humans are needed to determine if the neuroprotective benefits seen in animal models will be confirmed in humans.

Melatonin

Melatonin, a low-molecular-weight hormone secreted by the pineal gland, best known for its role in regulation of circadian rhythm, also has important roles in normal neurodevelopment. Because melatonin readily crosses the placenta and the blood–brain barrier, it has drawn interest as a candidate treatment to reduce the risk of hypoxic-ischemic injury in high-risk deliveries. The role of its antioxidative, antiapoptotic, and antiinflammatory activities in protecting the developing brain has been studied in animal models of both premature and term brain injury.[80] In rodent models of HIE, melatonin is neuroprotective when given either prophylactically or immediately after an hypoxic-ischemic insult. In sheep models of both term and preterm brain injury, prophylactic melatonin was neuroprotective, with effects that were specific for gestational age, such as preservation of mature oligodendrocytes in the preterm model and reduced neuronal death and astrogliosis in the term model. In a piglet model of HIE, animals treated with melatonin (5 mg/kg/hour for 5 hours starting 10 minutes after resuscitation and repeated at 24 hours) in conjunction with therapeutic hypothermia for 24 hours had decreased histologic damage in both gray and white matter regions, and magnetic resonance spectroscopy demonstrated decreased lactate with preservation of cerebral ATP.[81]

One small trial randomized 15 infants to treatment with melatonin (10 mg/kg orally for 5 days) with hypothermia and 15 to hypothermia alone.[82] Melatonin was well tolerated without adverse effects and was associated with decreased white matter injury on MRI and increased survival with a normal neurologic examination at 6 months of age. The sample size was small, and long-term neurodevelopmental follow-up is not available. The optimal neuroprotective dose of melatonin is not yet known. An ongoing dose escalation study in infants with moderate to severe HIE receiving therapeutic hypothermia (TH) will randomize 30 patients and increase the dose from 0.5 to 5 mg/kg (NCT02621944).

Allopurinol

Allopurinol, a xanthine oxidase inhibitor, acts as a neuroprotectant by preventing formation of free radicals that trigger programmed cell death. Free radical production occurs after reperfusion and reoxygenation after an hypoxic-ischemic insult. Allopurinol was neuroprotective in a rodent model of hypoxic-ischemic injury but did not improve neurodevelopmental outcome in a small human study of neonatal HIE.[83] The study by Benders et al. enrolled only 32 of a planned 100 infants; all had severe HIE, and none were cotreated with hypothermia. The dose of allopurinol was 40 mg/kg within 4 hours after birth and then repeated at 12 hours of age. The study was stopped early due to the likelihood of not finding a difference in outcome between the groups. It is not known whether allopurinol may be more effective in moderate HIE, in conjunction with hypothermia, or with earlier initiation. One small RCT by Torrance et al. (n = 53) gave antenatal allopurinol to mothers with nonreassuring fetal heart rate patterns or fetal acidemia.[84] Cord blood was obtained and evaluated for lactate and S-100B, a marker of brain injury. Infants with measurable levels of allopurinol or its metabolite had lower S-100B levels, suggesting that early treatment with allopurinol should be further investigated. A proposed placebo-controlled, double-blinded trial of early allopurinol (20 mg/kg within 30 minutes of birth followed by a second dose at 12 hours of age) along with hypothermia, the ALBINO trial (NCT03162653), is not yet enrolling patients.

Magnesium Sulfate

The neuroprotective effects of magnesium sulfate are reviewed in the preterm section. Evidence regarding neuroprotective effects of magnesium sulfate in term infants with HIE is inconsistent.[85] In animal models, there appears to be some additive neuroprotection by combining magnesium with hypothermia. The results of the one small RCT to evaluate safety of magnesium sulfate plus hypothermia for HIE (MagCool Study, NCT01646619) have not yet been published.

Stem Cell Therapy

Stem cell–based therapy to prevent or repair perinatal brain injury is an area of active investigation.[86–89] Stem cell therapies may act by diverse mechanisms at different phases of brain injury. Early studies focused on the ability of stem cells to engraft and replace dying cells. In general, the net increase in cell numbers in the brain was negligible, despite significant functional improvements. This suggests that the key mechanism is the release of neurotropic and immune-modulatory factors. This is an attractive neuroprotectant for term infants with HIE, as often the etiology and precise timing of the brain injury are unclear.

Umbilical cord blood (UCB) contains a rich and diverse mixture of stem and progenitor cells with the potential to generate a variety of cell types. UCB is one of the most abundant sources of nonembryonic stem cells and has high engraftment rates when used for transplantation with low rates of graft-versus-host disease. UCB also contains a population of mesenchymal stem cells, which have a high potential for neural differentiation.[90] In animal models of stroke and hypoxia-ischemia, UCB decreases clinical sequelae and neuroimaging abnormalities.[91,92]

Investigators at Duke University studied the feasibility and safety of autologous cord blood in 23 newborns with moderate to severe HIE.[93] Infants were eligible if they were ≥35 weeks and met the National Institute of Child Health and Human Development criteria for therapeutic hypothermia. Cord blood was collected in deliveries of mothers who had previously consented for public banking or in deliveries where obstetric staff thought the infant might meet cooling criteria. The cord blood was volume and red blood cell reduced and divided into aliquots containing 1 to 5 $\times 10^7$ nucleated cells. All infants were treated with therapeutic hypothermia and, after pretreatment with hydrocortisone, given up to four UCB infusions. The first dose was given as soon as possible after birth and subsequent doses at 24, 48, and 72 hours of age (NCT00593242). In 2011 the FDA began regulation of UCB and the investigational new drug protocol was modified to administer only two doses in the first 48 hours. The volume of UCB collected varied, but even the lowest collected volumes provided cell numbers adequate for at least one dose containing the target cell number. No significant adverse events occurred, but oxygen saturation decreased by 1% to 2% after the third and fourth infusions ($P < 0.05$). One-year outcomes were compared with a cohort of 82 infants who did not have UCB available and were cooled. All newborns treated with autologous UCB and 87% in the comparison group survived to 1 year ($P = 0.12$). Bayley III testing was available for 18 (78%) treated infants and 46 (56%) in the comparison group; in these subgroups, 74% of the UCB group and 41% of the comparison group had Bayley III scores ≥85 in all three testing domains (cognitive, language, and motor development). Stem cell therapy remains an intriguing possibility for newborns identified to be at risk of brain injury. Additional research is needed to determine the most appropriate cell type, dose, timing, and mode of administration, as well as to provide sufficient data on safety and outcome.

REFERENCES

1. Jacobs SE, Berg M, Hunt R, et al. Cooling for newborns with hypoxic ischaemic encephalopathy. *Cochrane Database Syst Rev*. 2013;(1):CD003311.
2. Committee on F, Newborn, Papile LA, et al. Hypothermia and neonatal encephalopathy. *Pediatrics*. 2014;133:1146–1150.
3. Lynn S, Huang EJ, Elchuri S, et al. Selective neuronal vulnerability and inadequate stress response in superoxide dismutase mutant mice. *Free Radic Biol Med*. 2005;38:817–828.
4. Ferriero DM, Miller SP. Imaging selective vulnerability in the developing nervous system. *J Anat*. 2010;217:429–435.
5. Volpe JJ. Intraventricular hemorrhage and brain injury in the premature infant. Neuropathology and pathogenesis. *Clin Perinatol*. 1989;16:361–386.
6. Glass HC, Bonifacio SL, Chau V, et al. Recurrent postnatal infections are associated with progressive white matter injury in premature infants. *Pediatrics*. 2008;122:299–305.
7. Bonifacio SL, Glass HC, Chau V, et al. Extreme premature birth is not associated with impaired development of brain microstructure. *J Pediatr*. 2010;157:726–732.
8. Back SA, Luo NL, Borenstein NS, et al. Late oligodendrocyte progenitors coincide with the developmental window of vulnerability for human perinatal white matter injury. *J Neurosci*. 2001;21:1302–1312.
9. Back SA, Luo NL, Borenstein NS, et al. Arrested oligodendrocyte lineage progression during human cerebral white matter development: dissociation between the timing of progenitor differentiation and myelinogenesis. *J Neuropathol Exp Neurol*. 2002;61:197–211.
10. Haynes RL, Xu G, Folkerth RD, et al. Potential neuronal repair in cerebral white matter injury in the human neonate. *Pediatr Res*. 2011;69:62–67.
11. Kinney HC, Haynes RL, Xu G, et al. Neuron deficit in the white matter and subplate in periventricular leukomalacia. *Ann Neurol*. 2012;71:397–406.
12. Back SA, Rivkees SA. Emerging concepts in periventricular white matter injury. *Semin Perinatol*. 2004;28:405–414.
13. Chau V, McFadden DE, Poskitt KJ, et al. Chorioamnionitis in the pathogenesis of brain injury in preterm infants. *Clin Perinatol*. 2014;41:83–103.
14. Hagberg H, Mallard C, Ferriero DM, et al. The role of inflammation in perinatal brain injury. *Nat Rev Neurol*. 2015;11:192–208.
15. Back SA. Brain injury in the preterm infant: new horizons for pathogenesis and prevention. *Pediatr Neurol*. 2015;53:185–192.
16. McLendon D, Check J, Carteaux P, et al. Implementation of potentially better practices for the prevention of brain hemorrhage and ischemic brain injury in very low birth weight infants. *Pediatrics*. 2003;111:e497–e503.
17. Mercer JS, Vohr BR, McGrath MM, et al. Delayed cord clamping in very preterm infants reduces the incidence of intraventricular hemorrhage and late-onset sepsis: a randomized, controlled trial. *Pediatrics*. 2006;117:1235–1242.
18. Barton SK, Tolcos M, Miller SL, et al. Unraveling the links between the initiation of ventilation and brain injury in preterm infants. *Front Pediatr*. 2015;3:97.
19. Schmid MB, Reister F, Mayer B, et al. Prospective risk factor monitoring reduces intracranial hemorrhage rates in preterm infants. *Dtsch Arztebl Int*. 2013;110:489–496.
20. Sabir H, Jary S, Tooley J, et al. Increased inspired oxygen in the first hours of life is associated with adverse outcome in newborns treated for perinatal asphyxia with therapeutic hypothermia. *J Pediatr*. 2012;161:409–416.
21. Meinzen-Derr J, Poindexter B, Wrage L, et al. Role of human milk in extremely low birth weight infants' risk of necrotizing enterocolitis or death. *J Perinatol*. 2009;29:57–62.
22. Als H, McAnulty GB. The Newborn Individualized Developmental Care and Assessment Program (NIDCAP) with kangaroo mother care (KMC): comprehensive care for preterm infants. *Curr Womens Health Rev*. 2011;7:288–301.
23. Ballabh P. Intraventricular hemorrhage in premature infants: mechanism of disease. *Pediatr Res*. 2010;67:1–8.
24. Wei JC, Catalano R, Profit J, et al. Impact of antenatal steroids on intraventricular hemorrhage in very-low-birth weight infants. *J Perinatol*. 2016;36:352–356.
25. Liggins GC, Howie RN. A controlled trial of antepartum glucocorticoid treatment for prevention of the respiratory distress syndrome in premature infants. *Pediatrics*. 1972;50:515–525.

26. Roberts D, Brown J, Medley N, et al. Antenatal corticosteroids for accelerating fetal lung maturation for women at risk of preterm birth. *Cochrane Database Syst Rev.* 2017;(3):Cd004454.
27. Liebowitz M, Clyman RI. Antenatal betamethasone: a prolonged time interval from administration to delivery is associated with an increased incidence of severe intraventricular hemorrhage in infants born before 28 weeks gestation. *J Pediatr.* 2016;177:114–120.
28. Marret S, Doyle LW, Crowther CA, et al. Antenatal magnesium sulphate neuroprotection in the preterm infant. *Semin Fetal Neonatal Med.* 2007;12:311–317.
29. Bain E, Middleton P, Crowther CA. Different magnesium sulphate regimens for neuroprotection of the fetus for women at risk of preterm birth. *Cochrane Database Syst Rev.* 2012;(2):CD009302.
30. Hsieh EM, Hornik CP, Clark RH, et al. Medication use in the neonatal intensive care unit. *Am J Perinatol.* 2014;31:811–821.
31. Fredholm BB. Astra Award Lecture. Adenosine, adenosine receptors and the actions of caffeine. *Pharmacol Toxicol.* 1995;76:93–101.
32. Thurston JH, Hauhard RE, Dirgo JA. Aminophylline increases cerebral metabolic rate and decreases anoxic survival in young mice. *Science.* 1978;201:649–651.
33. Henderson-Smart DJ, Steer P. Methylxanthine treatment for apnea in preterm infants. *Cochrane Database Syst Rev.* 2001;(3):CD000140.
34. Schmidt B, Roberts RS, Davis P, et al. Caffeine therapy for apnea of prematurity. *N Engl J Med.* 2006;354:2112–2121.
35. Schmidt B, Roberts RS, Davis P, et al. Long-term effects of caffeine therapy for apnea of prematurity. *N Engl J Med.* 2007;357:1893–1902.
36. Schmidt B, Anderson PJ, Doyle LW, et al. Survival without disability to age 5 years after neonatal caffeine therapy for apnea of prematurity. *JAMA.* 2012;307:275–282.
37. Doyle LW, Schmidt B, Anderson PJ, et al. Reduction in developmental coordination disorder with neonatal caffeine therapy. *J Pediatr.* 2014;165:356–359.
38. Schmidt B, Roberts RS, Anderson PJ, et al. Academic Performance, Motor Function, and Behavior 11 Years After Neonatal Caffeine Citrate Therapy for Apnea of Prematurity: An 11-Year Follow-up of the CAP Randomized Clinical Trial. *JAMA Pediatr.* 2017;171:564–572.
39. Doyle LW, Cheong J, Hunt RW, et al. Caffeine and brain development in very preterm infants. *Ann Neurol.* 2010;68:734–742.
40. Fowlie PW, Davis PG, McGuire W. Prophylactic intravenous indomethacin for preventing mortality and morbidity in preterm infants. *Cochrane Database Syst Rev.* 2010;(7):CD000174.
41. Coyle MG, Oh W, Petersson KH, et al. Effects of indomethacin on brain blood flow, cerebral metabolism, and sagittal sinus prostanoids after hypoxia. *Am J Physiol.* 1995;269:H1450–H1459.
42. Ment LR, Stewart WB, Ardito TA, et al. Indomethacin promotes germinal matrix microvessel maturation in the newborn beagle pup. *Stroke.* 1992;23:1132–1137.
43. Gonzalez FF, Ferriero DM. Neuroprotection in the newborn infant. *Clin Perinatol.* 2009;36: 859–880, vii.
44. Juul SE, Pet GC. Erythropoietin and Neonatal Neuroprotection. *Clin Perinatol.* 2015;42:469–481.
45. Larpthaveesarp A, Georgevits M, Ferriero DM, et al. Delayed erythropoietin therapy improves histological and behavioral outcomes after transient neonatal stroke. *Neurobiol Dis.* 2016;93:57–63.
46. Patel S, Ohls RK. Darbepoetin Administration in Term and Preterm Neonates. *Clin Perinatol.* 2015;42:557–566.
47. Ohls RK, Christensen RD, Kamath-Rayne BD, et al. A randomized, masked, placebo-controlled study of darbepoetin alfa in preterm infants. *Pediatrics.* 2013;132:e119–e127.
48. Ohls RK, Kamath-Rayne BD, Christensen RD, et al. Cognitive outcomes of preterm infants randomized to darbepoetin, erythropoietin, or placebo. *Pediatrics.* 2014;133:1023–1030.
49. Ohls RK, Cannon DC, Phillips J, et al. Preschool Assessment of Preterm Infants Treated With Darbepoetin and Erythropoietin. *Pediatrics.* 2016;137:e20153859.
50. Natalucci G, Latal B, Koller B, et al. Effect of early prophylactic high-dose recombinant human erythropoietin in very preterm infants on neurodevelopmental outcome at 2 years: a randomized clinical trial. *JAMA.* 2016;315:2079–2085.
51. Reynolds LC, Duncan MM, Smith GC, et al. Parental presence and holding in the neonatal intensive care unit and associations with early neurobehavior. *J Perinatol.* 2013;33:636–641.
52. Pineda RG, Neil J, Dierker D, et al. Alterations in brain structure and neurodevelopmental outcome in preterm infants hospitalized in different neonatal intensive care unit environments. *J Pediatr.* 2014;164:52–60.
53. Filippa M, Panza C, Ferrari F, et al. Systematic review of maternal voice interventions demonstrates increased stability in preterm infants. *Acta Paediatr.* 2017;106:1220–1229.
54. Chirico G, Cabano R, Villa G, et al. Randomised study showed that recorded maternal voices reduced pain in preterm infants undergoing heel lance procedures in a neonatal intensive care unit. *Acta Paediatr.* 2017;106(10):1564–1568.
55. Vinall J, Miller SP, Bjornson BH, et al. Invasive procedures in preterm children: brain and cognitive development at school age. *Pediatrics.* 2014;133:412–421.
56. Zwicker JG, Miller SP, Grunau RE, et al. Smaller cerebellar growth and poorer neurodevelopmental outcomes in very preterm infants exposed to neonatal morphine. *J Pediatr.* 2016;172:81–87.
57. McPherson C, Haslam M, Pineda R, et al. Brain injury and development in preterm infants exposed to fentanyl. *Ann Pharmacother.* 2015;49:1291–1297.
58. Duerden EG, Guo T, Dodbiba L, et al. Midazolam dose correlates with abnormal hippocampal growth and neurodevelopmental outcome in preterm infants. *Ann Neurol.* 2016;79:548–559.

18

59. Creeley CE. From drug-induced developmental neuroapoptosis to pediatric anesthetic neurotoxicity-where are we now? *Brain Sci*. 2016;6(3).
60. Davidson JO, Wassink G, van den Heuij LG, et al. Therapeutic hypothermia for neonatal hypoxic-ischemic encephalopathy—where to from here? *Front Neurol*. 2015;6:198.
61. Westin B, Miller JA Jr, Nyberg R, et al. Neonatal asphyxia pallida treated with hypothermia alone or with hypothermia and transfusion of oxygenated blood. *Surgery*. 1959;45:868–879.
62. Azzopardi DV, Strohm B, Edwards AD, et al. Moderate hypothermia to treat perinatal asphyxial encephalopathy. *N Engl J Med*. 2009;361:1349–1358.
63. Thoresen M, Tooley J, Liu X, et al. Time Is brain: starting therapeutic hypothermia within three hours after birth improves motor outcome in asphyxiated newborns. *Neonatology*. 2013;104:228–233.
64. Gunn AJ, Laptook AR, Robertson NJ, et al. Therapeutic hypothermia translates from ancient history in to practice. *Pediatr Res*. 2017;81:202–209.
65. Shankaran S, Laptook AR, Pappas A, et al. Effect of depth and duration of cooling on deaths in the NICU among neonates with hypoxic ischemic encephalopathy: a randomized clinical trial. *JAMA*. 2014;312:2629–2639.
66. Sun Y, Zhang L, Chen Y, et al. Therapeutic targets for cerebral ischemia based on the signaling pathways of the GluN2B C terminus. *Stroke*. 2015;46:2347–2353.
67. Wu YW, Bauer LA, Ballard RA, et al. Erythropoietin for neuroprotection in neonatal encephalopathy: safety and pharmacokinetics. *Pediatrics*. 2012;130:683–691.
68. Wu YW, Mathur AM, Chang T, et al. High-Dose Erythropoietin and Hypothermia for Hypoxic-Ischemic Encephalopathy: A Phase II Trial. *Pediatrics*. 2016;137:e20160191.
69. Filippi L, Fiorini P, Catarzi S, et al. Safety and efficacy of topiramate in neonates with hypoxic ischemic encephalopathy treated with hypothermia (NeoNATI): a feasibility study. *J Matern Fetal Neonatal Med*. 2018;31:973–980.
70. Hobbs C, Thoresen M, Tucker A, et al. Xenon and hypothermia combine additively, offering long-term functional and histopathologic neuroprotection after neonatal hypoxia/ischemia. *Stroke*. 2008;39:1307–1313.
71. Ma D, Hossain M, Chow A, et al. Xenon and hypothermia combine to provide neuroprotection from neonatal asphyxia. *Ann Neurol*. 2005;58:182–193.
72. Martin JL, Ma D, Hossain M, et al. Asynchronous administration of xenon and hypothermia significantly reduces brain infarction in the neonatal rat. *Br J Anaesth*. 2007;98:236–240.
73. Thoresen M, Hobbs CE, Wood T, et al. Cooling combined with immediate or delayed xenon inhalation provides equivalent long-term neuroprotection after neonatal hypoxia-ischemia. *J Cereb Blood Flow Metab*. 2009;29:707–714.
74. Sabir H, Osredkar D, Maes E, et al. Xenon combined with therapeutic hypothermia is not neuroprotective after severe hypoxia-ischemia in neonatal rats. *PLoS ONE*. 2016;11:e0156759.
75. Dingley J, Tooley J, Liu X, et al. Xenon ventilation during therapeutic hypothermia in neonatal encephalopathy: a feasibility study. *Pediatrics*. 2014;133:809–818.
76. Rawat S, Dingley J. Closed-circuit xenon delivery using a standard anesthesia workstation. *Anesth Analg*. 2010;110:101–109.
77. Azzopardi D, Robertson NJ, Bainbridge A, et al. Moderate hypothermia within 6 h of birth plus inhaled xenon versus moderate hypothermia alone after birth asphyxia (TOBY-Xe): a proof-of-concept, open-label, randomised controlled trial. *Lancet Neurol*. 2016;15:145–153.
78. Dingley J, Liu X, Gill H, et al. The feasibility of using a portable xenon delivery device to permit earlier xenon ventilation with therapeutic cooling of neonates during ambulance retrieval. *Anesth Analg*. 2015;120:1331–1336.
79. Azzopardi D, Robertson NJ, Kapetanakis A, et al. Anticonvulsant effect of xenon on neonatal asphyxial seizures. *Arch Dis Child Fetal Neonatal Ed*. 2013;98:F437–F439.
80. Alonso-Alconada D, Alvarez A, Arteaga O, et al. Neuroprotective effect of melatonin: a novel therapy against perinatal hypoxia-ischemia. *Int J Mol Sci*. 2013;14:9379–9395.
81. Robertson NJ, Faulkner S, Fleiss B, et al. Melatonin augments hypothermic neuroprotection in a perinatal asphyxia model. *Brain*. 2013;136:90–105.
82. Aly H, Elmahdy H, El-Dib M, et al. Melatonin use for neuroprotection in perinatal asphyxia: a randomized controlled pilot study. *J Perinatol*. 2015;35:186–191.
83. Benders MJ, Bos AF, Rademaker CM, et al. Early postnatal allopurinol does not improve short term outcome after severe birth asphyxia. *Arch Dis Child Fetal Neonatal Ed*. 2006;91:F163–F165.
84. Torrance HL, Benders MJ, Derks JB, et al. Maternal allopurinol during fetal hypoxia lowers cord blood levels of the brain injury marker S-100B. *Pediatrics*. 2009;124:350–357.
85. Galinsky R, Bennet L, Groenendaal F, et al. Magnesium is not consistently neuroprotective for perinatal hypoxia-ischemia in term-equivalent models in preclinical studies: a systematic review. *Dev Neurosci*. 2014;36:73–82.
86. Bennet L, Tan S, Van den Heuij L, et al. Cell therapy for neonatal hypoxia-ischemia and cerebral palsy. *Ann Neurol*. 2012;71:589–600.
87. Liao Y, Cotten M, Tan S, et al. Rescuing the neonatal brain from hypoxic injury with autologous cord blood. *Bone Marrow Transplant*. 2013;48:890–900.
88. Sun JM, Kurtzberg J. Cord blood for brain injury. *Cytotherapy*. 2015;17:775–785.
89. Castillo-Melendez M, Yawno T, Jenkin G, et al. Stem cell therapy to protect and repair the developing brain: a review of mechanisms of action of cord blood and amnion epithelial derived cells. *Front Neurosci*. 2013;7:194.

90. Lim JY, Park SI, Oh JH, et al. Brain-derived neurotrophic factor stimulates the neural differentiation of human umbilical cord blood-derived mesenchymal stem cells and survival of differentiated cells through MAPK/ERK and PI3K/Akt-dependent signaling pathways. *J Neurosci Res*. 2008;86:2168–2178.
91. Pimentel-Coelho PM, Magalhaes ES, Lopes LM, et al. Human cord blood transplantation in a neonatal rat model of hypoxic-ischemic brain damage: functional outcome related to neuroprotection in the striatum. *Stem Cells Dev*. 2010;19:351–358.
92. van Velthoven CT, Dzietko M, Wendland MF, et al. Mesenchymal stem cells attenuate MRI-identifiable injury, protect white matter, and improve long-term functional outcomes after neonatal focal stroke in rats. *J Neurosci Res*. 2017;95:1225–1236.
93. Cotten CM, Murtha AP, Goldberg RN, et al. Feasibility of autologous cord blood cells for infants with hypoxic-ischemic encephalopathy. *J Pediatr*. 2014;164:973–979 e1.

18

CHAPTER 19

Pharmacologic Therapy for Neonatal Abstinence Syndrome

Prabhakar Kocherlakota, MD

- NAS increases morbidity and prolongs the length of stay among infants.
- Nonpharmacological measures should be implemented before the initiation of pharmacological measures.
- Breast feeding may decrease the need and duration of therapy.
- Protocolized management decreases the length of stay and the length of treatment.
- Morphine or methadone can be used to control severe signs of NAS.
- Adjunctive medications can be initiated when opioid therapy is not successful or when the maximum dose of opioid reached.

Neonatal abstinence syndrome (NAS) is a constellation of clinical signs that are a consequence of abrupt discontinuation of chronic fetal exposure to substances used, misused, or abused by a mother during pregnancy.[1] NAS can be due to various substances, which may be legal or illegal, prescribed or not prescribed, opioids or nonopioids. NAS due to opioids is more common and intense; hence, it is often referred as *neonatal opioid withdrawal syndrome.*[2] NAS is a generalized multisystem disorder primarily involving the central nervous, autonomic nervous, and gastrointestinal systems.

Incidence

Although NAS was first reported more than 150 years ago, a recent communiqué from the Centers for Disease Control and Prevention in the United States has noted a 300% increase over the last 15 years.[3] The incidence of hospital admissions due to NAS increased from 1.5 per 1000 hospital births to 7.3 per 1000 hospital births in the United States.[4] In some states, the incidence of NAS was as high as 33 per 1000 hospital births.[3] Similar increases of NAS were also seen in Canada, England, Europe, and Australia,[5–8] and are reported from all types of hospitals, whether teaching or nonteaching, rural or urban, and children's or community hospitals.[9] Though the NAS epidemic has affected all communities and all ethnicities, it is disproportionately seen in Caucasians. The percentage of infants with NAS born to Caucasian mothers increased from 64% in 2004–2005 to 69% in 2008–2009 and to 76% in 2012–2013.[10] In addition to increased incidence, the length of hospital stay for infants with NAS has increased,[10] leading to increased governmental cost, as the majority of NAS cases occur in a population that depends upon government-subsidized health care.[11]

Etiology

Historically, opium addiction increased from early in the 19th century, following commercial production of morphine and heroin.[12,13] Heroin use became illegal after the Harrison Act in 1914.[14] Because of concerns about addiction, physicians were restricted in prescribing opiates except for conditions of severe pain associated with terminal cancer.[15,16] However, pressure increased on physicians to control pain and decrease suffering, and nonopiate analgesics turned out to be either not as effective or associated with toxicity. The misconception that orally administered opioids are not associated with addiction led to increased prescription of oral opioid preparations by the physician community.[17–20] The increased availability of multiple prescription opioids, aggressive marketing techniques by the pharmaceutical industry, and liberal prescription practices among some physicians helped propagate the opioid epidemic. Increased cost and difficulty in obtaining prescription opioids, along with increased availability and decreased cost of heroin, may have led to the resurgence of heroin use and worsened the current opioid epidemic across the world (Fig. 19.1). Pregnant women are no exception to this phenomenon.

Methadone and buprenorphine maintenance treatment for opioid addiction, excessive use of prescription medications, and the continuous popularity of heroin among pregnant women have all contributed to the increased incidence of NAS in

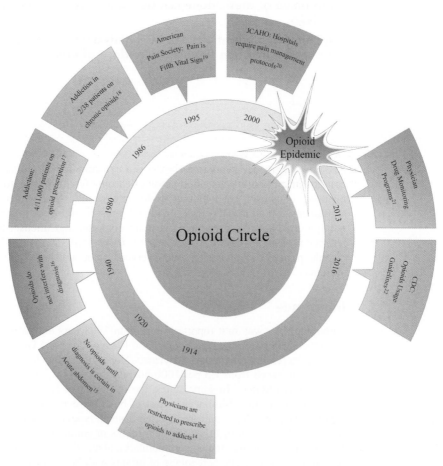

Figure 19.1 Opioid circle. Restriction of opioid use was introduced in the early 20th century due to social misuse of heroin and morphine.[14] That was followed by gradual relaxation of restrictions, and increased prescription opioid use and heroin use led to an opioid epidemic with severe consequences in the early 20th century,[15–20] which led to the reintroduction of restricted opioid use practices.[21,22]

infants. Self-medication is common among women with substance use disorders (SUDs), and anxiety and depression during pregnancy further complicate SUD. In a recent study by Tolia et al., of 4146 infants with NAS in the United States during 2012–2013, 31% of infants were exposed to methadone, 24% were exposed to a prescription opioid, and 15% were exposed to buprenorphine.[10] Among infants in the same study, 9% were also exposed to antidepressants and 8% to benzodiazepines.[10] Thus the spectrum of NAS worsened because of increased use of opioids, use of multiple opioids, and concurrent use of other legal (such as benzodiazepines and antidepressants) and illegal substances (such as cocaine and marijuana).

Pathophysiology

Opioid withdrawal is a complex phenomenon and is not completely understood in infants. Chronic opioid exposure is associated with desensitization and downregulation of opioid receptors, causing adaptation of a neuron-mediated altered normality state, and termination of opioid exposure leads to upregulation of opioid receptors with ripple effects on various counterregulatory pathways, causing massive neurotransmitter imbalances.[23] Opioid withdrawal causes increased production of norepinephrine from the locus coeruleus of the pons,[24] decreased production of dopamine from the ventral tegmental area of the midbrain and nucleus accumbens of the basal ganglia,[25] relative serotonin deficiency from the dorsal raphe nucleus of the brain stem,[26] and increased acetylcholine from the medial habenula of the thalamus and from autonomic and peripheral nervous systems.[27] In addition, withdrawal is associated with increased corticotrophin release, due to activation of the hypothalamic–pituitary–adrenocortical axis[28] and increased release of multiple other substances, including dynorphin, substance P, orexin, and others, which complicates the clinical picture of NAS.[29,30]

Clinical Presentation

NAS is a complex cluster of clinical signs involving multiple systems, including the central nervous, autonomic nervous, respiratory, and gastrointestinal systems.[1] The acute phase may last for 1 to 2 weeks and be followed by a subacute stage lasting another 2 to 6 weeks, with relapses and remissions, terminating with a long chronic stage of persisting symptoms that may last for 6 to 12 weeks or more.

Tremors and irritability may be the initial presenting features. Hyperirritability is the hallmark of NAS. Agitation and excessive crying, probably secondary to lack of sleep, are striking features of NAS. Abnormal movements, myoclonic jerks, and occasionally seizures are seen during the acute phase.[31] Gastrointestinal signs, including uncoordinated sucking, poor feeding, regurgitation, vomiting, and diarrhea, may lead to poor weight gain, electrolyte imbalance, and dehydration in infants affected by NAS. Autonomic nervous system signs, including tachycardia, tachypnea, sweating, sneezing, and skin mottling, may affect these infants for months.[32]

Many NAS signs may be mistaken for other conditions. Tachypnea and nasal flaring may be mistaken for respiratory distress in newborns. Temperature disturbance and sweating can be misdiagnosed as sepsis. Poor feeding, tremors, and sweating may be interpreted as hypoglycemia. Vomiting and diarrhea may be mistaken for formula intolerance. Hyperphagia is also often missed in infants with NAS.

NAS may manifest at different times with different substances. Heroin withdrawal is seen in NAS infants within the first day of life. Methadone and buprenorphine withdrawal are seen by the second and third day. NAS onset may be delayed in infants when barbiturates or benzodiazepines are used along with opioids by the mother. NAS due to nonopioids is usually less intense and rarely lasts a week.[1]

NAS can be severe and of long duration in full-term infants, in infants of polydrug-abusing mothers, and in infants with delayed drug metabolism. Preterm infants are less prone to NAS because their cumulative exposure is shorter and placental transmission in early pregnancy is lower. Immaturity of the nervous system, as well as decreased hepatic clearance of methadone, may play a role in decreased NAS in preterm infants. Preterm infants with NAS scored lower in sleep disturbances, tremors, muscle tone, sweating, nasal stuffiness, and loose stools compared with full-term controls.[33,34] Male gender, maternal smoking, and a high maternal methadone dose may be additional risk factors for more severe NAS.[1]

NAS is a clinical diagnosis, but toxicology confirmation is needed because the maternal history is often unreliable. It is important to identify the type of opioid the mother is using or misusing and to confirm or rule out other licit or illicit drug use during pregnancy. Urine testing is inexpensive, reproducible, and has a short turnaround time, but there is a short window of time of detection. Meconium testing is more sensitive and has a long window of time of detection, but it is costly, depends upon extraction technology, and has a longer turnaround time. Umbilical cord, hair, placenta, and amniotic fluids can also be tested for in utero substance exposure.[1,35] Earlier detection of substance exposure leads to better management of exposed infants.[36]

Management

NAS is a treatable disease that can cause morbidity and mortality in infants if untreated. NAS is a multisystem disorder, but management is symptomatic. There are wide variations in its management, and no evidence-based guidelines are available at present.

Management depends upon the severity of signs of substance withdrawal. A scoring system is essential—in the absence of other quantifiable assessment measures—to initiate, monitor, titrate, and terminate therapy in infants. Scoring needs to be performed every 3 to 4 hours, after infant feedings, and when the infant is awake, and the score should accurately represent the status of the infant not only at the time of scoring but also during the preceding 3 to 4 hours. An ideal NAS scoring system would be reliable, easy to implement, less time consuming, and consistent with minimal interobserver variability. In the absence of an ideal scoring system at present, the modified Finnegan scoring system continues to be a popular tool for monitoring withdrawal in infants.[37] Opinions differ about the specific scores required for initiating, increasing, decreasing, or terminating NAS treatment.[38]

Nonpharmacologic Management

Management of the infant includes both pharmacologic and nonpharmacologic measures. Nonpharmacologic measures often suffice for mild withdrawal and are also important for the success of pharmacologic measures. Nonpharmacologic measures are less costly, easy to implement, and should be tried on all infants with NAS before initiating pharmacologic therapy. The neonatal care team needs to practice a non-judgmental approach toward parents. Parental involvement is a crucial part of treatment of NAS. Parental presence was shown to decrease Finnegan scores and delay the need for pharmacologic therapy.[39] Rooming-in of mother and infant also encourages active parental participation in the care of the infant.[40]

Breastfeeding is recommended in infants with NAS. Multiple studies have demonstrated that breastfeeding decreases length of treatment (LOT), the amount of morphine needed, the length of hospital stay, and most importantly allows maternal participation in the management of the infant.[41–44] The amounts of methadone or buprenorphine in breast milk are too small to treat NAS, and sudden discontinuation of breast milk is not associated with worsening of NAS.[45,46] Mothers with SUD with no prenatal care and/or not in drug treatment programs are discouraged from breast-feeding.[47] Women with SUD are often treated for comorbid psychiatric conditions, such as anxiety or depression (which may themselves interfere with breastfeeding), but the safety of exposure of breastfeeding babies to many of the medications used for these conditions has not been established.[48] Lactation experts have differences of opinion regarding breastfeeding among mothers using marijuana.[49,50] Breastfeeding is contraindicated if the mother is using an illicit substance (such as cocaine, heroin, amphetamine, or phencyclidine) or is infected with HIV.

Gentle handling is the rule, and minimal stimulation is a priority. Frequent feedings and high-calorie formulas may be required to meet the increased metabolic demands of NAS infants.[51] Kangaroo care, pacifiers, rocking beds, water beds, acupuncture, and music therapy may also help soothe these babies.[52-55] It often helps to simply hold and cuddle infants with NAS. Staying alert to a newborn's irritability may be important in controlling the severity of symptoms. Continuous excellent supportive care may not only help to avoid pharmacologic intervention, but may also accelerate the infant's discharge from the hospital.[56]

Pharmacologic Management

Pharmacologic measures are required only if NAS cannot be contained with non-pharmacologic measures. Studies have shown that 27% to 91% of infants with NAS require medical intervention to control withdrawal symptoms.[57,58] More infants are now being treated with medications compared with 10 years ago.[10] In a study involving 10,327 infants, Tolia et al. noted that the proportion of infants with NAS who received pharmacotherapy increased from 74% in 2004-2005 to 87% in 2012-2013.[10] The complex nature of withdrawal, polysubstance use by pregnant women, and multiple substantiated or unsubstantiated nonpharmacologic interventions may complicate determination of advantages or disadvantages of pharmacologic management of NAS. Though drug withdrawal is a self-limiting process, medication treatment is essential when nonpharmacologic measures fail to control NAS signs, or when withdrawal is associated with serious complications such as seizures or severe dehydration due to diarrhea and vomiting. Delays in pharmacologic therapy are associated with higher morbidity and longer hospital stays.[59]

Protocol or No Protocol

In the absence of specific guidelines, the diagnosis and management of NAS were historically left to the discretion of individual physicians or hospitals. The number of hospitals with written NAS management protocols increased from 54% in 2006 to 72% in 2012.[60,61] The Joint Commission in the United States has advised hospitals to adopt practice guidelines for the management of NAS.[62] As the incidence of NAS has increased, along with increased time in neonatal intensive care units, multidisciplinary standardized protocols have been developed for the management of NAS. Many states in the United States have initiated statewide protocols.[63,64] These protocols include measures for screening, scoring, and nonpharmacologic as well as pharmacologic interventions, including addition of adjunct medications and weaning of medications. Consensus on uniform guidelines has not been achieved, however, because NAS is a complex cluster of signs and symptoms, scorings are mostly subjective, NAS is a self-limiting disorder, treatment can be continued in or out of the hospital, and there is no single criterion for effectiveness of any protocol.

The impacts of protocol implementations have been inconsistent (Table 19.1). Hall et al. found decreased LOT and length of stay (LOS) in infants who were managed with a stringent weaning protocol compared with infants who were managed without any protocol.[65] This difference persisted irrespective of medication used in the management of NAS. Asti et al. decreased LOS by half when a standardized protocol was used.[66] In a larger retrospective study, Hall et al. further showed that LOS and LOT decreased in hospitals that continue to practice the existing weaning protocols, as well as in the hospitals that started adopting new weaning protocols.[63] In a large multistate, multicenter collaborative quality study, Patrick et al. also showed that standardized protocol decreased LOT and LOS, but no decrease of LOS or LOT was achieved in the absence of regular reinforcements.[67] Standardization of the management protocol failed to produce any change in another study.[68] Successful implementation requires protocols that are simple, practical, and evidence based. All protocols require dedicated commitment from hospitals as well as staff.

Medications

Multiple recent studies demonstrated that an increasing number of infants are being treated with various medications in the management of NAS. In a study of 3458

Table 19.1 STUDIES WITH STANDARDIZED PROTOCOLS IN THE MANAGEMENT OF NEONATAL ABSTINENCE SYNDROME

Author	Protocol	Number	Results	Comments
Hall et al.[65] 2014	Protocol (guidelines for identification, scoring, initiation of pharmacologic treatment) 3 regions: Stringent weaning protocol 3 regions: No stringent weaning protocol	20 hospitals n = 547 No weaning protocol: 130 stringent weaning protocol: 417	No weaning protocol vs. stringent protocol LOT: 32.1 days vs. 17.7 days* LOS: 32.1 days vs. 22.7 days *	Retrospective Weaning protocol only Different treatment protocols Different medications 12% discharged home on opioid medication
Asti et al.[66] 2015	Communication between medical and nursing staff Finnegan scoring training Standard initiation and weaning protocol Collaboration with OB and addiction specialist	8 NICU n = 92 Control: 23 Study: 52	LOS: Controls: 36 days Study: 21 days	Retrospective Small study No statistics Infants of mothers on methadone ≥80 mg/day required adjunctive meds
Hall et al.[63] 2015	Identification, scoring Initiation of treatment Standardized inpatient weaning 3 protocol existing centers 3 protocol adopting centers	20 hospitals n = 981 Controls: 813 Study: 168	Adopting sites: LOT: Before: 34 days After: 23 days* LOS: Before: 31 days After: 23 days*	Retrospective study Nonpharmacologic measures not included 48% study patients followed protocol 11% patients discharged home on opioids Adjunct therapy decreased from 21%–5%* in the study group but not in the control group No difference if only inpatients were included
Rajbhandari et al.[68] 2016	Higher maximum dose of morphine Earlier initiation of phenobarbital Specific weaning criteria	Single hospital n = 66 Control: 49 Study: 17	LOS: Control: 35 Study: 41 LOT: Control: 30 Study: 30	Retrospective Single institution No significant difference No scoring education Nonpharmacologic measures not included
Patrick et al.[67] 2016	Identification Screening NAS scoring Nonpharmacologic treatment Pharmacologic treatment Breastfeeding Reinforcing training every 6 mo	199 hospitals n = 3458 83% morphine 15% methadone	LOT: 16 to 15 days* LOS: 21 to 19 days* Home medications at discharge decreased from 39.7%–26.5%	Retrospective No control group LOT decreased by 1 day only LOS decreased by 2 days only No change without reinforcements

*P < 0.05

LOS, Length of stay; *LOT,* length of treatment; *NAS,* neonatal abstinence syndrome; *NICU,* neonatal intensive care unit; *OB,* obstetric.

infants from 2012 to 2014, Patrick et al. noted that 83% of infants received pharmacotherapy in the management of NAS.[69] In another study, 87% of infants required medications to control NAS.[10] Though many medications are available to provide short-term amelioration of signs of NAS, none are approved by the US Food and Drug Administration (FDA) for use in NAS management. Most of these medications are also associated with potential harm to the developing brain. Morphine, methadone, and phenobarbital are the most commonly used medications.[69] Buprenorphine and clonidine are used occasionally. Opioid therapy, recommended by the American Academy of Pediatrics (AAP), is superior to other medications, as it is associated with less treatment failure. However, opioid therapy may prolong hospital stay.[51,70] Older medications like the paregoric or tincture of opium are no longer used or available now because of their toxic ingredients and high alcohol content.[71] Sedatives like diazepam and chlorpromazine were not shown to be useful because of prolonged half-lives and adverse side effects.[72,73] Other medications, such as ondansetron are in trials now. Major medications used in the management of NAS, their mechanisms of action, pharmacokinetic (PK) properties, doses, advantages, and disadvantages are listed in Table 19.2.

Morphine

Morphine, a natural μ-opioid receptor agonist, is the most commonly used medication in the treatment of NAS in the United States, England, Europe, and Australia.[51,87] Oral morphine decreases agitation, improves feeding, and controls severe withdrawal symptoms. Oral morphine solution is stable, free of alcohol, and has a short serum half-life (of approximately 8 hours in term infants[74,75]) that necessitates frequent administration. When an optimal response is not attained with the maximal dose, additional medications may be considered. Morphine dose can be increased or decreased depending upon the Finnegan scores. The concentration of commercially available oral preparations is too high for use in infants, so these solutions must be diluted further before dispensing for this indication; hence, caution should be exercised lest errors happen with morphine dilution or dose. Home treatment is not the preferred option with morphine. Kelly et al. showed that LOS could be decreased to 16 days in infants with home morphine treatment (n = 28) from 22 days in infants with hospital morphine treatment (n = 52), but the home treatment group required more adjunct treatment, had longer LOT, and had one death.[88] Morphine has become popular, as its safety is well established and dose adjustments can be easily managed (Fig. 19.2).

Methadone

Methadone, a semisynthetic complete μ-opioid receptor agonist, is an alternative to morphine in the treatment of NAS. It is more frequently used in the United States compared with other countries.[89] Methadone is more acceptable for administration to an infant if the mother is also on methadone treatment. The long half-life of methadone (median 26–41 hours[78,79]) facilitates reduced interdose variation in serum concentrations, but the correspondingly longer interval required for achievement of steady-state mandates less frequent dose adjustments and may make dose adjustment more difficult. Methadone dose also can be increased or decreased depending upon the Finnegan scores. Methadone is commercially prepared and does not require dilution. Caution should be exercised when methadone is used along with other medications like phenobarbital (phenobarbital may accelerate the metabolism of methadone) or antiretroviral medications (methadone may inhibit metabolism and clearance of zidovudine).[90] Infants can be discharged home on methadone[91]; however, multiple studies have reported increasing pediatrician concern for out-of-hospital methadone treatment.[66,84] Tolia et al. noted that the proportion of infants with NAS who were discharged home on medications decreased by 50% in the last 10 years.[10] Methadone labeling by the FDA carries a black box warning of prolonged QT interval.

Morphine or Methadone

Multiple studies compared the effectiveness of morphine to methadone. However, conclusions are difficult to draw from these studies, as seven of eight studies were retrospective, and six of eight studies were not based on a protocol. Of three large studies, two studies did not show a difference between morphine and methadone.[63,64] Another large study showed that methadone use decreased LOS, but methadone use decreased from 25% to 15% and morphine use increased from 49% to 72% during

Table 19.2   COMMON MEDICATIONS USED IN THE MANAGEMENT OF NEONATAL ABSTINENCE SYNDROME

Medication	Mechanism of Action	Pharmacokinetics	Treatment Dose	Maximum Dose	Advantages	Disadvantages
Morphine	Natural μ-receptor agonist Schedule II drug	Half-life: 8 hr[74,75] Bioavailability: 48%[76] Protein binding: 20% Hepatic glucuronidation	0.05–0.2 mg/kg/dose q3–4h Increase by 0.05 mg/kg q24–48h	1.3 mg/kg/day[83]	No alcohol Ease of titration	Sedation Apnea Constipation Frequent dosing
Methadone	Synthetic Complete μ-receptor agonist N-methyl-D aspartate antagonist Schedule II drug	Half-life: 26 hr[77–79] Bioavailability: 86% Protein binding: 85%–90% Hepatic demethylation	0.05–0.1 mg/kg/dose q12h Increase by 0.05 mg/kg q48h	1 mg/kg/day[84]	12-hr doses Ease of dosing	Alcohol 8% Longer duration of action Variable half-life Prolongation of QT interval
Buprenorphine	Semisynthetic Partial μ receptor agonist κ-receptor antagonist Schedule III drug	Half-life: 11 hr[80] Bioavailability: 7% (sublingual) Protein binding: 96% Hepatic N-dealkylation	4–5 μg/kg/dose q8h	60 μg/kg/day[85]	Sublingual route Ease of dosing	Alcohol 30% Respiratory depression Adjuvant medications may be required
Phenobarbital	γ-amino butyric acid agonist Schedule IV drug	Half-life: 45–100 hr[81] Bioavailability: 48% Protein binding: 35%–50% Hepatic hydroxylation	Loading dose: 16 mg/kg Maintenance dose: 1–4 mg/kg/dose q12h	Levels >40 μg/mL[81]	Monitor levels Well studied	Alcohol 15% Possible hyperactivity High treatment failure Drug–drug interactions Sedation
Clonidine	α-adrenergic receptor agonist	Half-life: 44–72 hr[82] Bioavailability: 90% Protein binding: 20%–40% Renal	Initial dose: 0.5–1 μg/kg followed by 0.5–1.25 μg/kg/dose q4–6h	12 μg/kg/day[86]	No sedation No alcohol Monitor levels	Hypotension Abrupt discontinuation may cause rapid rise of blood pressure and heart rate

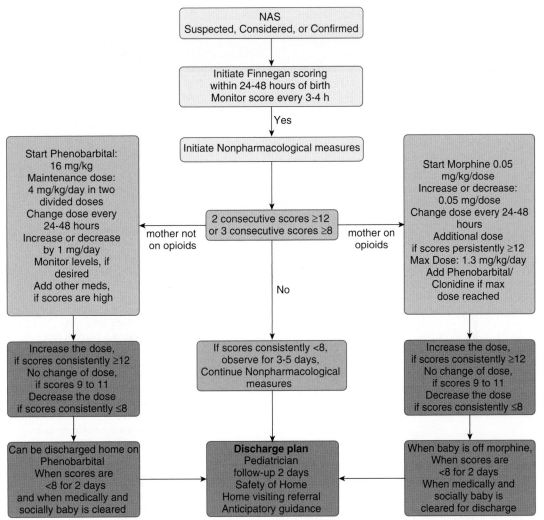

Figure 19.2   A management plan for neonatal abstinence syndrome in infants. Initial dose is based on weight, and further standard doses are based Finnegan NAS scores. Medications are increased, decreased, or discontinued depending on the scores. The morphine standard dose can be increased if scores are ≥12 for two consecutive times, decreased if <8 for two consecutive times, and not changed if scores are between 9 and 11. Methadone can be substituted for morphine for opioid withdrawal, and phenobarbital is usually initiated for nonopioid NAS. Cardiopulmonary monitoring of the infant is preferred during the acute stage.

the course of the study.[10] Similarly, another study showed that LOS was shorter with methadone use compared with morphine, but methadone use decreased from 44% to 11%, and morphine use increased from 49% to 53% in that study.[69] One study needed to discontinue methadone treatment because pediatricians in the community were reluctant to continue methadone intervention out of the hospital.[84] Hall et al. showed no difference in morphine and methadone with respect to LOT and LOS when a protocol is followed.[65] A preliminary study showed that genetic variations may decrease LOS with morphine and methadone treatment in infants with NAS.[96] Both morphine and methadone are associated with short-term side effects as well as long-term adverse neurologic affects (Table 19.3).

Morphine: Score-Based or Weight-Based Dosing

Morphine and methadone doses are usually based on weight, but an increasing number of studies have used dosing based on Finnegan score. However, as scores are subjective and observer dependent, it is difficult to compare these approaches.

Table 19.3 STUDIES COMPARING MORPHINE TO METHADONE IN THE TREATMENT OF NEONATAL ABSTINENCE SYNDROME

Author	Number of Patients	Results (Days) (Morphine vs. Methadone)	Comments
Lainwala et al.[92] 2005	Morphine: 17 Methadone: 29	LOS: (median) 36 (33–39) vs. 40 (30–51)	Retrospective, cohort study Small sample (two hospitals) No statistical significance Deodorized tincture of opium and morphine solution were grouped together
Napolitano et al.[84] 2013	Morphine: 139 Methadone: 154	LOS: 20 vs. 13	Retrospective No statistical inference 89% discharged home on methadone
Hall et al.[65] 2014	Morphine: 232 Methadone: 151	LOT: 15.6 vs. 16.2 LOS: 21.6 vs. 21.5	Retrospective Protocol driven No statistical significance
Patrick et al.[69] 2014	Morphine: 6 hospitals Methadone: 6 hospitals (Total = 1424)	LOT: 22.2 vs. 17.4* LOS: 25.0 vs. 21*	Retrospective, cohort study (14 hospitals) Wide variation in protocols and adjunct medication use Methadone use decreased from 44% to 11% No breastfeeding data, no nonpharmacologic measures Stand-alone children's hospital data (mostly)
Lee et al.[93] 2015	Morphine: 48 Methadone: 41	LOS: 21.6 vs. 11.4	Retrospective, cohort study Methadone has lowest LOS of all medications Wide variation of LOS within individual hospitals Inpatient treatment for morphine and combined inpatient and home treatment with methadone
Karna et al.[64] 2015	Morphine: 254 Methadone: 88	LOT: 16 ± 10 vs. 19 ± 23	Retrospective, cohort study State quality collaborative study No statistical significance Adjunct medicine required more with morphine
Young et al.[94] 2015	Morphine: 13 Methadone: 13	LOS: 12.08 vs. 44.23* LOT: 7.46 vs. 38.08*	Retrospective, small sample Morphine: score-based protocol Methadone: weight-based protocol Different scoring systems for morphine and methadone No difference in average score or need for adjunct therapy
Brown et al.[95] 2015	Morphine: 16 Methadone: 15	LOS: 21 vs. 14*	Prospective, randomized, double-masked study Single-center study Median maternal methadone dose is 160 mg in morphine group and 72 mg on methadone group

*$P < 0.05$
LOS, Length of stay; *LOT*, length of treatment.

In addition, different institutions have used different score-based regimens and different scoring systems.[97,98] A recent retrospective observational study failed to find any difference with regard to total cumulative dose of morphine or LOS between weight-based model (n = 18) or score-based model (n = 57).[99] When clonidine was included along with morphine in that study, the total cumulative dose of morphine and LOS were less in the weight-based model (n = 68) compared with the score-based model (n = 78).[99] Score-based treatments are in use for opioid medications and not for nonopioid medications. Because there are no large multicenter studies presently available that favor one over the other, this author is in favor of a weight-based initial dose followed by score-based increases or decreases in a standard dose (see Fig. 19.2).

Methadone: Standard Weaning or Pharmacokinetic Weaning

The standard weaning protocols managed methadone doses based on clinical response and dose of medication being used; however, a new protocol managed methadone dose based on PK modeling.[100] A recent study compared 267 infants on standard weaning protocol with 93 infants on a new PK model weaning protocol in the management of NAS.[101] Both LOS and LOT decreased by 3 days in the new PK modeling-based weaning protocol compared with the standard weaning protocol. However, the amount of methadone to treat NAS or the need for adjunct therapy did not decrease. This new weaning protocol can be tailored to individual patients and is physiologically sound, but it requires frequent blood sampling, requires advanced laboratory support, and may require 2 to 3 days before a steady-state is attained. Though this study's results are exciting, the PK model protocol should be considered experimental until a larger prospective study is carried out to validate these observations.

Buprenorphine

Buprenorphine, a semisynthetic partial μ-receptor agonist, is a new addition in NAS treatment. A long half-life (approximately 20 hours, based on limited data from premature infants[102]) is a major advantage for buprenorphine. There is also no cardiovascular toxicity associated with buprenorphine. Phenobarbital has minimal effect on buprenorphine clearance.[103] Kraft et al., in a prospective, randomized, open-label phase I study with buprenorphine in a dose of 4.4 μg/kg/dose every 8 hours, were unable to decrease either LOS or LOT in 12 infants compared with 13 infants treated with oral neonatal opium solution.[104] However, with a higher initial dose of buprenorphine (5.3 μg/kg/dose every 8 hours) and more aggressive dose advancement for high NAS scores, Kraft et al. were able to decrease LOT and LOS in a buprenorphine group (n = 12) compared with the oral neonatal opium solution group (n = 12) in another prospective phase I study.[85] Hall et al., in a retrospective study, had shown decreased LOT and LOS in 38 infants treated with a buprenorphine protocol compared with 163 infants treated with a methadone protocol.[105] Because buprenorphine must be given sublingually, further PK studies are needed to determine the absorption, bioavailability, and efficacy of buprenorphine in infants.[103] A large prospective study might further define the role of buprenorphine in the management of NAS.

Phenobarbital

Phenobarbital, a gamma-amino butyric acid receptor agonist, can be used as a first-line medication as well as an adjunct medication in NAS treatment. The half-life of phenobarbital is long at birth and decreases with postnatal age (114 hours at 1 week, and 67 hours after 4 weeks).[106] Phenobarbital levels can be monitored to prevent toxicity. However, phenobarbital does not prevent seizures at the doses administered for withdrawal, and it will not improve gastrointestinal manifestation of NAS.[107] Phenobarbital is the drug of choice in nonopioid NAS, and it is also preferred in polydrug abuse.[70] Use of phenobarbital as a primary treatment increased from 8% to 36% in a recent observation by Patrick et al.[69] Multiple studies compared phenobarbital with morphine with conflicting results. Jackson et al.[108] and Ebner et al.[109] concluded that morphine is superior to phenobarbital in the management of NAS. However, Finnegan et al.[110] and Nayeri et al.[111] drew opposite conclusions in their studies. Different loading doses, different management protocols, different scoring systems, and different maternal substance use all might have contributed to the different conclusions in these studies. The AAP favors opiates over phenobarbital in the treatment of opiate-induced NAS.[51]

Clonidine

Clonidine is a centrally acting alpha-adrenergic receptor agonist and can be used as a single replacement therapy or as an adjunct medication in the treatment of NAS.[112] Clonidine is a nonnarcotic medication; however, the theoretical risk of hypotension and bradycardia may prohibit increasing the dose. Clonidine can be administered every 4 to 6 hours, and it is possible to monitor clonidine level. Clonidine requires a loading dose to attain an early steady-state concentration. The half-life decreases with increasing age.[82] Hoder et al. successfully used clonidine as a monotherapy for NAS in earlier studies.[113,114] Bada et al. in a prospective, randomized, double-blind study decreased LOT to 28 days in 16 NAS infants treated with clonidine from 39 days in another 16 NAS infants treated with morphine.[86] However, there was no difference with regard to LOS between the two groups, as both in-hospital treatment and home treatment were used in this study, nor was there any difference in 1-year motor, cognitive, and language scores between the two groups.[86] Unless large studies prove beneficial effects of clonidine monotherapy, this therapy must be considered experimental only.

Adjunct Medications

Adjunct medications are used when an infant does not respond to a single opioid, when maximum dose of an opioid is reached, when side effects have developed with opioids, or when there is a relapse after withdrawal was adequately treated. Adjunct medications were required in 40% to 80% of infants with NAS.[65,69] Phenobarbital, clonidine, and clonazepam are commonly used adjunct medications.[96] Phenobarbital is the most common second-line drug. Once instituted, the infant can be discharged home and the phenobarbital dose can be titrated, or the infant can outgrow the dose. Although one study reported discharging infants home on clonidine, potential adverse cardiovascular effects may require discontinuation of clonidine treatment before the infant can be safely discharged home.[86] Effects of exposure on the developing brain is a concern with phenobarbital, whether used for long-term or for short-term treatment,[115] whereas no adverse long-term neurologic outcomes have been associated with clonidine. Phenobarbital is a sedative that may be administered twice a day. Clonidine is not a sedative and may be administered three times a day. Different authors have used different dosages for these drugs. Coyle et al. showed that when phenobarbital was combined with tincture of opium, LOS decreased.[116] Agthe et al. obtained similar results with clonidine.[117] Phenobarbital and morphine in combination increased LOS compared with a combination of phenobarbital and methadone in one study, but the results were exactly opposite in another study.[63,68] In the only prospective randomized study comparing phenobarbital with clonidine, there was no difference with respect to LOS; however, infants were discharged home on phenobarbital in that study[118] (Table 19.4). Adjunctive medications control the severity of neonatal withdrawal, but may prolong LOS.[73]

Discharge and Follow-up

Infants with NAS can be discharged home on medications, but there is a possibility of misuse of these medications in the home environment, so caution should be exercised before such a discharge. When an infant is feeding well, sleeping well, gaining weight, and not showing signs of withdrawal with minimal or no medication support, the infant can be safely discharged home. All infants, whether they received medication for NAS or not, need to be followed regularly after discharge from the hospital A multidisciplinary approach, along with parental participation, is extremely helpful in the management of these infants during their hospital stay and after discharge from the hospital because these infants are more prone to short-term as well as long-term problems.[119,120] Whether prenatal opioid exposure or postnatal opioid or nonopioid treatment has any long-term effects on the newborn brain is presently unknown, as there are few long-term follow-up studies beyond the first few years

Table 19.4 STUDIES WITH ADJUNCT MEDICATION USE IN THE TREATMENT OF NEONATAL ABSTINENCE SYNDROME

Author	Primary Medication	Adjunct Medication	Results	Comments
Coyle et al.[116] 2002	Deodorized tincture of opium (DTO)	Phenobarbital: 10 vs. Placebo: 10	LOS: 38 days vs. 79 days* Maximum daily dose (DTO): 4.7 ± 2.7 mL vs. 16.8 ± 3.7 mL*	Partial randomized study Duration of phenobarbital treatment: 3.5 months
Agthe et al.[117] 2009	Morphine (DTO)	Clonidine: 40 vs. Placebo: 40	LOS: 11 days vs. 15 days* Total dose of Morphine: 7.7 mg vs. 19.2 mg*	Prospective, randomized trial Three clonidine neonates died within 2 months of discharge
Hall et al.[65] 2014	Morphine: 37.1% of 232 vs. Methadone: 22.5% of 151	Phenobarbital	LOT: Morphine: 19.6 days Methadone: 12.0 days*	Retrospective Weaning protocol Multihospital study
Karna et al.[64] 2015	Morphine: 99 vs. Methadone:15	Phenobarbital	LOT: Morphine: 24 ± 15 days Methadone: 37 ± 10 days*	Retrospective State quality collaborative study Polydrug-exposed neonates
Surran et al.[118] 2013	Morphine	Phenobarbital: 34 vs. Clonidine: 32	Morphine treatment 12.4 days vs. 19.5 days* Total morphine dose: 3.8 vs. 6.7	Prospective, randomized Longer treatment with phenobarbital after discharge

*$P < 0.05$
LOS, length of stay; *LOT*, length of treatment.

of life.[121] NAS infants require neurodevelopmental, nutritional, social, environmental, and family assessments during follow-up after discharge.[122,123]

REFERENCES

1. Kocherlakota P. Neonatal abstinence syndrome. *Pediatrics*. 2014;134:e547–e561.
2. Sutter MB, Leeman L, Hsi A. Neonatal opioid withdrawal syndrome. *Obstet Gynecol Clin North Am*. 2014;41:317–334.
3. Ko JY, Patrick SW, Tong VT, et al. Incidence of neonatal abstinence syndrome—28 states, 1999–2013. *MMWR Morb Mortal Wkly Rep*. 2016;65:799–802.
4. Brown JD, Doshi PA, Pauly NJ, et al. Rates of neonatal abstinence syndrome amid efforts to combat the opioid abuse epidemic. *JAMA Pediatr*. 2016;170:1110–1112.
5. Patrick SW, Davis MM, Lehmann CU, et al. Increasing incidence and geographic distribution of neonatal abstinence syndrome: United States 2009 to 2012. *J Perinatol*. 2015;35:650–655.
6. Healy D, English F, Daniels A, et al. Emergence of opiate-induced neonatal abstinence syndrome. *Ir Med J*. 2014;107:46.
7. Allegaert K, van den Anker JN. Neonatal withdrawal syndrome: reaching epidemic proportions across the globe. *Arch Dis Child Fetal Neonatal Ed*. 2016;101:F2–F3.
8. Davies H, Gilbert R, Johnson K, et al. Neonatal drug withdrawal syndrome: cross-country comparison using hospital administrative data in England, the USA, Western Australia and Ontario, Canada. *Arch Dis Child Fetal Neonatal Ed*. 2016;101:F26–F30.
9. Patrick SW, Benneyworth BD, Schumacher R, et al. Variation in hospital type in treatment of neonatal abstinence syndrome in the United States. Presented at Pediatric Academic Societies; Annual Meeting May 4-May 7, 2013, Washington DC, Abstract 2922.
10. Tolia VN, Patrick SW, Bennett MM, et al. Increasing incidence of the neonatal abstinence syndrome in U.S. neonatal ICUs. *N Engl J Med*. 2015;372:2118–2126.
11. Patrick SW, Schumacher RE, Benneyworth BD, et al. Neonatal abstinence syndrome and associated health care expenditures: United States, 2000–2009. *JAMA*. 2012;307:1934–1940.
12. Merry J. A social history of heroin addiction. *Addiction*. 1975;70:307–310.
13. Courtwright D. *Dark paradise: Opiate addiction in America Before 1940*. Cambridge, Massachusetts: Harvard University Press; 1982.

19

14. The Harrison Narcotics Tax Act Ch. 1, 38 Stat. 785, The Opium and Coca Leaves Trade Restrictions Act, Enacted by 63 United States US Congress.

15. Cope Z. *Early Diagnosis of the Acute Abdomen.* New York: Oxford University Press; 1921.

16. Thomas SH, Silen W. Effect on diagnostic efficiency of analgesia for undifferentiated abdominal pain. *Br J Surg.* 2003;90:5–9.

17. Porter J, Jick H. Addiction rare in patients treated with narcotics. *N Engl J Med.* 1980;302:123.

18. Portenoy RK, Foley KM. Chronic use of opioid analgesics in non-malignant pain: report of 38 cases. *Pain.* 1985;25:171–186.

19. Campbell JN. APS 1995 Presidential address. *J Pain.* 1996;5:85–88.

20. Phillips DM. JCAHO pain management standards are unveiled. Joint Commission on Accreditation of Health Organizations. *JAMA.* 2000;284:428–429.

21. Worley J. Prescription drug monitoring programs, a response to doctor shopping: purpose, effectiveness, and directions for future research. *Issues Ment Health Nurs.* 2012;33:319–328.

22. Dowell D, Haegerich TM, Chou R. CDC guideline for prescribing opioids for chronic pain—United States, 2016. *MMWR Recomm Rep.* 2016;65:1–49.

23. Evans CJ, Cahill CM. Neurobiology of opioid dependence in creating addiction vulnerability. *F1000Res.* 2016;5:1748. doi:10.12688/f1000research.8369.1.

24. Little PJ, Price RR, Hinton RK, et al. Role of noradrenergic hyperactivity in neonatal opiate abstinence. *Drug Alcohol Depend.* 1996;41:47–54.

25. Spiga S, Puddu MC, Pisano M, et al. Morphine withdrawal induced neurological changes in nucleus accumbens. *Eur J Neurosci.* 2005;22:2332–2340.

26. Lunden J, Kirby LG. Opiate exposure and withdrawal dynamically regulate mRNA expression in the serotonergic dorsal raphe nucleus. *Neuroscience.* 2013;254:160–172.

27. Capasso A, Gallo C. Molecules acting on CB1 receptor and their effects on morphine withdrawal *in vitro. Open Biochem J.* 2009;3:78–84.

28. Nunez C, Folders A, Laorden ML, et al. Activation of stress related hypothalamic neuropeptide gene expression during morphine withdrawal. *J Neurochem.* 2007;101:1060–1071.

29. Koob GF, Volkow ND. Neurobiology of addiction: a neurocircuitry analysis. *Lancet Psychiatry.* 2016;3:760–773.

30. Korpi ER, den Hollander B, Farooq U, et al. Mechanisms of action and persistent neuroplasticity by drugs of abuse. *Pharmacol Rev.* 2015;67:872–1004.

31. Herzlinger RA, Kandall SR, Vaughan HG Jr. Neonatal seizures associated with narcotic withdrawal. *J Pediatr.* 1997;91:638–641.

32. Gaalema DE, Scott TL, Heil SH, et al. Differences in the profile of neonatal abstinence syndrome signs in methadone—versus buprenorphine—exposed neonates. *Addiction.* 2012;107:53–62.

33. Ruwanpathirana R, Abdel-Latif ME, Burns L, et al. Prematurity reduces the severity and need for treatment of neonatal abstinence syndrome. *Acta Paediatr.* 2015;104:e188–e194.

34. Allocco E, Melker M, Rojas-Miguez F, et al. Comparison of neonatal abstinence syndrome manifestations in preterm versus term opioid-exposed infants. *Adv Neonatal Care.* 2016;16:329–336.

35. Wright TE. Biochemical screening for *in utero* drug exposure. *Drug Metab Lett.* 2015;9:65–71.

36. Murphy-Oikonen J, Montelpare WJ, Southon S, et al. Identifying infants at risk for neonatal abstinence syndrome. A retrospective cohort comparison study of 3 screening approaches. *J Perinat Neonatal Nurs.* 2010;24:366–372.

37. Finnegan LP, Cannaoghton JF, Kron RE, et al. Neonatal abstinence syndrome: assessment and management. *Addict Dis.* 1975;2:141–158.

38. Bagley SM, Wachman EM, Holland E, et al. Review of the assessment and managment of neonatal abstinence syndrome. *Addict Sci Clin Pract.* 2014;9:19.

39. Howard MB, Muses J, Wolfgang T, et al. Impact of parental presence at bedside on neonatal abstinence syndrome. Presented at Pediatric Academic Societies; Annual Meeting April 30-May 3, 2016 Baltimore MD, PAS 2016, Abstract 1665.6.

40. Holmes AV, Atwood EC, Whalen B, et al. Rooming-in to treat neonatal abstinence syndrome: improved family-centered care at lower cost. *Pediatrics.* 2016;137:e20152929.

41. Cirillo C, Francis K. Does breast milk affect neonatal abstinence syndrome severity, the need for pharmacologic therapy, and length of stay for infants of mothers on opioid maintenance therapy during pregnancy? *Adv Neonatal Care.* 2016;16:369–378.

42. Short VL, Gannon M, Abatemarco DJ. The association between breastfeeding and length of hospital stay among infants diagnosed with neonatal abstinence syndrome: a population-based study of in-hospital births. *Breastfeed Med.* 2016;11:343–349.

43. Wellestrand GK, Skurtveit S, Jansson LM, et al. Breast feeding reduces the need for withdrawal treatment in opioid-exposed infants. *Acta Paediatr.* 2013;102:1060–1066.

44. Abdel-Latif ME, Pinner J, Clews S, et al. Effects of breast milk on the severity and outcome of neonatal abstinence syndromes among infants of drug dependent mothers. *Pediatrics.* 2006;117:e1163–e1169.

45. Bogen DL, Perel JM, Helsel JC, et al. Estimated exposure to enatiomer-specific methadone levels in breast milk. *Breastfeed Med.* 2011;8:377–384.

46. Lindemalm S, Nydert P, Svensson JO, et al. Transfer of buprenorphine into breast milk and calculation of infant drug dose. *J Hum Lact.* 2009;25:199–205.

47. Wachman EM, Saia K, Humphreys R, et al. Revision of breast feeding guidelines in the setting of maternal opioid use disorder: one institution's experience. *J Hum Lact.* 2016;32:382–387.

48. Jansson LM, Velez M. Lactation and the Substance-Exposed Mother-Infant Dyad. *J Perinat Neonatal Nurs.* 2015;29:277–286.

49. Reece-Stremtan S, Marinelli KA. ABM clinical protocol #21: guidelines for breastfeeding and substance use or substance use disorder, revised 2015. *Breastfeed Med.* 2015;10:135–141.
50. American College of Obstetricians and Gynecologists Committee on Obstetric Practice. Committee Opinion No. 637: Marijuana Use During Pregnancy and Lactation. *Obstet Gynecol.* 2015;126: 234–238.
51. Hudak ML, Tan RC; American Academy of Pediatrics Committee on Drugs and Committee on Fetus and Newborn. Clinical Report: neonatal drug withdrawal. *Pediatrics.* 2012;29:e540–e560.
52. D'Apolito K. Comparison of a rocking bed and standard bed for decreasing withdrawal symptoms in drug-exposed infants. *MCN Am J Matern Child Nurs.* 1999;24:138–144.
53. Caiola E. Swaddling young infants can decrease crying time. *J Pediatr.* 2007;150:320–321.
54. Raith W, Schmölzer GM, Resch B, et al. Laser acupuncture for neonatal abstinence syndrome: a randomized controlled trial. *Pediatrics.* 2015;136:876–884.
55. Oro AS, Dixon SD. Waterbed care of narcotic-exposed neonates. A useful adjunct to supportive care. *Am J Dis Child.* 1988;142:186–188.
56. Edwards L, Brown LF. Nonpharmacologic management of neonatal abstinence syndrome. An integrative review. *Neonatal Netw.* 2016;35:305–313.
57. Kuschel C. Managing drug withdrawal in the newborn infant. *Semin Fetal Neonatal Med.* 2007;12: 127–133.
58. Greig E, Ash A, Douiri A. Maternal and neonatal outcomes following methadone substitution during pregnancy. *Arch Gynecol Obstet.* 2012;286:843–851.
59. Finnegan L, Kaltenach K. Neonatal abstinence syndrome. In: Hoekalman R, Friedman S, Nelson N, et al, eds. *Primary Pediatric Care.* St. Louis, MO: Mosby-Year Book; 1992:1367–1378.
60. Sarkar S, Donn SM. Management of neonatal abstinence syndrome in neonatal intensive care units: a national survey. *J Perinatol.* 2006;26:15–17.
61. Mehta A, Forbes KD, Kuppala VS. Neonatal abstinence syndrome management from prenatal counseling to a post discharge follow-up care: results of a national survey. *Hosp Pediatr.* 2013;3: 317–323.
62. The Joint Commission. Quick Safety: Managing neonatal abstinence syndrome. Issue 27, September 2016.
63. Hall ES, Wexelblatt SL, Crowley M, et al. Implementation of a neonatal abstinence syndrome weaning protocol: a multicenter cohort study. *Pediatrics.* 2015;136:e803–e810.
64. Karna P. Pharmacologic treatment and duration of therapy for neonatal abstinence syndrome at Michigan State Quality Collaborative. Presented at Pediatric Academic Societies; Annual Meeting April 25-28, 2015, San Diego CA. Abstract 2909.
65. Hall ES, Wexelblatt SL, Crowley M, et al. A multicenter cohort study of treatments and hospital outcomes in neonatal abstinence syndrome. *Pediatrics.* 2014;134(2):e527–e534.
66. Asti L, Magers JS, Keels E, et al. A quality improvement project to reduce length of stay for neonatal abstinence syndrome. *Pediatrics.* 2015;135:e1494–e1500.
67. Patrick SW, Schumacher RE, Horbar JD, et al. Improving care for neonatal abstinence syndrome. *Pediatrics.* 2016;137:e20153835.
68. Rajbhandari S, Mehra K, Loona S, et al. Effect of standardizing neonatal abstinence syndrome treatment and weaning in a level III NICU. Presented at Pediatric Academic Societies; Annual Meeting April 30-May 3, 2016 Baltimore MD, Abstract 153.
69. Patrick SW, Kaplan HC, Passarella M, et al. Variation in treatment of neonatal abstinence syndrome in US children's hospitals, 2004-2011. *J Perinatol.* 2014;34:867–872.
70. Osborn DA, Jeffrey HE, Cole MJ. Opiate treatment for opiate withdrawal in newborn infants. *Cochrane Database Syst Rev.* 2010;(10):CD002059.
71. Bio LL, Siu A, Poon CY. Update on the pharmacologic management of neonatal abstinence syndrome. *J Perinatol.* 2011;31:692–701.
72. Peinemann F, Daldrup T. Severe and prolonged sedation in five neonates due to persistence of active diazepam metabolites. *Eur J Pediatr.* 2001;160:378–381.
73. Osborn DA, Jeffrey HE, Cole MJ. Sedatives for opiate withdrawal in newborn infants. *Cochrane Database Syst Rev.* 2010;(10):CD002053.
74. Scott CS, Riggs KW, Ling EW, et al. Morphine pharmacokinetics and pain assessment in premature newborns. *J Pediatr.* 1999;135:423–429.
75. Kart T, Christrup LL, Rasmussen M. Recommended use of morphine in neonates, infants and children based on a literature review: part 1–Pharmacokinetics. *Paediatr Anaesth.* 1997;7:5–11.
76. Liu T, Lewis T, Gauda E, et al. Mechanistic population pharmacokinetics of morphine in neonates with abstinence syndrome after oral administration of diluted tincture of opium. *J Clin Pharmacol.* 2016;56:1009–1018.
77. Ward RM, Drover DR, Hammer GB, et al. The pharmacokinetics of methadone and its metabolites in neonates, infants, and children. *Paediatr Anaesth.* 2014;24:591–601.
78. Rosen TS, Pippenger CE. Pharmacologic observations on the neonatal withdrawal syndrome. *J Pediatr.* 1976;88:1044–1048.
79. Mack G, Thomas D, Giles W, et al. Methadone levels and neonatal withdrawal. *J Paediatr Child Health.* 1991;27:96–100.
80. Ng CM, Dombrowsky E, Lin H, et al. Population pharmacokinetic model of sublingual buprenorphine in neonatal abstinence syndrome. *Pharmacotherapy.* 2015;35:670–680.
81. Marsot A, Brevaut-Malaty V, Vialet R, et al. Pharmacokinetics and absolute bioavailability of phenobarbital in neonates and young infants, a population pharmacokinetic modelling approach. *Fundam Clin Pharmacol.* 2014;28:465–471.

19

82. Xie HG, Cao YJ, Gauda EB, et al. Clonidine clearance matures rapidly during the early postnatal period: a population pharmacokinetic analysis in newborns with neonatal abstinence syndrome. *J Clin Pharmacol*. 2011;51:502–511.

83. Kraft WK, van den Anker JN. Pharmacological management of the opioid neonatal abstinence syndrome. *Pediatr Clin North Am*. 2012;59:1147–1165.

84. Napolitano A, Theophilopoulos D, Seng SK, et al. Pharmacologic management of neonatal abstinence syndrome in a community hospital. *Clin Obstet Gynecol*. 2013;56:193–201.

85. Kraft WK, Dysart K, Greenspan JS, et al. Revised dose schema of sublingual buprenorphine in the treatment of the neonatal opioid abstinence syndrome. *Addiction*. 2011;106:574–580.

86. Bada HS, Sithisarn T, Gibson J, et al. Morphine versus clonidine for neonatal abstinence syndrome. *Pediatrics*. 2015;135:e383–e391.

87. O'Grady MJ, Hopewell J, White MJ. Management of neonatal abstinence syndrome: a national survey and review of practice. *Arch Dis Child Fetal Neonatal Ed*. 2009;94:F249–F252.

88. Kelly LE, Knoppert D, Roukema H, et al. Oral morphine weaning for neonatal abstinence syndrome at home compared with in-hospital: an observational cohort study. *Paediatr Drugs*. 2015;17:151–157.

89. Oei J, Lui K. Management of the newborn infant affected by maternal opiates and other drugs of dependency. *J Paediatr Child Health*. 2007;43:9–18.

90. Kapur BM, Hutson JR, Chibber T, et al. Methadone: a review of drug-drug and pathophysiological interactions. *Crit Rev Clin Lab Sci*. 2011;48:171–195.

91. Backes CH, Backes CR, Gardner D, et al. Neonatal abstinence syndrome: transitioning methadone-treated infants from an inpatient to an outpatient setting. *J Perinatol*. 2012;32:425–430.

92. Lainwala S, Brown ER, Weinschenk NP, et al. A retrospective study of length of hospital stay in infants treated for neonatal abstinence syndrome with methadone versus oral morphine preparations. *Adv Neonatal Care*. 2005;5:265–272.

93. Lee J, Hulman S, Musci M Jr, et al. Neonatal abstinence syndrome: influence of a combined inpatient/outpatient methadone treatment regimen on the average length of stay of a medicaid nicu population. *Popul Health Manag*. 2015;18:392–397.

94. Young ME, Hager SJ, Spurlock D. Retrospective chart review comparing morphine and methadone in neonates treated for neonatal abstinence syndrome. *Am J Health Syst Pharm*. 2015;72(23 suppl 3):S162–S167.

95. Brown MS, Hayes MJ, Thornton LM. Methadone versus morphine for treatment of neonatal abstinence syndrome: a prospective randomized clinical trial. *J Perinatol*. 2015;35:278–283.

96. Wachman EM, Hayes MJ, Brown MS, et al. Association of OPRM1 and COMT single –Nucleotide polymorphisms with hospital length of stay and treatment of neonatal abstinence syndrome. *JAMA*. 2013;309:1821–1827.

97. Jones HE, Kaltenbach K, Heil SH, et al. Neonatal abstinence syndrome after methadone or buprenorphine exposure. *N Engl J Med*. 2010;363:2320–2331.

98. Kraft WK, Stover MW, Davis JM. Neonatal abstinence syndrome: pharmacologic strategies for the mother and infant. *Semin Perinatol*. 2016;40:203–212.

99. Chisamore B, Labana S, Blitz S, et al. A comparison of morphine delivery in neonatal opioid withdrawal. *Subst Abuse*. 2016;10:49–54.

100. Wiles JR, Isemann B, Mizuno T, et al. Pharmacokinetics of oral methadone in the treatment of neonatal abstinence syndrome: a pilot study. *J Pediatr*. 2015;167:1214–1220.

101. Hall ES, Meinzen-Derr J, Wexelblatt SL. Cohort analysis of a pharmacokinetic-modeled methadone weaning optimization for neonatal abstinence syndrome. *J Pediatr*. 2015;167:1221–1225.

102. Barrett DA, Simpson J, Rutter N, et al. The pharmacokinetics and physiological effects of buprenorphine infusion in premature neonates. *Br J Clin Pharmacol*. 1993;36:215–219.

103. Bell SG. Buprenorphine: a newer drug for treating neonatal abstinence syndrome. *Neonatal Netw*. 2012;31:178–183.

104. Kraft WK, Gibson E, Dysart K, et al. Sublingual buprenorphine for treatment of neonatal abstinence syndrome: a randomized trial. *Pediatrics*. 2008;122:e601–e607.

105. Hall ES, Isemann BT, Wexelblatt SL, et al. A cohort comparison of buprenorphine versus methadone treatment for neonatal abstinence syndrome. *J Pediatr*. 2016;170:39–44.

106. Pacifici GM. Clinical pharmacology of phenobarbital in neonates: effects, metabolism and pharmacokinetics. *Curr Pediatr Rev*. 2016;12:48–54.

107. Ward RM, Stiers J, Buchi K. Neonatal medications. *Pediatr Clin North Am*. 2015;62:525–544.

108. Jackson L, Ting A, Mckay S, et al. A randomized controlled trial of morphine versus phenobarbitone for neonatal abstinence syndrome. *Arch Dis Child Fetal Neonatal Ed*. 2004;89:F300–F304.

109. Ebner N, Rohrmeister K, Winklbaur B, et al. Management of neonatal abstinence syndrome in neonates born to opioid maintained women. *Drug Alcohol Depend*. 2007;87:131–138.

110. Finnegan LP, Mitros TF, Hopkins LE. Management of neonatal narcotic abstinence utilizing a phenobarbital loading dose method. *NIDA Res Monogr*. 1979;27:247–253.

111. Nayeri F, Sheikh M, Kalani M, et al. Phenobarbital versus morphine in the management of neonatal abstinence syndrome, a randomized control trial. *BMC Pediatr*. 2015;15:57.

112. Streetz VN, Gildon BL, Thompson DF. Role of clonidine in neonatal abstinence syndrome: a systematic review. *Ann Pharmacother*. 2016;50:301–310.

113. Hoder EL, Leckman JF, Ehrenkranz R, et al. Clonidine in neonatal narcotic-abstinence syndrome. *N Engl J Med*. 1981;305:1284.

114. Hoder EL, Leckman JF, Poulsen J, et al. Clonidine treatment of neonatal narcotic abstinence syndrome. *Psychiatry Res*. 1984;13:243–251.

115. Liu Y, Wang XY, Li D, et al. Short-term use of antiepileptic drugs is neurotoxic to the immature brain. *Neural Regen Res*. 2015;10:599–604.
116. Coyle MG, Ferguson A, Lagasse L, et al. Diluted tincture of opium (DTO) and phenobarbital versus DTO alone for neonatal opiate withdrawal in term infants. *J Pediatr*. 2002;140:561–564.
117. Agthe AH, Kim GR, Mathias KB, et al. Clonidine as an adjunct therapy to opioids for neonatal abstinence syndrome: a randomized controlled trial. *Pediatrics*. 2009;123:e849–e856.
118. Surran B, Visintainer P, Chamberlain S, et al. Efficacy of clonidine versus phenobarbital in reducing neonatal morphine sulfate therapy days for neonatal abstinence syndrome. A prospective randomized clinical trial. *J Perinatol*. 2013;33(12):954–959.
119. Conradt E, Sheinkopf SJ, Lester BM, et al. Prenatal substance exposure: neurobiological organization at 1 month. *J Pediatr*. 2013;163:989–994.
120. Hunt RW, Tzioumi D, Collins E, et al. Adverse neurodevelopmental outcome of infants exposure to opiate drugs *in utero*. *Early Hum Dev*. 2008;84:29–35.
121. Lester BM, Lagasse LL. Children of addicted women. *J Addict Dis*. 2010;29:259–276.
122. Walhovd KB, Bjørnebekk A, Haabrekke K, et al. Child neuroanatomical, neurocognitive, and visual acuity outcomes with maternal opioid and polysubstance detoxification. *Pediatr Neurol*. 2015;52: 326–332.
123. Mactier H. Neonatal and longer term management following substance misuse in pregnancy. *Early Hum Dev*. 2013;89:887–892.

19

CHAPTER 20

Therapies for Gastroesophageal Reflux in Infants

Ninfa M. Candela, MD, Jenifer R. Lightdale, MD, MPH

- Review the differentiating diagnostic criteria for gastroesophageal reflux (GER) and gastroesophageal reflux disease (GERD) in infants.
- Consider tests in infants with atypical presentations who may have GERD or other conditions with similar clinical signs.
- Recognize that dietary changes, rather than acid suppression, may often represent the best first-line therapy for infants with clinical signs consistent with GERD.
- Consider the limited role and risks of pharmacologic therapy in the treatment of GERD in infants.
- Inform parents about the etiology, treatment, and possible complications of GERD.
- Schedule clinical follow-up for all patients treated for GERD.
- Consider consultation with a gastroenterologist or other appropriate specialist when there is uncertainty of the diagnosis and/or potential complications of GERD.

Introduction

Gastroesophageal reflux (GER) is common in infancy, typically peaking in prevalence at 4 months of age in children born at full term and generally resolving between the ages of 12 and 24 months. The prevalence of clinically significant GER in premature infants is higher than in term infants and has been estimated to be as high as 22%.[1-4]

In term and preterm infants without clinical signs of reflux, physiologic passage of gastric contents into the esophagus (GER) occurs a few times a day, mostly after feeds, and is generally related to supine positioning and gut immaturity.[5] Reflux that is pathologic and consistent with disease (gastroesophageal reflux disease [GERD]) occurs when exposure of the esophagus to acidic and nonacidic gastric contents causes complications such as esophagitis, feeding difficulties, failure to gain weight, sleep disorders, respiratory issues, gastrointestinal (GI) bleeding, or apnea.[6] Fortunately, the occurrence of GER is far more common than GERD. Indeed, in one study of 119 premature infants who underwent pulmonary monitoring, there were 6255 episodes of GER.[7] Yet only 1% of episodes were associated with apnea lasting 15 seconds or longer; there was no difference in the apnea rate before, during, or after GER; and no difference in the incidence of apnea lasting >10 seconds before or during GER. These investigators found a decrease in apnea immediately after GER—a finding that underscores the complexity of the exact relationships between GER, apnea, and respiratory disease. Nevertheless, apnea remains one of several biologically plausible reported complications of reflux in infants, and investigators continue to work on delineating when and if apnea represents an indication for treatment of GER.

In most term and preterm infants with vomiting, a good history and physical examination are sufficient to reliably diagnose GERD. Diagnostic evaluation with other testing modalities is rarely necessary, but may be helpful and even critical to perform if there is concern for other pathology, such as intraventricular bleeding or intestinal obstruction.

It is important to recognize the lack of randomized, controlled trials that support pharmacotherapeutic management of infants to reduce gastric acid.[8] Conservative measures that employ nonpharmacologic interventions, such as prone positioning, dietary changes, and parental reassurance, are currently recommended by the North American Society for Pediatric Gastroenterology, Hepatology and Nutrition (NASP-GHAN) as the first steps in an evidence-based approach to management.[8] Nevertheless, neonatologists should have a working knowledge of currently available drug therapies, including histamine-2 receptor antagonists, PPIs, buffering agents, and prokinetic agents. This chapter will provide an evidence basis for when and if pharmacologic treatment of GERD in neonatal populations should be considered.

Pathogenesis of Reflux Disorders in Infants

Several pathophysiologic mechanisms are responsible for triggering GER in preterm and term infants, including transient relaxation of the lower esophageal sphincter (LES), a short esophagus and small gastric capacity, and air swallowing.[9] The LES is a barrier between the stomach and esophagus created by the crura of the diaphragm that encircles and provides support for the esophagus. The main components of the human "antireflux barrier" are the LES, the crural diaphragm, and the phrenoesophageal ligament. These work together to prevent GER by creating high pressures at the gastroesophageal junction.

Transient LES relaxations (TLESRs) are the predominant mode of GER in individuals of all ages. TLESR is defined as an inadequate response of LES tone to changes in intragastric pressure and is unassociated with normal peristalsis. Relaxation of the LES occurs via the brain stem, with afferent and vagal pathways using release of nitric oxide to achieve it.[10]

Acidification of the stomach and the esophagus may also contribute to GERD. Omari and colleagues have described various mechanisms of GER in the premature infant 33 to 38 weeks postmenstrual age and have found most to be associated with low esophageal pH. For example, TLESRs occur in response to decreases in esophageal pH, as well as to esophageal body contractions, to multiple swallows, and to peristaltic failure.[11] In their model of reflux disorders, Omari and colleagues demonstrated that premature infants have low LES pressure at baseline (<5 mm Hg), as well as delayed emptying of gastric contents. Premature infants also have a short and narrow esophagus, which can result in a slight misalignment of the LES above the diaphragm.[12] These factors contribute to poor clearance of refluxed contents from the esophagus of premature infants and may contribute to complications and GERD.[11]

Other research has found that GI motor innervation gradually develops as postmenstrual age increases. Esophageal motor responses to spontaneous intraluminal stimulation by refluxed contents usually first become evident after 33 weeks post-menstrual age.[13,14] Therefore clearance of refluxed contents in premature infants via primary peristalsis initiated by swallowing, as well as via secondary peristalsis stimulated by esophageal distention and upper esophageal sphincter reflexes, may be impaired. It is also postulated that ineffective peristalsis can contribute to mucosal damage and esophagitis, as well as other potential complications of GERD, including aspiration, apnea, and respiratory compromise. To date, there is limited evidence for this model, which remains to be validated.

Factors That Can Exacerbate Reflux in Infants

Beyond TLESRs and impaired motility, factors such as excessive crying and increases in intraabdominal pressure due to straining, coughing, or a seated position putting pressure on the abdomen are associated with GER and GERD. In addition, delayed gastric emptying may play a role in infant reflux disorders. Emptying of the stomach is dependent on characteristics of a meal composition, including volume, osmolality, and caloric density. In fact, it is the composition of a meal that induces the proximal stomach to relax, affecting the occurrence of TLESRs.[15] This receptive relaxation is thought to be minimal in infants, which may also explain the increase in reflux in this population.[15] Additionally, supine position as well as frequent feedings can contribute to gastric distention and increased GER.

Components of gastroesophageal refluxate can also determine pathogenicity to the esophageal mucosa. For example, production of pepsinogen by parietal cells in the gastric mucosa fully mature by 3 to 8 months postnatal age. Pepsinogen is activated to pepsin by gastric acid. When refluxed into the esophagus, this proteolytic enzyme can produce potentially irreversible injury of the esophageal squamous epithelium.

Gastric acid may also injure the mucosa. Gastric acid secretion is limited in premature infants, but generally doubles between the first week after birth and a postnatal age of 2 months.[16] Stomach acidity varies with feedings, in that gastric fluid pH is usually higher before and during meals and lower in the postprandial period. Generally, infants experience reflux most commonly after meals, likely in part due to ingestion of air in their stomach during feeds, which may potentially distend the esophagus and worsen the event.[17] The duration of postprandial esophageal acid exposure may also be longer in infants due to ineffective acid-clearing defenses.

Nonacid and gaseous reflux have not been well studied, but likely are important mediators in the pathogenesis of GERD. Endogenous acid-neutralizing mechanisms, including salivary secretions that may neutralize residual esophageal acid, also remain poorly understood in infants. Nevertheless, there has been a tendency to target acid suppression as a medical goal.

Clinical Presentation

Evaluation of infants for suspected reflux is often initiated because of clinical findings, which commonly include vomiting and regurgitation. In addition, fussiness after feedings and back arching are often believed to occur in response to discomfort and may be worrisome to parents and caregivers. From the clinician's perspective, both GER and GERD can be associated with similar presentations. The similarity of signs between physiologic GER and pathologic GERD has been well documented in the literature. In one study comparing 100 healthy infants with 35 infants diagnosed with GERD, healthy infants were found to have a high prevalence of signs of reflux, including daily regurgitation (40%), crying for more than 1 hour a day (17%), arching of the back (10%), and daily hiccups (36%).[18]

Reflux is more consistent with physiologic regurgitation than with vomiting.[10] Regurgitation does not involve a centrally mediated emetic reflex, but rather is an effortless movement of refluxed gastric contents into the mouth.[8,19] Regurgitation can be physiologically normal in infants and often does not cause discomfort. Infants with painless regurgitation consistent with GER are often characterized as "happy spitters" and have no complications of their reflux, including no evidence of discomfort with reflux episodes and no adverse effects on growth.

Associations Between GERD and Other Extraesophageal Signs

Most reflux in infants will not result in poor growth. However, at times continuous regurgitation or vomiting may be complicated by poor weight gain despite adequate caloric intake. In such situations, diagnoses other than physiologic reflux should be carefully considered, including pyloric stenosis and cow's milk protein allergy (CMPA). Additionally, a feeding history should be obtained that includes a thorough evaluation of infant swallowing and sucking behavior, frequency of feed, and type and amount of milk intake. Infants with GERD may be described as being averse to a feed.

Episodes of choking, gagging, or coughing with feeds should prompt concern for possible aspiration and further diagnostic evaluation.

Reported extraesophageal manifestations of GERD in infants have included apnea and apparent life-threatening events (ALTEs), bronchospasm, and respiratory distress. However, any association between these events and reflux disorders in infants remains debatable, as studies have not found a clear relationship between the occurrence of respiratory events and acid reflux detected by a pH probe,[20] nor between apneas and nonacid reflux recorded by multiple intraluminal impedance monitoring.[21] In premature infants with episodes of hypoxemia, feeding discoordination between sucking, swallowing, and breathing may be less due to acid reflux and more to an inability to clear the airway effectively because of immaturity.[22]

In severe cases of GERD, infants can be reported to present clinically with spasmodic and dystonic movements and exaggerated back arching. This uncommon presentation is known as *Sandifer syndrome*.[8,22] Nevertheless, infants described in this manner should be carefully evaluated for other neurologic causes of their posturing before this behavior is ascribed to acid reflux.

Differential Diagnosis

Potential signs of GER, such as unexplained fussiness, crying and irritability, sleep disturbance, and distressed behavior, are nonspecific and can be associated with both pathologic and nonpathologic conditions. More than 60% of infants <4 months of age have daily spit-ups, and they can experience as many as three to five regurgitation events per hour.[23,24] Reflux peaks in frequency and prevalence at 4 months of age and then typically resolves by 6 months of age. By 12 months, almost all infants with a history of GER have resolution of their symptoms. Accordingly, many infants with physiologic GER do not require medical treatment. Instead, parents can benefit greatly from reassurance that the natural course of reflux in newborns is that it almost always diminishes with increasing age. Individual variability in parental response to a distressed infant should be a consideration in the diagnosis and treatment of infants with reflux disorders. Infants vary in crying times, and some otherwise healthy infants can cry up to 6 hours per day. Other causes of distress and irritability in an infant should be noted. In addition, it is important to use parental reports to screen for potential associated conditions that range from rare midgut or diaphragmatic defects to much more common entities, including CMPA (Table 20.1).

Table 20.1   DIFFERENTIAL DIAGNOSIS OF GASTROESOPHAGEAL REFLUX DISEASE (GERD)

Disease	Characteristics
Colic	By definition, colic is self-limited crying for at least 3 hours a day, 3 days a week, and for 3 weeks in a row.
Eosinophilic esophagitis (allergic esophagitis)	Vomiting and abdominal pain. Symptoms improve with removal of offending food. Eosinophils seen on esophageal biopsy.
Cow's milk allergy	Symptoms of GERD, bloody or mucoid diarrhea, green watery stool. History of atopy common. Symptoms improve with extensively hydrolyzed or amino acid–based formula.
Candidal esophagitis	Vomiting and abdominal pain. Associated with immune deficiency.
Malrotation	Persistent vomiting, weight loss. Abdominal pain with volvulus, can be associated with decreased stooling. Check for other digestive system defects, heart defects, and abnormalities of the spleen or liver.
Pyloric stenosis	Projectile forceful vomiting, poor weight gain, metabolic alkalosis. May palpate an "olive" on abdominal examination.
Duodenal atresia, antral web	Vomiting after feeding. Associated with Down syndrome.
Anomalous subclavian artery	Vomiting after feeding.
Esophageal foreign body	Vomiting after feeding.

GERD, gastroesophageal reflux disease.

Therapies for Gastroesophageal Reflux in Infants 265

Cow's Milk Protein Allergy

Another condition to consider when an infant exhibits excessive irritability is the relatively common entity of CMPA, which occurs in up to 8% of infants.[25] CMPA is a non–IgE-mediated condition that generally resolves by age 2 and often involves cross-reactivity with other large-molecular-weight food proteins, including soy.[26] Mothers of breastfed infants should continue breastfeeding, while eliminating all milk and milk products, as well as soy, from their diet. If an infant receives supplemental feeding, these must also be free of cow's milk protein. In formula-fed infants, avoidance of cow's milk–based formula as well as other animal milk proteins (goat or sheep milk) should be initiated. Elimination diet in formula-fed infants starts with an extensively hydrolyzed formula (eHF). Most infants with CMPA tolerate an eHF with whey or casein with proven efficacy.

In one study of the relationship between GER and CMPA, 18 of 42 infants were found to have esophagitis on endoscopy and/or a reflux index >10% on pH/impedance studies. Within the subgroup of 10 patients diagnosed ultimately in this study with both acid-mediated GERD and CMPA there was a significantly higher reflux index compared with infants with primary GERD.[27] CMPA and GERD are believed to coexist in at least 50% of affected infants.[28,29]

Tools for Diagnosis

In most infants, history and physical examination alone are sufficient to make the diagnosis of physiologic GER. However, several questionnaires have been developed that may be used to organize the information collected for diagnosis.[30] To date, these have not been shown to correlate with disease severity, but they may be helpful in differentiating GER from GERD.

Radiologic Testing for GERD

A number of radiologic tests can be used to determine whether patients with atypical presentations may have GERD. None are necessary to diagnose GERD, but may be useful to obtain, depending on specific diagnostic questions. For example, an upper GI series should not be used to diagnose reflux, but rather to look for other pathologic and anatomic conditions, such as malrotation or duodenal strictures, which may be contributing to the severity or persistence of symptoms. An upper GI series may also be useful to evaluate for esophageal webs or strictures or tracheoesophageal fistula. Similarly, a modified barium swallow with feeding evaluation may be helpful to evaluate for pulmonary aspiration. Finally, nuclear scintigraphy provides information about gastric emptying and may help to identify postprandial reflux. However, as with all radiologic studies, this test can only be used to provide some evidence for the condition and does not, in and of itself, diagnose GERD.

Intraesophageal Monitoring for Acid and Nonacid Reflux

Intraesophageal pH monitoring can be used to quantify the acidity of refluxed stomach contents, as well as the reflux index (the percentage of time that the esophageal pH is <4.0). The reflux index is a valid measure that reflects overall esophageal acid exposure. In infants, a reflux index of ≥11% is considered abnormal. To ensure validity of a reflux index value, pH probe monitoring should be performed for 24 hours, as opposed to a shorter measurement period.[31]

pH probe monitoring for a minimum of 24 hours is also most useful for determining the effectiveness of therapy and symptom correlation. In one study, simultaneous 1-hour pH monitoring, gastroesophageal scintigraphy, and upper GI series were obtained in 49 infants with suspected GERD; 47 of these infants also were monitored subsequently with a 24-hour pH probe test.[32] In this study, all infants with a "positive" 1-hour pH monitoring result that confirmed acid reflux also had positive simultaneous scintigraphy results and reflux seen on upper GI series. When compared with results of 24-hour pH probe testing, reflux seen by gastroesophageal scintigraphy had a sensitivity of 79% and a specificity of 93% for predicting a reflux index ≥11%, whereas reflux seen by upper GI series had a sensitivity of 86% and a specificity of 21%.[32]

Combined pH and multiple intraluminal impedance monitoring (pH/MII) may be more useful for detecting reflux events than pH probe monitoring alone and may aid with clinical correlation to symptoms. pH/MII is a catheter-based method that can be used to determine bolus reflux, without regard for acidity, by measuring a change in resistance to electrical current flow between two sensors due to gas, liquid, or mixed reflux episodes. Advantages of pH/MII include the detection of nonacidic GER events often seen postprandially. It can also be used to differentiate reflux from swallows, to assess full column reflux, and to better correlate treatment response compared with pH probe alone.[33,34]

Endoscopy

Endoscopy with biopsies for histology is considered the most accurate method of demonstrating esophageal mucosal injury from reflux and for ruling out other conditions. However, there are known risks associated with endoscopy, including bleeding, perforation, and infection, as well as anesthesia risks.[35] Histologic criteria of reflux esophagitis involve basal hyperplasia, increased papillae length, and presence of intraepithelial eosinophils. Nevertheless, it is important to recognize that infants have a normal thickening of the mucosa, as well as erythema, due to increased vascularity of the basal zone in the distal esophagus (Fig. 20.1). In addition, it is widely accepted that there is insufficient evidence to support the routine use of endoscopy to diagnose or exclude GERD, except perhaps to differentiate eosinophilic esophagitis, which rarely occurs in infants. This is in part because there is no clear relationship between esophagitis and symptom severity, including extraesophageal manifestations.[8]

Treatment

Nondrug Management

In many cases, physiologic GER and uncomplicated GERD in infants can be managed empirically and with minimal intervention. Nevertheless, parental education and reassurance of normal and healthy findings on physical examination, including documentation of normal growth, is of utmost importance if overuse of medications

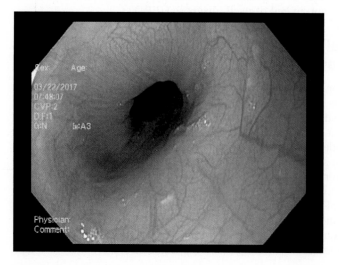

Figure 20.1 Normal esophagus with well-visualized vascular pattern.

is to be avoided. Indeed, the treatment of infants with reflux disorders should always focus first and foremost on parental education, reassurance, and support. In particular, a discussion around soothing maneuvers, as well as feeding techniques and positioning, may be helpful for frustrated parents.[36] Ideally, infants with GERD should not be placed in a position that increases abdominal pressure, but rather held upright after feeds. Burping an infant several times after feedings may also reduce GER.

It is well known that infant positioning can play a role in reflux disorders. For example, infant car seats and cot elevation (unsupported upright posture) may be associated with worsening symptoms, perhaps due to increased abdominal pressure.[37] Other studies have found that left lateral positioning after feeds can significantly reduce TLESRs, thereby reducing reflux episodes.[38,39]

In one clinical trial of positioning, 18 premature infants with clinically significant GER were studied prospectively using 24-hour esophageal pH monitoring. Infants were randomly assigned to be nursed in three positions (prone, left lateral, and right lateral) for 8 consecutive hours.[37] In this study, the median reflux index for the group was 13.8% (study subject range: 5.8%–40.4%), but did vary by position. The prone and left lateral positions significantly reduced the number and duration of GER episodes.

Nevertheless, an increased risk of sudden infant death syndrome is associated with sleeping in the prone position.[40,41] Therefore prone positioning of infants <12 months of age is not recommended, and infants should always be placed in the supine position for sleep, regardless of clinical signs suggestive of GER.[41]

Thickening Feeds to Treat GER

The 2009 Pediatric Gastroesophageal Reflux Clinical Practice Guidelines issued by NASPGHAN recommended a change to thickened formula as a first-line therapy for uncomplicated reflux disorders in formula-fed infants.[8] However, benefits of thickened feedings have not been observed in premature infants.[42,43] Current commonly used thickeners include rice cereal, carob bean gum (St. John's bread), carob-seed flour, and sodium alginate. Prethickened formulas are also commercially available and may be convenient and well tolerated by some infants. In 2011 the US Food and Drug Administration (FDA) warned against the use of a commercially available thickening agent, "SimplyThick," in infants born <37 weeks gestation who required hospitalization, as its use was associated with an increased risk of necrotizing enterocolitis.[44]

In term infants, thickened formula appears to significantly reduce regurgitation frequency and amount, as reflected in reduction in the number of nonacid (pH >4) GER episodes and a decrease in the mean height of reflux in the esophagus. However, the occurrence of acid GER is not reduced.[45] In fact, although thickening with rice cereal increases the viscosity of feeds, it also appears to increase the acidity of stomach contents.[45]

Dry rice cereal ($\frac{1}{2}$ to 1 tablespoon per ounce of formula) is a common thickener associated with easy digestibility. Nevertheless, it also increases the caloric density of formula and can cause constipation as well as weight gain. Coughing has also been found to occur more frequently after thickened feedings than after unthickened feedings.[46]

In infants, reflux becomes more apparent with gastric distention and delayed gastric emptying. Breastfed infants have shorter episodes of GER and faster gastric emptying compared with formula-fed infants.[47] The occurrence of GER also correlates with greater volumes per feed as well as the osmolality of feeds.[17] Maneuvers in the preterm infant to minimize these changes include feeding smaller volumes and providing more frequent bolus feeds in gavage-fed infants to decrease gastric distention. It is also often helpful to avoid use of hyperosmolar oral medications.

Dietary Changes

According to guidelines from NASPGHAN, use of an extensively hydrolyzed or amino acid–based formula is effective in reducing signs of GERD. This recommendation is based primarily on the previously noted overlap in clinical findings between CMPA and GERD in approximately 50% of infants, which can include spitting up, fussiness, and poor weight gain.[28,29] In one study by Corvaglia et al., extensively hydrolyzed formula administered to premature infants reduced the number of GER episodes and decreased the reflux index noted on pH/MII studies.[48]

When choosing formulas, a stepwise approach is suggested, first trialing an extensively hydrolyzed protein formula and then changing to the amino acid–based formula if improvement in symptoms is inadequate. The NASPGHAN guidelines advocate for adequate time between formula changes—ideally 2 weeks—to monitor for treatment effect.

Transpyloric Feeds

In infants with severe GERD refractive to nondrug and medical therapies, it has become common to use transpyloric feedings. A reduction in apnea and bradycardia has been observed after initiation of transpyloric feeds with breast milk.[49] Both nasoduodenal and nasojejunal feeds in the premature infant reduce the incidence of reflux by minimizing gastric volume.[24] Although use of transpyloric feeds is an alternative to gastric fundoplication to treat GERD, complications may occur, including persistent reflux, dislodgement, and intestinal perforation.[50]

Fundoplication

The role of fundoplication as another therapeutic option in infants remains understudied and unclear. Extrapolated data from older children with GERD suggest fundoplication may be associated with improvement in GERD symptoms in neurologically impaired children, as well as those with esophageal atresia.[51] Children who have undergone fundoplication may also have improvement in pulmonary symptoms and quality of sleep. However, fundoplication in infants is associated with complications, including dumping syndrome.[8] Fundoplication is not advised for otherwise healthy infants, who by definition will acquire increased esophageal and gastric capacity during their first year.[8,44] Young infants are also likely to develop improved esophageal motility and reflux barrier function over a relatively short period, making an invasive surgery inappropriate if temporizing measures can be used without harm.

Other Lifestyle Changes

It may be helpful to identify other risk factors for GER to ensure the success of a treatment plan. In particular, limiting environmental exposure to tobacco smoke in infants has been clearly shown to reduce symptoms of GER.[52] In one study of otherwise healthy infants with a history of ALTEs, a strong correlation was found between pH study parameters and environmental tobacco smoke exposure.[52] There was also a linear relationship between the number of cigarettes smoked per day by caregivers and infants' reflux index values and episodes of reflux lasting longer than 5 minutes. Other aggravating factors in premature infants include oropharyngeal suctioning, percussive chest therapy, use of caffeine, and betamimetic agents, which increase LES relaxation.[17]

Medications to Treat Gastroesophageal Reflux in Infants

Currently available medications that can be used to treat GERD in infants include acid-buffering agents, mucosal surface protectors, antisecretory agents, and prokinetic agents. According to NASPGHAN and other guidelines, medications should only be considered for infants with GERD when conservative lifestyle measures, including dietary changes, do not produce effective results. Nevertheless, in recent years, there has been widespread use of empirical antireflux medications in infants, including premature infants.[53] This trend has occurred despite the lack of specific studies of these agents in infants. In addition, there is increasing evidence that antireflux medications are not without serious adverse effects. In particular, prokinetic agents may be associated with antipyramidal effects, whereas antisecretory agents have been associated with an increased incidence of infections.[54] A careful approach that assesses risks and benefits for each drug should be considered before initiating drug therapy.

Acid-Buffering Agents

Acid-buffering agents, known as *antacids,* directly neutralize gastric acid and may limit exposure of acid in the stomach to the esophagus during a reflux event. Most products contain magnesium and aluminum hydroxide or calcium carbonate. Side effects associated with antacids vary. For example, aluminum in antacids used in infants can be associated with toxicity, causing osteopenia, neurotoxicity, and anemia.[55] Both aluminum- and calcium-containing antacids can lead to constipation, and products containing magnesium can promote diarrhea.

Mucosal Surface Protectors

Alginate-based formulations, such as sucralfate, act as a surface barrier against acid effects on the gastric mucosa and are also commonly used to treat GERD in both adult and pediatric populations. Sucralfate consists of sucrose, sulfate, and aluminum, which combine together to form a gel in the presence of acid. Mucosal surface–protecting preparations often have a combination of sodium alginate and sodium bicarbonate, which work together to coat the mucosa. Specifically, sodium alginate precipitates to form a viscous gel in the presence of gastric acid, whereas sodium bicarbonate converts to a carbon dioxide–based foam. During a reflux event, the coating created by alginate-based formulations is carried into the esophagus, where it may alleviate the acid injury.[56]

Despite limited data regarding safety and efficacy of alginate-based medications, they are used as antireflux therapy in symptomatic premature infants.[2,57] This use has at least some evidence basis. For example, Infant Gaviscon (formulated by Reckitt Benckiser Healthcare, Inc., and containing sodium and magnesium alginate) has been found in a placebo-controlled, randomized, double-blind study to reduce the height of gastric contents refluxate in infants.[22] However, it is important to note that no differences in the number of acid and nonacid events were found on pH/MII. Instead, the mechanism of this formulation may rely on an increased viscosity of feeds.

There is also evidence that drugs containing sodium alginate and potassium bicarbonate may reduce acidic refluxate and contribute to decreased vomiting, while increasing weight gain with minimal side effects in preterm infants.[58] However, alginate formulations have also been associated with bezoar formation and with aluminum toxicity in infants.[22] There is increasing concern that these medications may not be appropriate for use in neonatal populations.

Antisecretory Agents

Two main classes of medications can be used to suppress acid secretion by the parietal cells in the gastric mucosa: histamine-2 (H_2) blockers and PPIs. H_2-blockers decrease acid secretion by competing with histamine at the H_2 receptor in parietal cells, thereby increasing intragastric pH.[59] PPIs act by blocking the Na^+–K^+–ATPase-driven gastric proton pump, which performs the final phase of the acid secretory process. PPIs inhibit the basal and stimulated secretion of acid, regardless of parietal cell stimulation.[22]

Histamine-2 (H_2) Blockers

Several reports support effectiveness of H_2 blockers (i.e., cimetidine, ranitidine, famotidine, and nizatidine) in children and infants affected by GER esophagitis.[60–62] Ranitidine is the most common H_2 blocker prescribed in neonatal intensive care units (NICUs). However, its use is off-label in premature infants, in whom evidence for its efficacy at treating GERD remains controversial. One important consideration is the frequent development of tachyphylaxis that may limit long-term use. Indeed, tolerance to H_2 blockers can be seen within 2 weeks and is associated with a decline in acid suppression.[44,63]

Dosing adjustment of H_2 blockers may be required in renal impairment.[53,64] In addition, significantly lower doses of ranitidine (e.g., 0.5 mg/kg bid) are needed to maintain a gastric pH >4 in preterm infants compared with those required for term infants (e.g., 1.5 mg/kg tid).[64] In infants >1 month of age, oral doses required to maintain a nonacidic gastric pH range between 4 and 10 mg/kg/day divided twice daily, and the intravenous dosage is reported to be 2 to 4 mg/kg/day, divided twice daily.[63] See Table 20.2 for comparable doses of cimetidine, famotidine, and nizatidine.

The safety profile of H_2 blockers, as with all antisecretory agents, has recently been called into question.[65–67] In particular, it has been noted that the inhibition of gastric acid secretion in premature infants can increase exposure to unwanted microorganisms due to the elimination of the acid barrier.[68] There may also be a higher load of bacteria in the distal intestine.[16]

Association of H_2 blockers with an increased incidence of necrotizing enterocolitis and infections in very low birth weight preterm infants has been reported.[69] H_2 blockers have also been associated with irritability, abnormal liver function, abnormal leukocyte function, pneumonia, and bacteremia in premature infants.[70,71] Cimetidine has been associated with infantile gynecomastia.[72]

Proton-Pump Inhibitors (PPIs)

A number of PPIs, including omeprazole and lansoprazole, are currently approved for use in children >1 year of age. Esomeprazole is approved for use in infants with GERD ≥1 month of age. PPIs have an excellent safety profile and are mostly well tolerated. Common side effects include headache, diarrhea, rash, nausea, and constipation.[73] To date, PPIs have not been associated with cancers or with cardiac arrhythmias. Nevertheless, as with the H_2 blockers, it is their tremendous success at acid suppression that may be associated with significant risks. PPIs decrease gastric mucosal viscosity, reduce GI motility, and delay gastric emptying; these effects may promote the growth of pathogenic bacteria and clearly lead to alteration in gut microbiota.[4]

Several studies have demonstrated the efficacy of PPIs at suppressing acid in infants, thereby treating erosive esophagitis.[22] However, the effectiveness of PPIs for reducing symptoms in infants with reflux is less clear. One randomized, placebo-controlled trial demonstrated that omeprazole and placebo produced similar improvement in irritability despite a reduction in acid in the esophagus in the PPI group.[74] Similarly, GERD symptoms were ineffectively relieved in the presence of a decreased frequency and duration of esophageal acid exposure.[75] The largest trial of lansoprazole assessed its efficacy versus placebo in 162 symptomatic infants and showed no advantage of lansoprazole over placebo in reducing crying, regurgitation, feeding refusal, back arching, or respiratory symptoms associated with GERD.[76]

In children where acid-suppressing therapy with either PPIs or H_2 blockers has been used, there is a growing appreciation for increased risks for community-acquired pneumonia and gastroenteritis.[77] The proposed mechanisms by which acid suppression might lead to these complications include bacterial overgrowth and altered GI function. In NICU populations, infants on these therapies have a sixfold increase in the risk of necrotizing enterocolitis.[54,78] At this time, we believe the use of these medications should be reserved for infants with severe symptoms, and ideally would be limited to a short 2-week course.

Promotility Agents

Promotility (prokinetic) agents work to improve reflux disorders by exerting their effects on LES pressure, esophageal peristalsis, and gastric emptying. Unfortunately, almost all involve unintended side effects, including prolongation of the QT interval, cardiac arrhythmias, and dystonia. The 2009 Pediatric Gastroesophageal Reflux Clinical Practice Guidelines issued by NASPGHAN stated that potential adverse effects of prokinetic agents currently available for the treatment of pediatric GERD, including metoclopramide and erythromycin, outweigh their potential benefits.[8]

Erythromycin is a macrolide antibiotic that acts as a prokinetic agent by acting on motilin receptors and inducing phase III activity of the migratory motor complex (MMC), propagating contents from the stomach to the small intestine.[79] Erythromycin has no effect on esophageal motility, but it has been selectively used in infants with feeding intolerance. The oral dose of erythromycin is 1 to 3 mg/kg three times a

Table 20.2 DRUG TREATMENT OF INFANTS FOR GERD

Drug or Drug Class	Dosing	Side Effects	Precautions
H$_2$ receptor antagonists		Headache, diarrhea, agitation, tolerance. Rare: allergic reactions, AV block, hepatotoxicity, hematologic toxicity	May increase risk of pneumonia. Risk of seizures with renal impairment.
Cimetidine	Neonates: 10 mg/kg PO total daily dose, dosed q6–12 hr	Gynecomastia	Decrease dose with severe hepatic disease. Decrease dose with CrCl <30. Inhibits CYPs 1A2, 2C19, 2D6, 3A4 (many drug interactions).
Famotidine	Neonates and infants <3 mo: 0.5 mg/kg/dose PO qd Infants >3 mo: 0.5 mg/kg/dose PO bid		If CrCl <50, decrease dose by 50%. Caution with theophylline.
Nizatidine	Neonates, infants, children <12 years: 2.5–5 mg/kg/dose PO bid	Vomiting, cough, nasopharyngitis, pyrexia	Decrease dose with CrCl <50
Ranitidine	Preterm infants: 0.5 mg/kg/dose PO bid Term infants: 1.5 mg/kg/dose PO tid Neonates >1 mo: 4–8 mg/kg PO total daily dose, dosed bid–tid	Nausea	If CrCl <50, decrease dose by 50%. Caution with: hepatic disease, theophylline.
Proton pump inhibitors	Take 30–60 minutes before a meal	Abdominal pain, diarrhea, nausea, flatulence, headache, arthralgia, myalgia. Long-term use: hypomagnesemia, vitamin B$_{12}$ deficiency. Rare: allergic reactions, hepatotoxicity, hematologic toxicity.	May increase risk of pneumonia, bone fracture, CDAD. Caution with clopidogrel. Substrates of CYPs 2C19, 3A4. Inhibitors of CYP2C19 to varying degrees.
Esomeprazole	Not labeled for use in neonates		Avoid with clopidogrel. Caution with severe hepatic disease. Moderate–strong inhibitor of CYP2C19.
Lansoprazole	Neonates, infants <10 wk: 0.2–0.3 mg/kg/days PO Infants >10 wk: 1–2 mg/kg/days PO		Consider decreased dose with severe hepatic disease, Asian patients. Substrate and inhibitor of P-gp.
Omeprazole	Neonates: 0.7 mg/kg PO qd Infants: 0.5 mg/kg PO qd	Rare: acute interstitial nephritis	Avoid with clopidogrel. Consider decreased dose with severe hepatic disease. Substrate and inhibitor of P-gp. Moderate–strong inhibitor of CYP2C19.
Pantoprazole	Infants >1 mo: 1.2 mg/kg/day PO	Rare: acute interstitial nephritis	Limited data with severe hepatic disease. Substrate and inhibitor of P-gp.
Rabeprazole	Children 1–11 years and <15 kg: 5 mg PO qd		Limited data with severe hepatic disease.
Prokinetic agent			
Erythromycin	Infants and children: 1–3 mg/kg/dose PO tid	Risk of infantile hypertrophic pyloric stenosis in the newborn period	Can prolong QT interval, can develop tachyphylaxis.

Continued

Table 20.2   DRUG TREATMENT OF INFANTS FOR GERD—cont'd

Drug or Drug Class	Dosing	Side Effects	Precautions
Metoclopramide	Infants and children: 0.1–0.3 mg/kg/dose PO tid–qid	Irritability, drowsiness, and extrapyramidal reactions	
Additional agent Sucralfate	40–80 mg/kg PO total daily dose, dosed qid, or 500 mg PO qid, on empty stomach	Constipation, hypersensitivity reactions	Caution with CKD, diabetes. Do not give concomitant aluminum-containing antacids. Binds with some drugs—separate dosing by 2 hr.

AV, Atrioventricular; *bid,* twice daily; *CDAD, Clostridium difficile*–associated diarrhea; *CKD,* chronic kidney disease; *CrCl,* creatinine clearance; *CYP,* cytochrome P450 isoenzyme; *GERD,* gastroesophageal reflux disease; *P-gp,* P-glycoprotein; *PO,* oral; *qd,* once daily; *qid,* four times daily; *tid,* three times daily.

day. Decreased effectiveness has been observed in preterm infants, possibly due to gut immaturity.[80] Adverse effects of erythromycin include an increased risk of infantile hypertrophic pyloric stenosis, especially with use in the first 2 weeks after birth.[81] At this time, there is insufficient evidence to support the use of erythromycin in premature infants.[82]

Metoclopramide is a dopamine agonist that improves peristalsis, gastric emptying, and LES tone in infants.[83] It has been widely used in the treatment of GER in infants and children, despite a lack of evidence of efficacy. Nonreversible adverse effects, including tardive dyskinesia, can be seen in children treated with metoclopramide, prompting the FDA to publish a black box warning in 2009.[22] The NASPGHAN guidelines counsel against using metoclopramide to treat pediatric GERD. Any use in infants should be approached with extreme caution and attention to side effects.

A number of other promotility agents have been removed from the market due to significant safety concerns. For example, cisapride, a nondopamine receptor–blocking, anticholinergic, antiserotoninergic agent, was briefly available in the late 1990s, but was associated with cardiac side effects, including QTc interval prolongation, arrhythmia, and sudden death.[84,85] Because of these toxicities, cisapride is no longer available as an approved therapy for GER. Nevertheless, its ability to enhance motility of the lower esophagus, stomach, and small intestine via the release of acetylcholine from the mesenteric plexus has led to use of this medication for compassionate use to treat refractory GERD in select patients.[86,87]

Similarly, domperidone, a peripheral dopamine D_2-receptor antagonist that enhances esophageal motility and gastric emptying, is associated with extrapyramidal signs. Due to immaturity of the nervous system and blood–brain barrier, infants may be at increased risk for this toxicity.[4,88,89] Immaturity of the cytochrome P450 system, which mediates metabolism of both domperidone and cisapride, may lead to higher concentrations of drug and enhanced toxicity in infants.

Bethanechol increases muscarinic cholinergic activity, increasing LES tone and esophageal peristaltic amplitude and velocity. However, as a muscarinic agonist, it also increases salivary and bronchial secretions and may induce bronchospasm. Furthermore, no clinical benefits were demonstrated in a study of 20 infants.[22,90,91]

Finally, baclofen is a gamma-aminobutyric acid B receptor agonist that inhibits TLESR occurrence. In one randomized, double-blinded, placebo-controlled trial in children with GERD, baclofen significantly accelerated gastric emptying.[92] Unfortunately, clinically significant common side effects of baclofen include drowsiness and lowered seizure threshold. There have been no trials of baclofen in infants to support its safety or use for GERD.

Figure 20.2 Erosive esophagitis with erythema, exudate, and loss of vascular pattern.

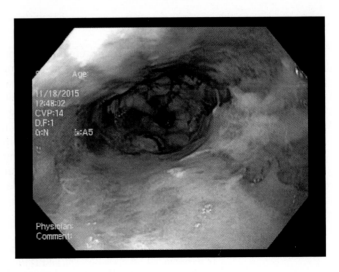

Counseling and Follow-Up

A key aspect of reflux treatment in infants is parent education and reassurance that the natural course of both physiologic GER and pathologic GERD is improvement over the first year of life. Reflux disorders peak in incidence and severity at 4 months of age and resolve by 8 to 12 months—often without need for medical therapy—with infant growth and maturation of gut motility. On the other hand, potential complications and long-term sequelae of infant GERD with peptic injury can include erosive esophagitis (Fig. 20.2), poor weight gain, and swallowing difficulties. Additional aerodigestive complications of GER can include reactive airway disease, apnea, bradycardia, and oxygen desaturation. It may be equally important to educate parents about benefits of acid-reducing medications and the importance of discontinuing these medications when they are no longer indicated.[93] Scherer et al. reported that utilizing the word *disease* when diagnosing reflux disorders in an otherwise healthy infant increased the parents' interest in using medication to treat the infant.[94]

Although little is known about the natural history of untreated esophagitis in infants, at least one PPI randomized trial reported on outcomes at 12 months of age of infants who had been assigned to the placebo arm after diagnosis of esophagitis. The investigators of this secondary analysis found that 10 of the 19 infants had completed the trial without rescue; of the 9 others, 3 had withdrawn and 6 had required drug therapy. Among the 10 patients who completed the trial without rescue, 9 were rated "completely well" and 1 was rated "improved" on the parent global score. Comparing 12-month symptoms with baseline symptoms, infants who completed the trial without rescue generally had resolution of the problematic regurgitation, inconsolable crying, arching spells, or hiccups that they had experienced before enrollment. However, although symptoms improved over 1 year without drug therapy, histology remained abnormal.[95]

At this time, it remains incumbent upon clinicians to use objective data to identify those infants who require pharmacologic treatments for reflux disorders and to follow infants carefully until signs of GER resolve and medications are discontinued, to minimize complications of both GERD and its therapies.[93] At follow-up visits, it is important to identify continued vomiting, weight loss, or continued irritability. If symptoms persist, the clinician should assess infant growth and development, reassess the appropriateness of diet, and consider positioning during feeding. Beyond adjusting drug therapy, it may also be appropriate to consider referral to a gastroenterologist or need for endoscopy. Symptoms of GERD will cease in most infants by 1 year of age; however, parents should be aware of possible signs of continued GER, such as hematemesis and reactive airway disease.

Conclusion

Although reflux disorders remain common among infants and may often resolve with the tincture of time, their management in preterm infants and infants may also involve lifestyle and dietary changes, as well as medications. Most infants do not require diagnostic testing to differentiate physiologic GER from pathologic GERD. Instead, methodical medical history taking and a stepwise therapeutic approach are advisable. When conservative measures fail or clinical complications arise, a short trial of pharmacologic therapy should be considered. Concomitantly, there are growing imperatives to devise plans for discontinuation when medications are no longer indicated. Indeed, known and emerging data on risks of medications to treat reflux disorders in infants should give all providers and patients pause to ensure that they are being appropriately and wisely used.

REFERENCES

1. Jadcherla SR, Slaughter JL, Stenger MR, et al. Practice variance, prevalence, and economic burden of premature infants diagnosed with GERD. *Hosp Pediatr*. 2013;3:335–341.
2. Dhillon AS, Ewer AK. Diagnosis and management of gastro-oesophageal reflux in preterm infants in neonatal intensive care units. *Acta Paediatr*. 2004;93:88–93.
3. Slaughter JL, Stenger MR, Reagan PB, et al. Neonatal histamine-2 receptor antagonist and proton pump inhibitor treatment at United States children's hospitals. *J Pediatr*. 2016;174:63–70.
4. Corvaglia L, Monari C, Martini S, et al. Pharmacological Therapy of Gastroesophageal Reflux in Preterm Infants. *Gastroenterol Res Pract*. 2013;2013:714564.
5. Newell SJ, Booth IW, Morgan M, et al. Gastroesophageal reflux in preterm infants. *Arch Dis Child*. 1989;64:780–786.
6. Birch JL, Newell SJ. Gastrooesophageal reflux disease in preterm infants: current management and diagnostic dilemmas. *Arch Dis Child*. 2009;94:F379–F383.
7. Di Fiore JM, Arko M, Whitehouse M, et al. Apnea is not prolonged by acid gastroesophageal reflux in preterm infants. *Pediatrics*. 2005;116:1059–1063.
8. Vandenplas Y, Rudolph CD, Di Lorenzo C, Hassall E, et al. Pediatric gastroesophageal reflux clinical practice guidelines: joint recommendations of the North American Society for Pediatric Gastroenterology, Hepatology, and Nutrition (NASPGHAN) and the European Society for Pediatric Gastroenterology, Hepatology, and Nutrition (ESPGHAN). *J Pediatr Gastroenterol Nutr*. 2009;49:498–547.
9. Poets CF, Brockmann PE. Myth: gastroesophageal reflux is a pathological entity in the preterm infant. *Semin Fetal Neonatal Med*. 2011;16:259–263.
10. Vanderplas Y. Gastroesophageal Reflux. In: Wyllie R, Hyams JS, Kay M, eds. *Pediatric Gastrointestinal and Liver Disease*. Netherlands: Saunders Elsevier; 2006:[Chapter 20]:305–325.
11. Omari TI, Barnett CP, Benninga MA, et al. Mechanisms of gastro-oesophageal reflux in preterm and term infants with reflux disease. *Gut*. 2002;51:475–479.
12. Schurr P, Findlater CK. Neonatal mythbusters: evaluating the evidence for and against pharmacological and non-pharmacological management of gastroesophageal reflux. *Neonatal Netw*. 2012;31:229–241.
13. Henry SM. Discerning differences: gastroesophageal reflux and gastroesophageal reflux disease in infants. *Adv Neonatal Care*. 2004;4:235–247.
14. Jadcherla SR, Duong HQ, Hoffmann RG, et al. Esophageal body and upper esophageal sphincter motor responses to esophageal provocation during maturation in preterm newborns. *J Pediatr*. 2003;143:31–38.
15. Di Lorenzo C, Mertz H, Alvarez S, et al. Gastric receptive relaxation is absent in newborn infants (abstract). *Gastroenterology*. 1993;104:A498.
16. Neu J, Li N. The neonatal gastrointestinal tract: developmental anatomy, physiology, and clinical implications. *NeoReviews*. 2003;4:e7–e12.
17. Jadcherla SR. Gastroesophageal reflux in the neonate. *Clin Perinatol*. 2002;29:135–158.
18. Orenstein SR, Shalaby TM, Cohn JF. Reflux symptoms in 100 normal infants: diagnostic validity of the infant gastroesophageal reflux questionnaire. *Clin Pediatr*. 1996;35:607–614.
19. Brown P. Medical management of gastroesophageal reflux. *Curr Opin Pediatr*. 2000;12:247–250.
20. Corvaglia L, Zama D, Gualdi S, et al. Gastro-oesophageal reflux increases the number of apnoeas in very preterm infants. *Arch Dis Child*. 2009;94:F188–F192.
21. Corvaglia L, Mariani E, Aceti A, et al. Combined oesophageal impedance-pH monitoring in preterm newborn: comparison of two options for layout analysis. *Neurogastroenterol Motil*. 2009;21:1027–e81.
22. Czinn SJ, Blanchard S. Gastroesophageal reflux disease in neonates and infants. *Pediatr Drugs*. 2013;15:19–27.
23. Peter CS, Sprodowski N, Bohnhorst B, et al. Gastroesophageal reflux and apnea of prematurity: no temporal relationship. *Pediatrics*. 2002;109:8–11.
24. Duncan DR, Rosen RL. Current insights into the pharmacologic and nonpharmacologic management of gastroesophageal reflux in infants. *NeoReviews*. 2016;17:e203–e212.
25. Vandenplas Y, Brueton M, Dupont C, et al. Guidelines for the diagnosis and management of cow's milk protein allergy in infants. *Arch Dis Child*. 2007;92:902–908.

26. Koletzko S, Niggemann B, Arato A, et al. Diagnostic Approach and Management of Cow's-Milk Protein Allergy in Infants and Children: ESPGHAN GI Committee Practical Guidelines. *J Pediatr Gastroenterol Nutr.* 2012;55:221–229.

27. Nielsen RG, Bindslev-Jensen C, Kruse-Andersen S, et al. Severe gastroesophageal reflux disease and cow milk hypersensitivity in infants and children: disease association and evaluation of a new challenge procedure. *J Pediatr Gastroenterol Nutr.* 2004;39:383–391.

28. Tighe MP, Afazal NA, Bevan A, et al. Pharmacological treatment of children with gastro-esophageal reflux. *Cochrane Database Syst Rev.* 2014;(11):CD008550.

29. Tovar JA, Luis AL, Encinas JL, et al. Pediatric surgeons and gastroesophageal reflux. *J Pediatr Surg.* 2007;42:277–283.

30. Kleinman L, Revicki DA, Flood E. Validation Issues in Questionnaires for Diagnosis and Monitoring of Gastroesophageal Reflux Disease in Children. *Curr Gastroenterol Rep.* 2006;8:228–234.

31. Salvatore S, Hauser B, Vandemaele K, et al. Gastroesophageal reflux disease in infants: how much is predictable with questionnaires, pH-metry, endoscopy and histology? *J Pediatr Gastroenterol Nutr.* 2005;40:210–215.

32. Seibert JJ, Byrne WJ, Euler AR, et al. Gastroesophageal reflux—the acid test: scintigraphy or the pH probe? *Am J Roentgenol.* 1983;140:1087–1090.

33. Rosen R, Hart K, Nurko S. Does reflux monitoring with multichannel intraluminal impedance change clinical decision making? *J Pediatr Gastroenterol Nutr.* 2011;52:404–407.

34. Wenzl TG. Investigating esophageal reflux with the intraluminal impedance technique. *J Pediatr Gastroenterol Nutr.* 2002;34:261–268.

35. Sun LS, Li G, Miller TL, et al. Association between a single general anaesthesia exposure before age 36 months and neurocognitive outcomes in later childhood. *JAMA.* 2016;315:2251–2253.

36. Shalaby TM, Orenstein SR. Efficacy of telephone teaching of conservative therapy for infants with symptomatic gastroesophageal reflux referred by pediatricians to pediatric gastroenterologist. *J Pediatr.* 2003;142:57–61.

37. Ewer AK, James ME, Tobin JM. Prone and left lateral positioning reduce gastro-oesophageal reflux in preterm infants. *Arch Dis Child Fetal Neonatal Ed.* 1999;81:F201–F205.

38. Omari TI, Rommel N, Staunton E, et al. Paradoxical impact of body position on gastroesophageal reflux and gastric emptying in the premature neonate. *J Pediatr.* 2004;145:194–200.

39. Van Wijk MP, Benninga MA, Dent J, et al. Effect of body position changes on post prandial gastro-esophageal reflux and gastric emptying in the healthy premature neonate. *J Pediatr.* 2007;151:591–596.

40. Moon RY, Darnall RA, Goodstein MH, et al. SIDS and other sleep-related infant deaths: expansion of recommendations for a safe infant sleeping environment. *Pediatrics.* 2011;128:1030–1039.

41. American Academy of Pediatrics Task Force on Sudden Infant Death Syndrome. The changing concept of sudden death syndrome: diagnostic coding shifts, controversies regarding the sleeping environment, and new variables to consider in reducing risk. *Pediatrics.* 2005;116:1245–1255.

42. Corvaglia L, Ferlini M, Rotatori R, et al. Starch thickening of human milk is ineffective in reducing the gastroesophageal reflux in preterm infants: a crossover study using intraluminal impedance. *J Pediatr.* 2006;148:265–268.

43. Corvaglia L, Aceti A, Mariani E, et al. Lack of efficacy of a starch-thickened preterm formula on gastro-oesophageal reflux in preterm infants: a pilot study. *J Matern Fetal Neonatal Med.* 2012;25: 2735–2738.

44. Lightdale JR, Gremse DA, Heitlinger LA, et al. Gastroesophageal reflux: management guidance for the pediatrician. *Pediatrics.* 2013;131:1684–1695.

45. Wenzl TG, Schneider S, Scheele F, et al. Effects of thickened feeding on gastroesophageal reflux in infants: a placebo-controlled crossover study using intraluminal impedance. *Pediatrics.* 2003;111: e355–e359.

46. Orenstein SR, Shalaby TM, Putnam PE. Thickened feedings as a cause of increased coughing when used as therapy for gastroesophageal reflux in infants. *J Pediatr.* 1992;121:913–915.

47. Heacock HJ, Jefrey HE, Baker JL, et al. Influence of breast versus formula milk on physiological gastroesophageal reflux in healthy, newborn infants. *J Pediatr Gastroenterol Nutr.* 1992;14:41–46.

48. Corvaglia L, Mariani E, Aceti A, et al. Extensively hydrolyzed protein formula reduces acid gastro-esophageal reflux in symptomatic preterm infants. *Early Hum Dev.* 2013;89:453–455.

49. Malcolm WF, Smith PB, Mears S, et al. Transpyloric tube feeding in very low birthweight infants with suspected gastroesophageal reflux: impact on apnea and bradycardia. *J Perinatol.* 2009;29:372–375.

50. Campwala I, Perrone E, Yanni G, et al. Complications of gastrojejunal feeding tubes in children. *J Surg Res.* 2015;199:67–71.

51. Kristensen C, Avitsland T, Emblem R, et al. Satisfactory long-term results after Nissen fundoplication. *Acta Paediatr.* 2007;96:702–705.

52. Alaswad B, Toubas PL, Grunow JE. Environmental tobacco smoke exposure and gastroesophageal reflux in infants with apparent life-threatening events. *J Okla State Med Assoc.* 1996;89:233–237.

53. Malcolm WF, Gantz M, Martin RJ, et al. Use of medications for gastroesophageal reflux at discharge among extremely low birth weight infants. *Pediatrics.* 2008;121:22–27.

54. Terrin G, Passariello A, De Curtis M, et al. Ranitidine is associated with infections, necrotizing enterocolitis, and fatal outcome in newborns. *Pediatrics.* 2012;129:e40–e45.

55. Tsou VM, Young RM, Hart MH, et al. Elevated plasma aluminum levels in normal infants receiving antacids containing aluminum. *Pediatrics.* 1991;87:148–151.

56. Zentilin P, Dulbecco P, Savarino E, et al. An evaluation of the antireflux properties of sodium alginate by means of combined multichannel intraluminal impedance and pH-metry. *Aliment Pharmacol Ther.* 2005;21:29–34.

20

57. Corvaglia L, Spizzichino M, Zama D, et al. Sodium Alginate (Gaviscon) does not reduce apnoeas related to gastro-oesophageal reflux in preterm infants. *Early Hum Dev*. 2011;87:775–778.

58. Atasay B, Erdeve O, Arsan S, et al. Effect of sodium alginate on acid gastroesophageal reflux disease in preterm infants: a pilot study. *J Clin Pharmacol*. 2010;50:1267–1272.

59. Kelly EJ, Chatfield SL, Brownlee KG, et al. The effect of intravenous ranitidine on the intragastric pH of preterm infants receiving dexamethasone. *Arch Dis Child*. 1993;69:37–39.

60. Cucchiara S, Minella R, Iervolino C, et al. Omeprazole and high dose ranitidine in the treatment of refractory reflux oesophagitis. *Arch Dis Child*. 1993;69:655–659.

61. Orenstein SR, Gremse DA, Pantaleon CD, et al. Nizatidine for the treatment of pediatric gastroesophageal reflux symptoms: an open-label, multiple-dose, randomized, multicenter clinical trial in 210 children. *Clin Ther*. 2005;27:472–483.

62. Orenstein SR, Shalaby TM, Devandry SN, et al. Famotidine for infant gastro-oesophageal reflux: a multi-centre, randomized, placebo-controlled, withdrawal trial. *Aliment Pharmacol Ther*. 2003;17:1097–1107.

63. Mallet E, Mouterde O, Dubois F, et al. Use of ranitidine in young infants with gastro-oesophageal reflux. *Eur J Clin Pharmacol*. 1989;36:641–642.

64. Kuusela AL. Long term gastric pH monitoring for determining optimal dose of ranitidine for critically ill preterm and term neonates. *Arch Dis Child*. 1998;78:F151–F153.

65. Bilali A, Galanis P, Bartsocas C, et al. H_2-blocker therapy and incidence of necrotizing enterocolitis in preterm infants: a case-control study. *Pediatr Neonatol*. 2013;54:141–142.

66. More K, Athalve-Jape G, Rao S, et al. Association of inhibitors of gastric acid secretion and higher incidence of NEC in preterm VLBW infants. *Am J Perinatol*. 2013;30:849–856.

67. Carrion V, Egan EA. Prevention of neonatal necrotizing enterocolitis. *J Pediatr Gastroenterol Nutr*. 1990;11:317–323.

68. Martinsen TC, Bergh K, Waldum HL. Gastric juice: a barrier against infectious diseases. *Basic Clin Pharmacol Toxicol*. 2005;96:94–102.

69. Guillet R, Stoll BJ, Cotton CM, et al. Association of H_2-blocker therapy and higher incidence of necrotizing enterocolitis in very low birth weight infants. *Pediatrics*. 2006;117:e137–e142.

70. Ribeiro JM, Lucas M, Baptista A, et al. Fatal hepatitis associated with ranitidine. *Am J Gastroenterol*. 2000;95:559–560.

71. Garcia Rodriguez LA, Wallander MA, Stricker BH. The risk of acute liver injury associated with cimetidine and other acid-suppressing anti-ulcer drugs. *Br J Clin Pharmacol*. 1997;43:183–188.

72. Garcia Rodriguez LA, Jick H. Risk of gynecomastia associated with cimetidine, omeprazole and other antiulcer drugs. *BMJ*. 1994;308:503–506.

73. Stedman CAM, Barclay ML. Review article: comparison of the pharmacokinetics, acid suppression and efficacy of proton pump inhibitors. *Aliment Pharmacol Ther*. 2000;14:963–978.

74. Moore DJ, Tao BS, Lines DR, et al. Double-blind placebo controlled trial of omeprazole in irritable infants with gastroesophageal reflux. *J Pediatr*. 2003;143:219–223.

75. Omari TI, Haslam RR, Lundborg P, et al. Effect of omeprazole on acid gastroesophageal reflux and gastric acidity in preterm infants with pathological acid reflux. *J Pediatr Gastroenterol Nutr*. 2007;44:41–44.

76. Orenstein SR, Hassall E, Furmaga-Jablonska W, et al. Multicenter, double-blind, randomized, placebo controlled trial assessing the efficacy and safety of proton pump inhibitor lansoprazole in infants with symptoms of gastroesophageal reflux disease. *J Pediatr*. 2009;154:514–520.

77. Canani RB, Cirillo P, Roggero P, et al. Therapy with gastric acidity inhibitors increases the risk of acute gastroenteritis and community-acquired pneumonia in children. *Pediatrics*. 2006;117(5):e817–e820.

78. Gupta RW, Tran L, Norori J, et al. Histamine-2 receptor blockers alter the fecal microbiota in premature infants. *J Pediatr Gastroenterol Nutr*. 2013;56:397–400.

79. Ng SCY, Gomez JM, Rajadurai VS, et al. Establishing enteral feeding in preterm infants with feeding intolerance: a randomized controlled study of low-dose erythromycin. *J Pediatr Gastroenterol Nutr*. 2003;37:554–558.

80. Chen CM. Erythromycin for the treatment of feeding intolerance in preterm infants. *Pediatr Neonatol*. 2012;53:2–3.

81. Mahon BE, Rosenman MB, Kleiman MB. Maternal and infant use of erythromycin and other macrolide antibiotics as risk factors for infantile hypertrophic pyloric stenosis. *J Pediatr*. 2001;139:380–384.

82. Ng E, Shah VS. Erythromycin for the prevention and treatment of feeding intolerance in preterm infants. *Cochrane Database Syst Rev*. 2008;(3):CD001815.

83. Hibbs AM, Lorch SA. Metoclopramide for the treatment of gastroesophageal reflux disease in infants: a systematic review. *Pediatrics*. 2006;118:746–752.

84. Khongphatthanayothin A, Lane J, Thomas D, et al. Effects of cisapride on QT interval in children. *J Pediatr*. 1998;133:51–56.

85. Bernardini S, Semama DS, Huet F, et al. Effects of cisapride on QTC interval in neonates. *Arch Dis Child*. 1997;77:F241–F243.

86. Dubin A, Kikkert M, Mirmiran M, et al. Cisapride associated with QTc prolongation in very low birth weight preterm infants. *Pediatrics*. 2001;107:1313–1316.

87. Maclennan S, Augood C, Cash-Gibson L, et al. Cisapride treatment for gastro-oesophageal reflux in children. *Cochrane Database Syst Rev*. 2010;(4):CD002300.

88. Pritchard DS, Baber N, Stephenson T. Should domperidone be used for the treatment of gastro-oesophageal reflux in children? Systematic review of randomized controlled trials in children aged 1 month to 11 years old. *Br J Clin Pharmacol*. 2005;59:725–729.

89. Grill BB, Hillemeier C, Semeraro LA, et al. Effects of domperidone therapy on symptoms and upper gastrointestinal motility in infants with gastro-oesophageal reflux. *J Pediatr*. 1985;106:311–316.

90. Levi P, Marmo F, Saluzzo C, et al. Bethanechol versus antiacids in treatment of gastroesophageal reflux. *Helv Paediatr Acta*. 1985;40:349–359.

91. McCallum RW, Kline MM, Curry N, et al. Comparative effects of metoclopramide and bethanechol on lower esophageal sphincter pressure in reflux patients. *Gastroenterology*. 1975;68:1114–1118.

92. Omari TI, Benninga MA, Sansom L, et al. Effect of baclofen on esophagogastric motility and gastroesophageal reflux in children with gastroesophageal reflux disease: a randomized controlled trial. *J Pediatr*. 2006;149:468–474.

93. Poets CF. Gastroesophageal reflux: a critical review of its role in preterm infants. *Pediatrics*. 2004;113: e128–e132.

94. Scherer LD, Zikmund-Fisher BJ, Fagerlin A, et al. Influence of "GERD" label on parents' decision to medicate infants. *Pediatrics*. 2013;131:839–845.

95. Orenstein SR, Shalaby TM, Kelsey SF, et al. Natural history of infant reflux esophagitis: symptoms and morphometric histology during one year without pharmacotherapy. *Am J Gastroenterol*. 2006;101: 628–640.

20

Index